£32·00   WO SOO EUL

KU-267-789

Essential Anesthesia

Second Edition

WITHDRAWN

Shrewsbury Health Library

SHR02902

Essential Anesthesia

From Science to Practice

Second Edition

T. Y. Euliano
J. S. Gravenstein
N. Gravenstein
D. Gravenstein
University of Florida
College of Medicine,
Gainesville, Florida, USA

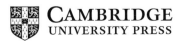
CAMBRIDGE
UNIVERSITY PRESS

CAMBRIDGE UNIVERSITY PRESS
Cambridge, New York, Melbourne, Madrid, Cape Town,
Singapore, São Paulo, Delhi, Tokyo, Mexico City

Cambridge University Press
The Edinburgh Building, Cambridge CB2 8RU, UK

Published in the United States of America by Cambridge University Press, New York

www.cambridge.org
Information on this title: www.cambridge.org/9780521149457

© Cambridge University Press 2011

This publication is in copyright. Subject to statutory exception
and to the provisions of relevant collective licensing agreements,
no reproduction of any part may take place without the written
permission of Cambridge University Press.

First published 2011

Printed in the United Kingdom at the University Press, Cambridge

A catalogue record for this publication is available from the British Library

Library of Congress Cataloguing in Publication data
Essential anesthesia : from science to practice / T.Y. Euliano … [et al.]. – 2nd ed.
    p. ; cm.
  Includes bibliographical references and index.
  ISBN 978-0-521-14945-7 (pbk.)
  1. Anesthesiology.   2. Anesthesia.   I. Euliano, T. Y. (Tammy Y.), 1966–
  [DNLM: 1. Anesthesia–methods.   2. Anesthetics–administration & dosage.
  3. Perioperative Care. WO 200]
  RD81.E83 2011
  617.9′6–dc22
  2011008029

ISBN 978-0-521-14945-7 Paperback

Cambridge University Press has no responsibility for the persistence or
accuracy of URLs for external or third-party internet websites referred to in
this publication, and does not guarantee that any content on such websites is,
or will remain, accurate or appropriate.

Every effort has been made in preparing this book to provide accurate and up-to-date information which is in accord with
accepted standards and practice at the time of publication. Although case histories are drawn from actual cases, every effort
has been made to disguise the identities of the individuals involved. Nevertheless, the authors, editors and publishers can
make no warranties that the information contained herein is totally free from error, not least because clinical standards are
constantly changing through research and regulation. The authors, editors and publishers therefore disclaim all liability for
direct or consequential damages resulting from the use of material contained in this book. Readers are strongly advised to pay
careful attention to information provided by the manufacturer of any drugs or equipment that they plan to use.

For Neil, Alix, Galey, DeeAnn and JS who was our
co-author, mentor and father

Contents

Foreword

The most recognizable part of the anesthesiologist's work consists of maintaining the stability of the patient's multiple and complex organ systems during surgical operations while providing freedom from pain. To accomplish these sometimes opposing goals, the anesthesiologist must have detailed knowledge of the diseases affecting the patient and must be able to base all therapeutic decisions on an astute understanding of physiology and pharmacology. Emphasizing the serious nature of the anesthetic state, anesthesia has been described as "a controlled overdose of drugs requiring continuous intensive care of the patient." Understandably then, many founders of critical care medicine were anesthesiologists and, by the same token, much material in this book is immediately applicable to the intensive care of critically ill patients.

The authors had set out to write a book to introduce medical students to the complexities of anesthetic practice including compassionate pre- and post-operative care. However, this little book rapidly grew beyond that early goal. Physicians and nurses outside of anesthesia will discover in these pages wonderful reviews of physiology and pharmacology and clinical pearls helpful in preparing a patient for anesthesia and surgery. That Drs Euliano and Gravenstein have a wealth of teaching experience shows on every page. They successfully present very complex subjects in a lively manner and in relatively simple terms. I am confident that the reader will find this text not only thorough but also – how rare for a medical text – pleasant to read. This book offers answers to many questions, while simultaneously stimulating the reader to consult one of the many voluminous specialty texts that provide details, requiring much more space than is available in a volume of this size.

Jerome H. Modell, M.D.

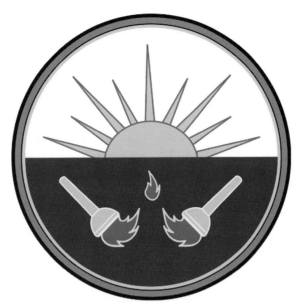

In Greek mythology, the night has twin sons, Thanatos (death) and Hypnos (sleep), who carry flaming torches pointing toward the floor, to light a path through the dark. Juan Marín, a Latin American anesthesia pioneer, designed this image to represent anesthesia. He placed a small light between Thanatos and Hypnos indicating the flame of life the anesthesiologist must guard. The upper half of the emblem shows the rising or setting sun of consciousness. The Confederación Latinoamericana de Anestesiología and the Revista Colombiana de Anestesiología have adopted this beautiful emblem, which in the past had been used by the World Federation of Societies of Anaesthesiologists.

Preface to the first edition

"What should I read in preparation for a rotation through the anesthesia service?" – so have asked not only students, but also other medical and non-medical visitors to the operating room. In response to this often posed question, we could recommend several wonderful and exhaustive texts, but such tomes demand an investment of time and effort only the dedicated specialist could muster. An introductory text should be easy to read, and it should be short enough to be completed in a few hours. It has to be a sketch instead of a full painting, yet it must clearly show the features of the subject. This we have striven to accomplish but, occasionally, we succumbed and included a bit of trivia. We hope the reader will forgive us for that.

We have divided the little book into three parts. The first part presents the equivalent of a miniature operating manual covering pre-, intra- and post-anesthesia tasks and the tools of the profession. In the second part, we give a synopsis of cardiovascular and respiratory physiology and pharmacology of importance to perioperative clinical practice. The third part places the reader into the operating room looking over the shoulder of a busy anesthesiologist taking care of patients with special problems. Here, we have chosen common clinical situations, and we have incorporated difficulties – some of them avoidable – in order to highlight challenges faced in daily practice. A reader who had started at the beginning of the book and now looks at the clinical examples should be able to apply much of the information presented in the first and second sections of the book to the problems arising in the clinical cases. Of course, some might prefer to read about the cases first – perhaps in preparation for a visit to the operating room – in order to get a preview of the extraordinary world of clinical anesthesia and surgery. Such an approach should raise many questions in the reader's mind, topics we hope to have touched on in the first two sections of the book.

Our hope is that this little text will intrigue some into further investigation of the fascinating field of anesthesiology, provide insight into the subspecialty for our colleagues in other areas, and improve the understanding of physiology, pharmacology, and perioperative medicine for all our readers.

T. Y. Euliano, J. S. Gravenstein July, 2004

Preface to the second edition

The goals of the second edition have not changed. The book, however, has been augmented with some new material and trimmed of some excess, in an effort to keep it light reading but still contemporary and reflective of modern anesthesia.

T. Y. Euliano, D. Gravenstein, N. Gravenstein

Acknowledgments

We are grateful to the many people who helped in the preparation of this text. In particular we thank Dr. Barys Ihnatsenka, Dr. Nicole Dobija, Kendra Kuck, Kelly Spaulding, and Frederike Gravenstein for lending their expertise, as well as Katie James and Cambridge University Press for providing direction in completing this edition. And finally, we are grateful to the medical students, who prompted the project in the first place, and continue to keep us on our toes.

About the authors

Dr. Tammy Euliano, Associate Professor of Anesthesiology and Obstetrics & Gynecology, received her M.D. from the University of Florida and continued there throughout residency and fellowship. She has received numerous awards for her dedication to teaching and is a member of the Society of Teaching Scholars. Her research in simulator technology and patient safety has been recognized by the American Society of Anesthesiologists.

The late **Dr. J. S. Gravenstein** was formerly the Graduate Research Professor of Anesthesiology, Emeritus, University of Florida College of Medicine. Dr. Gravenstein received his Dr. med. from the University of Bonn in Germany and his M.D. from Harvard University School of Medicine. Dr. Gravenstein was known worldwide for his work in patient monitoring, patient safety, and simulation technology. His numerous awards included the Massachusetts General Hospital Trustees' Medal, and an honorary doctorate in medicine from the University of Graz, Austria.

Dr. Dietrich Gravenstein is Associate Professor of Anesthesiology and a Physician Director of Quality at the University of Florida. He completed his medical training and neuroanesthesia fellowship at the University of Florida College of Medicine. He has been recognized by residents for his devotion to teaching. A biomedical engineer by training, his research interests have focused on instrumentation development, where he has numerous awards and patents.

Dr. Nikolaus Gravenstein is Professor of Anesthesiology, Neurosurgery and Periodontics at the University of Florida College of Medicine, where he also completed his anesthesiology training and fellowship. He has a longstanding interest in medical education, patient monitoring and safety.

Introduction

A *very* short history of anesthesia

Every now and then, you run into a high-school student who did a paper on the history of anesthesia, or the teacher who assigned it. Here are a few facts and dates that should keep you out of acute embarrassment.

God was first: "And the Lord God caused a deep sleep to fall upon Adam, and he slept." (Genesis 2:21). A date is not given.

Anesthesia as we know it started in the early to mid 1840s.

Crawford Long of Jefferson, Georgia, removed a small tumor from a patient under diethyl ether anesthesia. That was in 1842. Crawford Long failed to publish this event, and he was denied the fame of having been the first to use diethyl ether as a surgical anesthetic. Ether was not unknown; students inhaled it during the so-called ether frolics.

Horace Wells had used nitrous oxide in his dental practice. In 1844, he failed to demonstrate the anesthetic effects of N_2O in front of a critical medical audience. The patient, a boy, screamed during the extraction of a tooth, and the audience hissed. Later, the boy said that he had not felt anything. Excitement under light nitrous oxide anesthesia is common. Horace Wells died young and by his own hand.

William T. G. Morton, another dentist in anesthesia's history, successfully etherized a patient at the Massachusetts General Hospital in Boston on *October 16, 1846*. The news of this event spread worldwide as rapidly as the communication links permitted. Morton tried to patent his discovery under the name of Letheon. An English barrister later wrote: "a patent degrades a noble discovery to the level of a quack medicine."[1]

Oliver Wendell Holmes, only 2 months after Morton's epochal demonstration of surgical anesthesia, suggested the term "anesthesia" to describe the state of sleep induced by ether. Holmes was a physician, poet, humorist and, fittingly, finally dean of Harvard Medical School.

John Snow, from London, became the first physician to devote his energies to anesthetizing patients for surgical operations. His earliest experiences with ether anesthesia date to late 1846. In 1853, he administered chloroform to Queen Victoria for the delivery of her son Prince Leopold. This shook the acceptance of the divine command: "in sorrow thou shalt bring forth children" (Genesis 3:16) and thus powerfully furthered the use of anesthesia to alleviate the pain of childbirth. Incidentally, while anesthesiologists admire John Snow for his publications and the design of an etherizer, epidemiologists claim him as one of their own because he had recognized the source of a cholera epidemic, which he traced to a public pump. By removing the pump's handle, he stopped the spread of the infection. That was in 1854.

Those were the beginnings. By now, the two earliest anesthetic vapors, diethyl ether and chloroform, have been modified hundreds of times. Many descendants have come and gone, but their great-grandchildren still find daily use. Intravenous drugs have secured an increasingly prominent place in anesthesia, among them neuromuscular blockers – hailing back to South American Indians and their poisoned arrows shot from blowguns. A steadily growing pharmacopeia of analgesics, hypnotics, anxiolytics, and cardiovascular drugs now fill the drug cabinets.

We still listen for breath sounds, we still watch color and respiration, and we still feel the pulse, but today we are helped by the most subtle techniques of sensing invisible signals and the most invasive methods, with tubes snaking through the heart.

When we reduce the history of anesthesia to a few dates and facts, we do not do justice to the stories of the age-old and arduous struggle to alleviate pain. In one of the more comprehensive books on the genesis of surgical anesthesia, you will find a superb description of the interesting personalities and the many events that eventually paved the way to one of the greatest advances in medicine, the discovery of anesthesia.[2] The book brims with anecdotes, for example the story of a woman in 1591 accused of witchcraft. One of the indictments was for her attempt to ease the pain of childbirth. She was sentenced to be "bund to ane staik and brunt in assis (ashes), quick (alive) to the death." Why society's acceptance of pain relief changed and how obstetrical anesthesia eventually developed is the subject of another great historical book by Donald Caton.[3]

Notes

1   You will find this quotation in one of the three delightful volumes entitled *Essays of the First Hundred Years of Anaesthesia* by W. Stanley Sykes, who relates the most wonderful stories having to do with anesthesia. For example, did you know that to be eaten alive by a lion and the like might not be painful? Sykes, W. S. (1961). *Essays on the First Hundred Years of Anaesthesia.* Volume 2, pp. 75–79, E&S Livingstone Ltd, Edinburgh.

2   Norman A. Bergman (1998). *The Genesis of Surgical Anesthesia.* Wood Library – Museum of Anesthesiology, Park Ridge, Illinois.

3   Donald Caton (1999). *What a Blessing She Had Chloroform.* Yale University Press, New Haven and London.

Safety and quality in anesthesia

The specialty of anesthesiology came about in large part to reduce the unacceptable risk of death associated with the provision of surgical anesthesia by someone who wasn't specially trained in the field. Our goal is to shepherd each patient safely from pre-operative optimization, through intra-operative management and into a comfortable post-operative recovery. Thus it makes sense to begin our journey into the essentials of anesthesia by putting safety and quality in modern healthcare in perspective.

Safety in medicine has an illustrious history, of which we are reminded during medical school graduation ceremonies with the traditional recitation of the Hippocratic Oath (or perhaps a contemporary version). One of its central tenets, "abstain from doing harm", remains a core principle for physicians even 24 centuries later. But, alas, we are only human and errors, either gross ones – like injecting potassium too quickly or removing the wrong leg, or subtle ones – like antibiotics administered a few minutes after incision (instead of before) or an i.v. stopcock left uncapped inviting infection, do occur. Unfortunately these errors are not rare. In 1999 the Institute of Medicine estimated that almost 100 000 patients annually lost their lives in the USA due to medical errors; the equivalent of a fully loaded passenger jet crashing every day![1] Before this report pulled it all together we really had no idea of the magnitude of the opportunity for improvement. This report was in effect a call to arms and framed for us all the challenge that avoidable harm should and must be eliminated.

Anesthesia errors contribute only a small part to this staggering measure of harm inflicted on patients. This "success" is in large part due to the "early" (1980s) recognition by anesthesia leaders that the agents we administer, the procedures we perform, and monitoring lapses can have lethal consequences. The Anesthesia Patient Safety Foundation (APSF) was founded in 1985 with a vision "that no patient will be harmed by anesthesia." Its multidisciplinary approach (including physicians, equipment manufacturers, drug companies, and others) focused on preventing adverse clinical outcomes, especially those involving human error. The following year the American Society of Anesthesiology became the first medical society to adopt professional guidelines, and then standards, for its members.[2]

With a quiver full of assorted guidelines and standards to bring to bear on behalf of our patients, the anesthesiologist steps into the role of "patient protector." Our concerns for his safety start well before induction of anesthesia. We are very aware of the patient's fears and we use reassurance and, if necessary, drugs to prepare him for the trip to the operating room. Indeed, we administer potent drugs not only to allay fear and pain, but for induction and maintenance of sleep. As soon as we apply these drugs, safety concerns escalate. All the medications in our arsenal have potentially nasty side effects. We monitor a host of signals that tell us about the patient's well-being. We compensate as best we can for disturbances induced by the very drugs we use, as well as the often drastic perturbations triggered by the underlying pathophysiology of the patient, the operation, and operator. The transitions from awake to asleep (induction of anesthesia) and from anesthetized to self-sufficient (emergence) represent critical phases. We recognize the threat of latent problems during the recovery phase by using a post-anesthesia care unit (PACU, formerly called recovery room) where patients are closely watched. Indeed, we often care for patients even once they have left the operating room/PACU suite.

Clearly, we cannot hope for *certainty* of safety. We must make do with *relative* safety because all too many agents under defined (and some not defined) conditions can render unsafe the state in which the patient finds himself.

How safe is safe enough?

You might skip the discussion of this question as we have no good answers to offer. All too much depends on the shifting expectations of society and on the highly variable resources society makes available. As human beings we are not entirely "risk-averse," as we happily exchange certain safety for the risk of breaking bones or even killing ourselves while schussing down a black diamond slope, eschewing our seatbelt, jumping out of a perfectly good airplane, riding a motorcycle, or smoking or overeating. We also voluntarily face risks while working in a mine or serving in the military or living in a house exposed to radon. The list is long and interesting and ranges from minimal to dangerously high risks.

Societal assessment of risks and safety changes over time. In 1938 the March of Dimes was founded to fight poliomyelitis, with an incidence of 1 in 13 600. At that time anesthetic deaths garnered little or no attention. Even 16 years later when Beecher and Todd reported a death rate of about one in 2000 anesthetics, society paid little attention, yet annually more people died from anesthesia than from polio. Yet no march or even rally to reduce anesthetic mortality was held.

Advance the calendar three decades and enter the era of costly malpractice suits brought against anesthesiologists and companies (the deep pocket) supplying drugs and equipment to the anesthesia profession. The cost of malpractice insurance rose steeply as huge awards were paid to plaintiffs representing patients who had died during or soon after anesthesia or who had suffered permanent damage, often to the brain. Now the risks associated with anesthesia were widely discussed.

How safe is anesthesia?

The job of the anesthesiologist has often been compared to that of a pilot. In terms of safety, the pilots have it hands down. According to one government report,[3] *"a passenger who randomly chose a U.S. domestic jet flight between 1967 and 1976 would have a one in two million chance of dying. This death risk fell to one in seven million in the decades 1977–1986 and 1987–1996. Using data from 1990 to the present, the death risk falls to one in eight million."* Compare that to the best statistics for anesthesia that list one death in 200 000 anesthetics. Of course, flying and undergoing anesthesia have little in common except that both are not entirely safe, that in both the victim does not contribute to a disaster, and that in both the passenger or patient has every right to expect that he or she will not be harmed by the trip – be it a flight or anesthetic.

How much money are we prepared to invest in safety?

The question is not easy to answer as we are looking at a spectrum ranging from inexpensive prophylactic vaccination with benefits that last years to acute interventions, as exemplified in the following story:

During the 1990s war in Bosnia, Captain Scott O'Grady, an American fighter pilot, was shot down over enemy territory. He survived the crash. The rescue operation to bring him back to safety involved two CH-53 E Sea Stallions (cost: $26 million apiece), two AH-1W Sea-Cobra gunships ($12.5 million apiece), four AV-8B Sea Harriers ($24 million apiece), F/A-18 fighter bombers ($30 million apiece), F-16s ($20 million apiece), F-15Es ($35 million apiece), EF-111s ($60 million), and AWACs ($250 million apiece). The investment of resources and funds to save one life was enormous and it was spectacularly successful. Afterward no one publicly suggested that to expend millions of dollars and risk many millions more to rescue Captain O'Grady was fiscally irresponsible, even though it was impossible to predict whether the effort would be successful.

Contrast that with the efforts to make anesthesia safe. Hospital administrators are likely to reckon the cost of investing in measures designed to enhance safety and then bemoan the fact that their balance sheet does not show good fiscal return for their investment.

Human error and the system

Whether we look at train wrecks, atomic energy catastrophes, shipping collisions, air traffic disasters, automobile crashes or anesthesia accidents, overwhelmingly human errors rather than mechanical failures are responsible for the calamity. In the olden days a single physician took care of a patient. If he (it was usually a "he" in those days) made an error, it was his error alone. The evolution of medicine has replaced that lone physician with today's healthcare team comprising many physicians (often working a shift schedule) with narrow but highly specialized skills working with uncounted nurses, technicians, and assistants caring for thousands of patients.

Paracelsus, a 16th-century physician, said of medicine: "Does not a lover go far to see a beautiful woman? How much further for a beautiful art?" Contrast that with the terminology heard all too often, particularly from hospital administrators, using the vernacular of manufacturers: We have a healthcare *industry* in which healthcare *providers* sell *services* to healthcare *consumers*. Gone is the image of a beautiful art. Instead we sense in the ugly phrases an industry and the hum (and intermittent squeaks) of a factory.

Over the clanking of the engines in the healthcare industry we hear ever-louder calls for lower cost AND increased safety and a higher quality of care. "Quality" measures not only safety, but also the cost, effectiveness, efficiency, and equitableness of care rendered. In light of increasing costs and limited resources we strive to provide the greatest value (= quality/cost) to our patients. To this end we adopt clinical care pathways, treatment guidelines, care bundles, and standards of care, all formulated from evidence-based medicine. Now pervasive protocols, procedure manuals, and checklists encourage us to adhere to management prescriptions rather than rely on judgments based on narrow personal experience and memory. Ideally, broad adoption of evidence-based guidelines will minimize deviations from "best practice" care and, when applied over a population, will improve overall outcomes. Detractors argue prescribed regimens fail to consider the uniqueness of each patient, potentially compromising the care of some. Therein lies the kernel for disagreement between advocates of policies promoting regulated versus individualized care. "Practice to achieve best outcomes" presents the more modern view. Physicians or centers that exceed defined quality of care benchmarks present a valuable resource to define "best practices" for adoption by those struggling to achieve the same benchmark.

Complications

The sizeable efforts to reduce errors and accidents and promote safety and quality have resulted in a multi-layered and complex system of modern medical care. Despite this, complications still occur (although with substantially reduced frequency). As in the past, most complications have multi-factorial roots. For example: A fatigued physician at the end of a 24-hour shift writes an order for a potent narcotic drug, eg., morphine sulfate. She intends 2.0 mg for the dose, but the decimal is buried in the number. She fails to write an order specifying when she wants to be called in case of problems. A junior pharmacist, uncertain of the drug's potency, sees a hint of a decimal point on the fax, but knows it is improper to use a decimal point followed by a zero (for this very reason) and therefore fills the prescription for 20 mg. A student nurse questions her supervisor about the dose. The supervisor checks the prescription and says: "if that's what the doctor ordered, we give it. She must have had a good reason to use such a large dose." The drug is administered. The patient falls asleep and a concerned visitor calls the nurse to check on the patient when the pulse oximeter sounds an alarm. The nurse administers oxygen, which improves the saturation but she fails to alert a physician. Oxygen pinks the patient's skin but does nothing to reverse the respiratory depression. The CO_2 continues to rise until it causes a respiratory arrest. It takes another minute for the oximeter to chime in again, by which time the accumulated CO_2 has caused an acidosis and hypertension so severe that the patient's heart stops. By the time anyone can respond to the alarm, evaluate the patient, call a code, and collect the equipment to institute mask–ventilation and start cardiopulmonary resuscitation, the patient has become another casualty of poor care.

As soon as possible after the event we start a "root cause analysis" in which every link in the system is examined. Several flaws are identified:

The physician made two mistakes: one of **com**mission – using a trailing decimal point (medication errors are most common among the causes of medical disasters); the other of **o**mission – failing to identify thresholds for action. The system (i.e., administrators and service chiefs) had accepted a staffing pattern that caused a physician to work without the necessary breaks. The "system" often allows fiscal more than safety considerations to drive staffing decisions.

The pharmacist, uncertain about the prescribed dosage, dispensed the drug instead of checking on recommended dosages – a matter of protocols and education.

The student nurse was the next safety net. She almost succeeded in preventing the death. However, her supervisor, a senior nurse trained overseas in a hierarchical culture, was not prepared to challenge a physician's order. This failure can be attributed to the all too common hurdles of communicating between specialties and ranks of seniority. In the medical pecking order a cleaning woman is unlikely to call out when she sees the professor making a mistake. And yet, that's exactly what the patient, whose life was at stake, would expect her to do and the professor to appreciate. Every member of the system must feel personally responsible for the patient's safety.

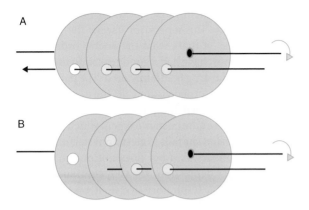

A

B

Fig. 1 Safety is sought by interposing layers of defenses. The first disk represents the physician erring in writing a prescription, the second the pharmacist, the third the student nurse, and the last the nurse administering oxygen without recognizing respiratory depression. The holes in these spinning disks have to be superimposed to allow the initial error to ripple through the system (A). Many more holes per disk and many more disks are required to represent the complexity of modern medical care. In B the disks have spun so that the propagation of the error has been stopped.

A nurse was called because the patient's oxygen saturation had dropped. Had she recognized this as an indication of hypoventilation, she could have called for help and avoided the disaster. Instead, she treated a symptom without correcting the problem. Adherence to a protocol spelling out the conditions that call for consultation would have prevented the problem, as would have appreciation of the ongoing pathophysiology.

The metaphor of slices of Swiss cheese or spinning disks has been used to illustrate that many serious complications in anesthesia, and medicine in general, have multiple roots. The holes in the disks line up so that an arrow (an error) can pass through (Fig. 1A). But when the wheels are spinning it takes a bit of bad luck to have the holes superimpose long enough for an error to sneak through (Fig. 1B).

Each error raises the question of what went wrong. When identifying the "holes in the disks" and linking it to a human error we are discouraged from pouncing on a wrongdoer. By focusing on the single culprit we can fail to deal with "upstream" errors, for example staffing decisions. Fear of punishment can inhibit the reporting of errors that must be identified before they cause harm.

The World Health Organization (WHO) has published a Surgical Safety Checklist. It establishes protocols designed to prevent the occasional, but recurring errors that have led to harm. The Safety Checklist

applies from the time before induction of anesthesia (sign in), through just before skin incision (time-out, i.e., a momentary halt of all activities) and on to the time before the patient leaves the operating room (sign out). Table 1 shows, slightly modified, the WHO document. Importantly, the protocol involves in most instances the entire team. Safety depends on teamwork. An alert team has a better chance of blocking the propagation of an error than the individual, isolated practitioner (see the spinning disk metaphor). To paraphrase Atul Gawande[4]: with the knowledge to do things properly comes the responsibility to do so and do so reliably. Using checklists provides an efficient and effective means to increase reliability and safety (Table 1).

Safety in anesthesia

Safety concerns start long before induction and extend well after anesthesia wears off. In the operating room we often marvel at the wonderful (in the literal sense of the word) workings of the human body. As best we can, we describe the system by assessing parameters we might call indicators of health (see Chapter 7 on monitoring). We put thresholds around these parameters and cause our instruments to sound alarms when these thresholds are violated. Safety for our patients during anesthesia is achieved if we can manage to keep these parameters within the desired limits in the face of an onslaught of perturbations, be they a disease process, the effect of anesthetic drugs, mechanical ventilation, the surgical intervention, or changes in the patient's fluid status or temperature.

Many of the parameters we monitor have been elevated by national professional organizations to "minimal monitoring standards," even though we lack scientific proof of their efficacy. The Federal Aviation Administration does no less. It also issues rules that are based on analysis by experts rather than experimental proof.

An ancient Greek may have viewed someone undergoing a modern anesthetic as being escorted by Hypnos (the god of sleep) down to the river of Lethe (for forgetfulness and oblivion). And nearby, perhaps only briefly, enjoying the blooming poppy fields of Morpheus, the god of dreams (and Hypnos's son), before comfortably re-awakening. But we can never deliver anesthesia with the guaranteed safe outcomes such divine guidance would assure. So we embrace all the devices and strategies that help us conduct a safe anesthetic. Safety is not, however, simply a measure of

Table 1: The World Health Organization Surgical Safety Checklist (slightly modified)

Sign in	Pre-incision time-out	Sign out
Confirm: The patient's identity Site of operation Procedure Consent given by patient	Confirm that all team members have introduced themselves by name and role	The nurse verbally confirms with the team: The name of the procedure recorded in the record That instrument, sponge, and needle counts are correct (or not applicable) How the specimen is labeled (including the patient's name) Whether there are any equipment problems to be addressed
Site marked if applicable	Surgeon, anesthesia professionals, and nurse verbally confirm: Patient identity Operative site Planned procedure	Surgeon, anesthesia professional, and nurse review the key concerns for the recovery and management of the patient
Anesthesia Safety Check completed	Is the patient's current and – if appropriate – old medical record available?	
Pulse oximeter applied and working	Anticipate critical events Surgeon reviews: What are the: critical or unexpected steps, operative duration, anticipated blood loss? Anesthesia team reviews: What are patient-specific concerns? Nursing team reviews: Has sterility (including indicator results) been confirmed? Are there equipment issues or other concerns?	
Does the patient have a: Known allergy? Yes No Difficult airway or risk of aspiration? No Yes, and is equipment and assistance available? Risk of more than 500 mL blood loss (7 mL/kg in children)? No Yes, and adequate intravenous access and fluids planned?	Has antibiotic prophylaxis been given within the last 60 minutes? Yes Not applicable	

how much data or how many monitors are available to the clinician. Safety begins with a caring physician who is knowledgeable about her patient's conditions and their anesthetic implications. Because we are all fallible (remember "to err is human"), redundant safety features provide added protection. This redundancy is familiar to all who give anesthesia; we simultaneously use pulse oximetry, an oxygen delivery sensor, and breathed gas oxygen analysis. Similar redundancy occurs with heart function (ECG, pulse oximetric plethysmography, capnometry, and precordial or esophageal stethoscope). We equally depend on those around us; a nurse who will remind about redosing antibiotics or a surgeon who notifies "anesthesia" about unexpected bleeding. Protocols and checkpoints help insure that steps critical for the delivery of a safe anesthetic are not overlooked.

Our very own APSF has become the model for safety foundations in other countries and for national (not limited to anesthesia) safety foundations. Safety and quality are a joint effort across the spectrum of healthcare providers and deserve to remain in the forefront. There is much opportunity for improvement.

In the chapters that follow it will quickly become apparent (and repetitively so) that the *why* for virtually everything we do is to minimize risk and improve safety for our patients.

Notes

1   This ground-breaking IOM report, "To Err is Human," was followed two years later by "Crossing the Quality Chasm." These reports focused attention on issues of healthcare quality defining six aims – care should be safe, effective, patient-centered, timely, efficient, and equitable. The redesign of healthcare delivery continues with numerous initiatives and increasing regulation at every level. Subsequent outcome data will certainly be scrutinized as we all focus on quality and safety in medicine.

2   The distinction between standards and guidelines warrants mention. Both come from a medical society, for anesthesiologists this is the ASA (American Society of Anesthesiologists), but differ in their weight: standards define rules or minimum requirements, which should be followed except in extreme circumstances; guidelines present expert recommendations and are modified over time; for completeness, Statements may be released representing opinions and best medical judgments of the society, but these lack the formal scientific review of Standards and Guidelines. Attorneys may refer to all three.

3   www.anest.ufl.edu/ea.

4   Atul Gawande, a surgeon and writer, and Director of the WHO's Global Challenge for Safer Surgical Care, as of this writing has researched and written extensively on safety. The interested reader, and we sincerely hope it is nearly all, will benefit greatly from his books which currently include: *Complications*, *Better*, and *The Checklist Manifesto*.

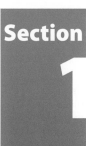

Section 1

Clinical management

Pre-operative evaluation

Surgery and anesthesia cause major perturbations to a patient's homeostasis. The risk of potentially life-threatening complications can be reduced with appropriate pre-operative evaluation and therapy. For those patients admitted prior to surgery, we take the opportunity to meet and evaluate them the evening before their operation. Because cost concerns have virtually eliminated pre-operative hospital admission, today the visit may occur just moments before the operation in the case of an emergency or a healthy outpatient, but is better managed in pre-anesthesia clinics to which patients report one or several days before their operation. Surgeons and primary-care physicians can do much to avoid operative delays and cancellations, as well as to reduce the patient's cost and risk by identifying patients who need a pre-operative anesthesia consultation and by sending all pertinent information, e.g., recent ECG, echocardiography and stress study reports, etc., with the patient. The pre-anesthetic evaluation appears to be just another routine of eliciting a history, reviewing all systems, performing a physical examination, and checking laboratory studies. However, this traditional approach provides the structure that enables us to ferret out information that can affect anesthetic preparation and management. A widely accepted shorthand, the famous ASA Physical Status classification (Table 1.1), summarizes a thorough patient evaluation into a simple scheme, found on every anesthesia record. In fact assigning an ASA Physical Status classification is an expected standard of care component of every pre-anesthetic evaluation by an anesthesia provider. The six Physical Status classes do *not* address risk specifically, but do provide a common nomenclature when discussing patients in general. That much more than the ASA Physical Status classification need be known will become apparent from the following.

History

We begin with the "H" in "H&P," obtaining a medical and surgical history. We are particularly concerned with the cardiopulmonary system, and exercise tolerance is a very good measure of current status. We also search for evidence of chronic diseases of other systems. For elective procedures, patients should be in the best condition possible, e.g., no exacerbation of chronic bronchitis or unstable angina. Below, we describe the pre-operative evaluation of some common medical conditions. When patients with these, or other rarer, conditions require an anesthetic, a pre-anesthesia clinic visit a week or so in advance of anesthesia allows time to seek additional information such as study results from the patient's private physician, perform studies such as cardiac pacemaker interrogation, or obtain consultation from a specialist. Such planning helps keep the operating schedule running smoothly.

We inquire about any previous anesthetics, particularly any untoward events such as bleeding or airway management difficulties. It is reassuring to learn a patient has tolerated previous anesthetics without complications or symptoms of a challenging airway (e.g., severe sore throat, chipped tooth). Next, we ask specifically about any family history of anesthetic complications. A patient might not realize that a remote event, such as his Aunt Edna dying with a raging fever soon after an anesthetic many years ago, might mean that malignant hyperthermia runs in his family. We need to ask specific questions to learn about inherited conditions, including those related to plasma cholinesterase (see discussion of succinylcholine in Chapter 12).

Medications

With surprising frequency, review of the patient's current medications reveals previously unmentioned medical problems: "Oh, the atenolol? Well I don't have high blood pressure *now*." Many medications influence the anesthetic, particularly those with cardiovascular or coagulation-related effects. Some need to be discontinued for some period prior to surgery (see below); others must be converted from oral to parenteral form

Table 1.1. ASA Physical Status classification

I A normal healthy patient

II A patient with mild systemic disease

III A patient with severe systemic disease

IV A patient with severe systemic disease that is a
constant threat to life

V A moribund patient who is not expected to survive
without the operation

VI A declared brain dead patient whose organs are
being removed for donor purposes

We append an "E" if the patient comes in as an emergency.
ASA = American Society of Anesthesiologists.

Table 1.2. Considerations in the latex-allergic/sensitive patient

Latex-free gloves!

Confirm latex-free equipment:

   manual breathing bag

   ventilator bellows, tourniquets, tape

   blood pressure cuff

   esophageal/precordial stethoscope tubing

   intravenous tubing access ports

   epidural access port

   syringe plunger caps (LF [latex free] should appear on
   the top of the plunger)

to continue their effect. Many patients do not think of herbal compounds when asked about their use of medicines and drugs. Therefore, we need to ask specifically about herbals, some of which may present us with problems.[1]

Allergies

Common are patients with allergies to latex and to drugs. Questions about such sensitivities need to be asked of every patient lest we get confronted with a life-threatening anaphylaxis during anesthesia. A distinction must be made, however, between sensitivities and true allergies. For example, a patient who "thought he was going to die" in the dentist's chair is probably not allergic to local anesthetics; rather, he likely had an intravascular injection, or rapid absorption of epinephrine contained in the local anesthetic mixture. Similarly, a patient who gets hives from morphine can still receive fentanyl, which is chemically quite different from the morphine-derived drugs. When an allergy is reported to a particular class of drug, there are often other classes available to accomplish the same task. We benefit our patients when we investigate these agents for potential cross-reactivity. For example, a penicillin-allergic patient with a mild reaction in childhood *likely may* receive a cephalosporin safely (about 1% risk of reaction); when determining the risk:benefit ratio, you must take into consideration their reaction and the indication for the cephalosporin.

Latex allergy deserves special mention as its recognition has grown substantially in recent years. The allergy to this natural rubber[2] occurs after repeated exposure (as in the spina bifida patient who must frequently catheterize his bladder). Its sudden rise in healthcare workers coincides with the 1980s admonition of "Universal Precautions" by the US Occupational Safety and Health Administration – healthcare workers were required to wear gloves to prevent transmission (as well as acquisition) of AIDS and other viral illnesses.

While some patients merely note skin irritation from rubber gloves (probably not a real allergy, but a precursor), of great concern is the patient who has experienced throat swelling, for example when blowing up a balloon or painting a room with latex paint. Latex is found in much of our medical equipment – from breathing bags, to syringe plungers, to Foley catheters. Since 1998 the US Food and Drug Administration (FDA) has required that all medical products containing latex be so-labeled, and many hospitals utilize non-latex alternatives wherever possible. In a patient with latex allergy, we must eliminate all latex-containing products from contact with the patient (Table 1.2).

We mentioned that healthcare workers are at risk. In fact, about one-third will develop a contact dermatitis to latex gloves, while 10% or more may develop a full-blown allergy, even more frequent in those who have other allergies, the so-called atopic individual. In particular those with allergy to chestnuts, bananas, kiwi, potatoes and tomatoes more commonly develop latex allergy. We can reduce our risk of developing this allergy by using non-latex gloves, or at least avoiding latex gloves containing cornstarch. While the cornstarch makes the glove easier to don and remove, it solubilizes the latex protein, increasing the chances of making its way through the skin – particularly through skin already irritated by the cornstarch; it also helps the latex protein become aerosolized (and breathed in) upon glove removal.

Habits

Moderate tobacco and alcohol intake are not of great concern, but the chronic alcoholic patient who has experienced delirium tremens, or the smoker who suffers severe pulmonary disease confronts us with serious problems. Patients who take street drugs also challenge us. On the one hand, they may not tell the truth about their habits; on the other hand, if they do take drugs, their response to anesthetics can be quite abnormal and troubling. These street drugs are known by colorful names to some of their devotees. Anesthesia affects the respiratory and cardiovascular systems; therefore, street drugs that depress the central nervous system (CNS) can exaggerate respiratory depression, while CNS stimulants such as cocaine can cause fatal cardiac complications.

Physical examination

In addition to the cardiopulmonary examination, we carefully evaluate the patient's airway in an attempt to predict whether it will be easily intubated (see Chapter 2). The physical examination should also seek pre-existing neurologic deficits, particularly if regional anesthesia, for example spinal, epidural, or nerve plexus block, is considered, and any limitations to flexibility that may present difficulties with positioning the patient. If we plan on regional anesthesia, we need to inspect the anatomy; for example, does the patient have a scoliosis that would make a lumbar puncture difficult, or is his skin infected over the site where we would place the needle?

Laboratory evaluations and studies

Here we must ask the question, "Can the results from additional tests influence my anesthetic and post-anesthetic management?" In the majority of cases, the answer turns out to be "No," but there are many exceptions. Among them might be a determination of serum potassium if we fear that the patient is hyperkalemic, in which case a superimposed succinylcholine-induced release of potassium would be dangerous. Coagulation studies would be needed if we plan regional anesthesia AND have reason to worry about a bleeding diathesis or thrombocytopenia. Uncontrolled bleeding into the nerve plexus can cause permanent damage. In general, laboratory and other studies should be ordered as indicated from the medical history, and only if they might have an effect on intra- or post-operative management,

or perhaps if the risk analysis may suggest canceling or altering the procedure itself. For example, suppose we detect a carotid bruit during the pre-anesthetic evaluation of a patient scheduled for elective hip replacement. While an asymptomatic bruit may not be an indication for operative repair, a significant carotid stenosis would temper our tolerance for any hypotension.

NPO status

During induction of general anesthesia, the gag reflex is necessarily abolished. Should the patient "choose" that most inopportune time to suffer gastroesophageal reflux (or worse yet, regurgitation), there is a high likelihood the stomach contents could end up in the lung, causing a chemical pneumonitis or even acute suffocation from the lodging of solid particles in the bronchial tree. In addition to pharmacologic means (see Pharmacology), we minimize this risk by having the patient report for surgery with an empty stomach. Patients are asked to refrain from eating solid foods for 6–8 hours prior to elective surgery. Recent guidelines[3] recommend a fasting period of 2 hours for clear liquids due to their rapid clearance and tendency to raise the pH of stomach contents above the pH 2.5 danger zone. Despite this it remains customary to tell patients who are scheduled for an elective operation in the morning not to eat or drink anything for at least 6 hours (for infants about 4 hours) before the operation. This convention remains in part because we worry that some patients might confuse eggs and bacon for clear liquids, but also because operating room (OR) schedules are fluid (no pun intended) and what was reported to the patient the night before as a 2 p.m. start, might suddenly move to 8 a.m. If the patient is already in the hospital, we write the order "NPO after midnight"[4] to achieve the same results. Here, we can also order "maintenance i.v. fluids" overnight to keep the patient hydrated. Therefore, on the day of surgery we ask every patient about their most recent intake of food and liquids. Avoid asking: "When did you have your last meal?" If the patient's history identifies risk factors for aspiration, e.g., frank gastroesophageal reflex disease (GERD) with frank reflux, diabetes with history suggestive of gastroparesis, or bowel obstruction, and we plan general anesthesia, we use a rapid or modified rapid-sequence induction (see Chapter 5 on general anesthesia). Pre-operatively we also consider pharmacologic means to raise gastric pH such as oral sodium citrate (distasteful to most, but instantly effective), or an H_2 blocker or proton pump inhibitor (30-minute onset, but may be effective at emergence even if induction cannot wait).

Many patients have not been fasting for several hours, or their stomach did not have time to empty. Labor pains, narcotics, or trauma can stop gastric peristalsis for hours on end. Of course, in the presence of an ileus, we always assume the stomach not to be empty even if the patient has had nothing by mouth for many hours or even days.

Planned procedure

The planned surgical, diagnostic, or therapeutic procedure influences the anesthetic management, sometimes producing problems for which we must be prepared. For example, the neurosurgeon may trigger a wild release of catecholamines when destroying the trigeminal ganglion in a percutaneous procedure that lasts only minutes. How are we going to protect the patient from the expected sympathetic storm? Or, how can we guard against a sudden and substantial rise in peripheral arterial resistance when the surgeon clamps the aorta in preparation for the resection of an aortic aneurysm? The planned procedure also has implications for, among other things, intra-operative positioning of the patient, potential need for blood replacement, anticipated severity of post-operative pain (is a regional anesthetic an option?), and need for intensive care after surgery.

Anesthetic choice

In addition to the above assessment, the anesthetic plan must consider the wishes of both patient and surgeon, as well as *our* individual skill and experience. Does the patient have special requests that need to be taken into account? For example, some patients would like to be awake (maybe the President so he doesn't have to pass control of the USA to the Vice-President), others asleep, and others do not want "a needle in the back."

Some patients present special problems, for example Jehovah's Witnesses who do not accept blood transfusions, based on their interpretation of several passages in the Bible (for example Acts 15:28, 29). A thoughtful and compassionate discussion with the patient usually finds the physician agreeing to honor the patient's wishes, an agreement that may not be violated. The caring for children of Jehovah's Witnesses brings an added concern and may require ethics consultation and perhaps even referral to a court. Again, these issues are best brought out days prior to surgery at a scheduled pre-anesthetic evaluation.

Numerous studies have failed to demonstrate that a particular inhalation anesthetic, muscle relaxant, or narcotic made for a better outcome than an alternative. Yet, over the years, actual or perceived differences and conveniences have caused some drugs to disappear and others to establish themselves. Given an array of options, we can often consider different approaches to anesthesia, which we can discuss with the patient. We should always recommend the approach with which we have the greatest experience and which we would select for ourselves or a loved one.

The choices depend on several factors, first of which is the surgical procedure. For example, the site of the operation, such as a craniotomy, can rule out spinal anesthesia. The nature of the operation, e.g., a thoracotomy, can compel us to use an endotracheal tube. For the removal of a wart or toenail or the lancing of a boil, we would not consider general anesthesia – unless the patient's age or psychological condition would make it preferable. The preferences of the surgeon might also be considered.

This introduces the patient's condition as a factor in the choice of anesthesia. For example, a patient in hemorrhagic shock depends on a functioning sympathetic nervous system for survival and therefore cannot tolerate the sympathetic blockade induced by spinal or epidural anesthesia. Vigorous coughing at the end of an eye operation might cause extrusion of vitreous humor and must be avoided. Respiratory depression and elevated arterial carbon dioxide levels can increase intracranial pressure with potentially devastating effects in patients with an intracranial mass or hemorrhage. In obstetrical anesthesia, mother *and* child have to be considered. Here, we do not wish to depress uterine contraction nor cause prolonged sedation of the newborn child. Some agents used in anesthesia rely on renal excretion, others on hepatic metabolism, thus tilting our choice of drugs in patients with renal or hepatic insufficiency.

In the majority of patients, however, it makes little difference what we pick. We could choose one or the other technique for general anesthesia, using one or the other intravenous induction drug and neuromuscular blocker, and relying on one or the other inhalation anesthetic. We can supplement such a technique with one of a number of narcotic drugs available to us, or we can use total intravenous anesthesia. When we use general anesthesia, we can intubate the patient's

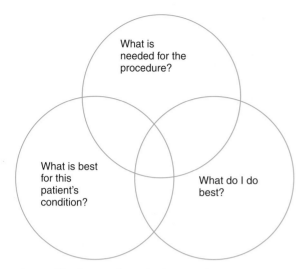

Fig. 1.1 The diagram shows the factors to be considered in the choice of anesthesia. In many instances the three circles coincide or greatly overlap, in others the choice is narrowed by the listed factors.

trachea and let the patient breathe spontaneously, or we can artificially ventilate the patient's lungs. Instead of an endotracheal tube, we have available the laryngeal mask airway (LMA), preferably used in spontaneously breathing patients or, in the very old-fashioned approach, we might use only a face mask.

In summary, many factors can influence the choice of anesthesia. In the majority of patients, however, we have the luxury of making the choice influenced by our own preference and routine (Fig. 1.1).

Common disorders

We encounter many patients with pre-existing medical conditions. Anesthetic and operative procedures constitute a physiologic trespass with which the patient can deal better if not simultaneously challenged by correctable derangements that sap his strength and threaten his homeostasis. Ideally, the surgeon would already have addressed these questions. However, that is not always the case, and the anesthesiologist needs to assess the medical condition of the patient. The answers to the question, "Is the patient in the optimal condition to proceed with anesthesia and operation?" are not always clear-cut. For example, a patient with transient ischemic attacks is scheduled for a carotid endarterectomy. The patient also has coronary artery disease and unstable angina. Should we risk the possibility of a stroke by first putting the patient through a heart operation, or should we risk a myocardial infarction by first

doing a carotid endarterectomy? Consultations with other experts help in resolving such difficult issues.

Trauma emergency

Rapid assessment of the airway and fluid status precedes, or coincides with, the most urgent: stemming of hemorrhage. Once we have secured an airway and established a route for administering fluids, we can contemplate anesthesia. A trauma patient in hemorrhagic shock will tolerate very little anesthesia, but we must keep in mind this makes him vulnerable to intra-operative awareness with recall. The mechanism of the trauma may suggest additional studies (Table 1.3).

Diabetes

We focus on the many end-organ effects of diabetes, as well as the patient's glucose control (HbA1c). Those with very poor control should be considered for pre-admission. Pre-operative studies should include assessment of metabolic, renal, and cardiac status. In general, diabetic patients should be scheduled early in the day.

Because of the 30% incidence of gastroparesis in this population, diabetics are often pretreated with metoclopramide to speed gastric emptying and are induced with a "rapid-sequence induction" (see Chapter 5). Intra-operative management aims to match insulin requirements, recognizing the fasting state and the effects of surgical stress.

Coronary artery disease

In 2007, the American College of Cardiology and the American Heart Association (ACC/AHA) published updated guidelines for the peri-operative cardiovascular evaluation of patients for non-cardiac surgery. These so-called "Eagle criteria" (named for the first author of the original guidelines) recommend further evaluation of active serious clinical conditions (e.g., unstable coronary syndromes, decompensated heart failure, significant arrhythmias, and severe valvular disease) prior to non-emergent surgery. We should always ask the patient about his exercise tolerance; the ACC/AHA recommendations attempt to quantify this by using metabolic equivalents (METs), which enables us to classify patients on a MET scale of 1 (take care of yourself around the house) to 10+ (participate in strenuous sports). A very useful dividing line is 4 METs (climb a flight of stairs). In general, patients unable to accomplish the equivalent of 4 METs physical activity

Table 1.3. Studies in the trauma patient

Study	Indication	Comments
Cervical spine radiographs	Trauma, especially with neck tenderness	Traditional direct laryngoscopy can further compromise the cervical spinal cord
Chest radiograph	Any chest trauma or motor vehicle accident	Potential for pneumothorax (avoid nitrous oxide, consider chest tube); pulmonary contusion
Echocardiography	Direct trauma to chest, for example, forceful contact with steering wheel	Cardiac contusion, pericardial effusion, aortic dissection, and pneumothorax may also be seen
Abdominal ultrasound	Direct trauma or motor vehicle accident	Potential for hemorrhage, ruptured spleen or fractured liver; replaces diagnostic peritoneal lavage (DPL)
Angiography	Chest or abdominal trauma	Aortic dissection

represent a group at high risk of cardiovascular complications. The algorithm in Figure 1.2 helps in assigning risks and identifying those patients who require additional cardiac evaluation. In addition to functional capacity, the algorithm incorporates the active cardiac conditions and clinical risk factors listed in Table 1.4 as well as the procedure planned (Table 1.5). Should we discover a potential issue that does not compel a delay in surgery, we advise the patient to follow up this finding post-operatively. For example, isolated ECG abnormalities or a heart murmur with normal exercise tolerance have potential significance and may require a long-term therapeutic strategy.

Pacemaker/AICD

Pacemakers are life-saving for many patients with heart rhythm disturbances. There are many types available, with a range of functionality (see Table 1.6). We come across more and more patients with them every year. The addition of an automated implantable cardioverter defibrillator (AICD) goes one step further and also suggests a more significant underlying cardiac history (often an ejection fraction <0.4). Unfortunately, these life-saving devices may fail to function properly in the presence of electrical devices routinely encountered in an operating suite, e.g., electrocautery. Many patients carry a card identifying the pacemaker make and model. Some can also provide a report from a recent electronic interrogation that specifies proper function and remaining battery life. But all too often, that information is not available. A chest radiograph can reveal pacer make and model, as well as lead location. In symptomatic (lightheaded spells, palpitations, hypotension) or in pacer-dependent patients, a pacemaker

interrogation (by a specialist with proprietary communication equipment) may be necessary. If this is not an option, a current ECG *might* be helpful, if it demonstrates pacer spikes in appropriate locations. To determine if a pacemaker is rate-responsive, i.e., adapts its rate to the patient's activity, gently shake the pacemaker and see if the heart rate increases. For all but the most minor procedures, we disable the AICD function to prevent electrocautery-induced confusion of the algorithms and ill-advised defibrillation attempts, which may succeed in just the opposite result.

Chronic hypertension

One-quarter of adults, and a much higher percentage of elderly people, present with hypertension. Of these, only a third are adequately treated. Add to that the "white coat hypertension" of anticipated surgery, and the confusion over which medications to discontinue the morning of surgery, and frequently we confront hypertension-range blood pressures (>140/90) in the pre-operative patient. Severe hypertension (>200/115) or evidence of significant end-organ damage prompts a delay of elective surgery. Rapid control of hypertension may compromise organ perfusion; for example, cerebral blood flow autoregulates around the prevailing pressure and can be reduced to a dangerous level with an acute drop in blood pressure even to "normal" levels. We encourage our patient to continue his chronic antihypertensive medications through the morning of surgery, with the possible exception of diuretics if we plan conscious sedation (and no bladder catheter), and angiotensin system blockers (see below). Intra-operatively we strive to maintain blood pressure within 30% of normal for the patient; a value best determined

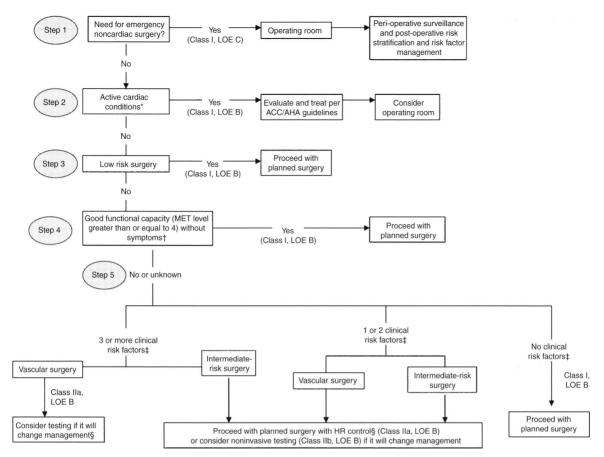

Fig. 1.2 ACC/AHA cardiac evaluation and care algorithm for non-cardiac surgery based on active clinical conditions, known cardiovascular disease, or cardiac risk factors for patients 50 years of age or greater. A stepwise approach to the risk assessment of patients with pre-existing cardiac disease, scheduled for surgery. Clinical predictors refer to Table 1.4. Subsequent care may include cancellation or delay of surgery, coronary revascularization followed by non-cardiac surgery, or intensified care. ACC/AHA: American College of Cardiology/American Heart Association; HR: heart rate; LOE: level of evidence; MET: metabolic equivalent. *Unstable coronary syndromes, decompensated heart failure, significant arrhythmias, severe valvular disease. †4 METs is roughly the activity equivalent of climbing a flight of stairs or walking on level ground at 4 miles per hour. ‡Clinical risk factors include history of ischemic heart disease, congestive heart failure, cerebrovascular disease, diabetes, and renal insufficiency. §Consider peri-operative beta-blockade. (Reprinted with permission. Circulation 2007;116:1971–1996. ©2007, American Heart Association, Inc.)

Table 1.4. Cardiac and clinical risk factors associated with increased peri-operative cardiovascular risk

Active cardiac conditions

- Unstable coronary syndromes (unstable or severe angina, recent MI [<30 days])
- Decompensated heart failure
- Significant arrhythmias
- Severe valvular heart disease

Clinical risk factors

- History of ischemic heart disease
- History of compensated or prior heart failure
- History of cerebral vascular disease
- Diabetes mellitus
- Renal insufficiency

by patient report from drug-store tests or by reviewing clinic notes from a lower-stress environment.

Congestive heart failure

As noted in the Eagle criteria above, heart failure increases the risk of complications from surgery, and only under extreme conditions would we anesthetize a patient with uncompensated failure. For a patient with a history of congestive heart failure (CHF), pre-operatively we inquire about current symptoms and compliance with his medication regimen. We check electrolytes if he reports diuretic use, and consider an echocardiogram and/or brain natriuretic peptide (BNP) test if he reports concerning symptoms that might significantly alter the risk:benefit ratio of the planned operation/anesthetic. There is little evidence

Table 1.5. Cardiac risk[a] stratification for non-cardiac surgical procedures

Vascular (reported cardiac risk often more than 5%)

- Aortic and other major vascular surgery
- Peripheral vascular surgery

Intermediate (reported cardiac risk generally 1–5%)

- Intraperitoneal and intrathoracic surgery
- Carotid endarterectomy
- Head and neck surgery
- Orthopedic surgery
- Prostate surgery

Low[b] (reported cardiac risk generally less than 1%)

- Endoscopic procedures
- Superficial procedures
- Cataract surgery
- Breast surgery
- Ambulatory surgery

[a] Combined incidence of cardiac death and non-fatal myocardial infarction.
[b] These procedures do not generally require further pre-operative cardiac testing.

Table 1.6. Pacemaker generators

Cardiac chamber paced	Cardiac chamber sensed	Response to sensed R and P
V-Ventricle	V-Ventricle	T-Triggering
A-Atrium	A-Atrium	I-Inhibited
D-Dual	D-Dual	D-Dual
	O-None (asynch)	

A fourth letter, "R" for rate-responsive, denotes a pacemaker that recognizes patient activity and responds by increasing its rate. Shivering or fasciculations may erroneously cause an increased pacing rate.
VVI: Stimulation and sensing occurs in the ventricle. "I" indicates that the pacemaker does not fire if it detects a native R wave. Depending on the patient's intrinsic heart rate, an ECG will show either ventricular pacing or no pacing.
VVIR: As above but responds to patient motion by increasing heart rate.
DDD: Stimulates atrium and ventricle, senses P and R waves.
VOO: Asynchronous ventricular pacing. This can cause a problem if a paced R wave occurs during the T wave of a native beat (R-on-T phenomenon).

recommending regional versus general anesthesia, but if the patient reports severe orthopnea, regional anesthesia and supine positioning may not be practical. Intra-operatively we maintain the tenets of CHF management: maintain preload without over-hydration, reduce afterload, and maintain inotropic support (e.g., limit myocardial depressants).

Pulmonary disease

The patient with pre-operative pulmonary disease faces risks of intra-operative and post-operative pulmonary complications including pneumonia, bronchospasm, atelectasis, respiratory failure with prolonged mechanical ventilation, and exacerbation of pre-existing lung disease. The risk of these complications depends on both the patient and the procedure.

- *Chronic pulmonary disease*. Both chronic obstructive pulmonary disease (COPD) and asthma can increase the risk. Therefore, well before anesthesia and surgery, we should treat the patient to bring him into the best possible condition, given his lung disease.
- *Smoking*. Even without evident lung disease, smoking increases the risk of pulmonary complications up to four times over that of non-smokers. Eight weeks of smoking cessation is required to reduce that risk, though carboxyhemoglobin will virtually vanish after only 24 smoke-free hours.
- *General health*. There are general risk indices that predict pulmonary complications well. In fact, exercise tolerance alone is an excellent predictor of post-operative pulmonary complications.
- *Obesity*. Obese patients present more airway management difficulties for several reasons: (i) mechanical issues related to optimal positioning; (ii) redundant pharyngeal tissue complicating laryngoscopy; (iii) many suffer from obstructive sleep apnea (and its sequelae: pulmonary hypertension/cor pulmonale); and (iv) in obese patients it can be extremely difficult or impossible to mask–ventilate the lungs due to the weight of the chest wall. Obesity also increases the risk for thromboembolic phenomena. Post-operatively, however, obesity has not proven to increase the risk of pulmonary complications.
- *Surgical site*. Proximity of the surgical site to the diaphragm is the single most important predictor of pulmonary complications. Thoracic and upper

abdominal operative sites confer a 10–40% incidence. This can be reduced perhaps 100-fold with laparoscopic techniques.

- *Surgery duration.* Operations lasting <3 hours are associated with fewer complications.
- *Intra-operative muscle relaxants.* Pancuronium, specifically, has been associated with an increased incidence of pulmonary complications; this is related to its long half-life and risk of residual muscle weakness.
- *Results of pre-operative testing.* Routine pre-operative pulmonary function tests (PFTs) are not indicated, unless the patient is undergoing a major lung resection. If available, however, the risk of complications increases when the forced expiratory volume in 1 second (FEV_1) or forced vital capacity (FVC) are <70% predicted, or when the FEV_1/FVC is <65%.

Asthma

Pre-operatively, our goals are to reverse bronchospasm and inflammation, prevent an asthma exacerbation, clear secretions, and treat any infection. We specifically ask about any increased inhaler use, recent hospitalizations or Emergency Department visits for bronchospasm, a recent change in sputum amount or color, or a recent cold. All of these factors increase the risk of peri-operative bronchospasm. If the patient is scheduled for thoracic or upper abdominal surgery (with a very high risk of pulmonary complications), spirometry can identify patients at greatest risk. Spirometry will also reveal any benefit to bronchodilator therapy pre- or post-operatively.

Glucocorticoids may be helpful in those patients who do not respond adequately to β_2 agonists. Patients who are steroid-dependent occasionally have suppressed adrenal cortical function and require supplemental steroids in the peri-operative period.

Chronic renal failure

Chronic renal failure (CRF) involves both the excretory and synthetic functions of the kidney. When the kidney fails to regulate fluids and electrolytes, the net result is acidosis, hyperkalemia, hypertension, and edema. Meanwhile, the lack of synthetic function results in anemia (due to decreased production of erythropoietin) and hypocalcemia from a lack of active vitamin D_3 (this also leads to secondary hyperparathyroidism, hyperphosphatemia, and renal osteodystrophy). Azotemia can cause platelet dysfunction.

Medications that are renally excreted will be affected by CRF, and most should be avoided. In particular, meperidine (pethidine, Demerol®) should not be given as its metabolite (normeperidine) can accumulate and cause seizures. The preferred muscle relaxant is one that does not primarily depend on renal function for its metabolism (atracurium, cisatracurium, or vecuronium for surgical relaxation).

We check electrolytes on these patients pre-operatively and prefer they undergo dialysis within the preceding 24 hours. We must resist the temptation to hydrate a patient who is intravascularly "dry" following dialysis, as they cannot excrete excess fluids. Useful information includes the patient's pre- and post-dialysis weight, quantifying the volume of fluid removed. Comparison with current weight can help infer volume status. Replacement fluids should not contain potassium (normal saline is preferred over Ringer's lactate) as these patients are at risk for hyperkalemia. CRF patients are also at increased risk for coronary artery and peripheral vascular disease.

Pre-operative medication management

Peri-operative beta-blockade

The last few years have seen increasing interest in the prophylactic use of beta-blockade to reduce peri-operative cardiac morbidity, particularly in patients already taking a beta-blocker or those at high risk for a cardiac event and undergoing major elective non-cardiac surgery. The target of this therapy is a heart rate of around 70 beats/min and systolic blood pressure of 110 mmHg – if tolerated by the patient. If a patient in the high-risk group is not currently on beta-blockers, a cardioselective agent (atenolol or metoprolol) is recommended. Use in lower-risk groups must balance the reduction in myocardial infarction with an increase in the incidence of stroke identified in recent analyses. If indicated, beta-blockade should be initiated *as early as possible* and maintained throughout the hospitalization and after discharge (at least 30 days and probably longer).

Antihypertensives

Angiotensin-converting enzyme (ACE) inhibitors (and angiotensin II receptor antagonists) have been linked

19

to severe and refractory intra-operative hypotension under anesthesia. Unless the patient has a history of congestive heart failure, cardiomyopathy (ejection fraction <45%), or very severe hypertension, many recommend discontinuation of these medications the day before surgery. Similarly, many advocate discontinuing diuretics the morning of surgery, both for the patient's comfort (if awake) and for intra-operative fluid management. If the diuretic is for acute CHF, however, it should be continued. Otherwise, antihypertensive drugs should be continued the morning of surgery. In particular, agents with a known rebound phenomenon, i.e., clonidine and beta-blockers, *must* be continued or refractory hypertension may result. Because patients are instructed to be fasting, we must actually *tell* them to take their antihypertensives or risk significant hypertension in the pre-operative holding area. We ask all patients, and especially those with hypertension, about their usual daily range of blood pressures. Most people can answer the questions, "What is the highest you have recently seen your blood pressure and what is the lowest?" This information guides us in setting intra-operative targets.

Anticoagulants

Many patients are on some form of platelet inhibitor. While single-agent therapy poses no problem for most operations, multi-modal platelet inhibition may increase the risk of peri-operative bleeding.

- *Non-steroidal anti-inflammatory agents (NSAIDs, including aspirin [ASA]).* These can be safely continued unless there are special surgical (aesthetic plastic surgery, neurosurgery) or anesthetic (nerve block) considerations, or the patient is on multi-modal therapy. Many surgeons, however, want ASA discontinued 10 days prior to surgery and other NSAIDs stopped for at least several days, even though we lack evidence that this alters the incidence of intra-operative blood loss. Actually, it may increase the incidence of thrombotic complications (deep vein thrombosis [DVT], coronary thrombosis, thrombotic stroke), and prevent the pre-emptive analgesia and opioid-sparing capacity of pre-operative NSAIDs. In patients with coronary stents (who are universally on at least one antiplatelet medication) aspirin should not be discontinued without involving a cardiologist. The type, number, and location of stent(s), as well as the time and circumstances of

stent placement all conspire to determine the need for anticoagulation.

- *Platelet-function inhibitors (ticlopidine [Ticlid®], clopidogrel [Plavix®]).* If the patient receives multi-modal therapy, consider switching to a single agent. We must weigh the risks of discontinuing anticoagulation against the risk of intra-operative or anesthetic-induced bleeding. Because of their prolonged half-lives, regional anesthesia would mandate discontinuing these agents for many days (ticlopidine: 14 days; clopidogrel: 7 days) prior to surgery.
- *GP IIb IIIa inhibitors (abciximab [Reopro®], eptifibatide [Integrilin®], tirofiban [Aggrastat®]).* These should be stopped prior to surgery and can be reversed with transfusion of platelets if thought necessary. However, patients on these agents usually *need* the anticoagulation. Continuation of these drugs represents a contraindication to regional anesthesia.
- *Heparin.* Subcutaneous prophylactic dosing (twice-daily dosing and total daily dose <10 000 units) need not be discontinued, but timed carefully if a regional anesthetic is to be administered; low-molecular-weight heparins should be stopped much earlier and subsequent doses administered well after the block.[5]

Monoamine oxidase inhibitors (MAOIs)

These agents interact with many drugs and may result in severe hypertension if indirect-acting vasopressors are administered. Even more worrisome are excitatory/depressive (central serotonin syndrome) reactions with administration of opioids. In particular, meperidine (Demerol®) is absolutely contraindicated in these patients. Some still advocate discontinuation of these agents for 2 weeks pre-operatively.

Herbal remedies

Public enthusiasm for herbal supplements has its drawbacks. The following are current considerations together with the recommended discontinuation period prior to surgery:

- Ephedra – works like ephedrine with direct and indirect sympathomimetic effects and all the consequent side effects including intra-operative hemodynamic instability from depletion of endogenous catecholamines; 24 hours.

- Garlic – inhibition of platelet aggregation and increased fibrinolysis; 7 days.
- Ginkgo – inhibition of platelet-activating factor; 36 hours.
- Ginseng – hypoglycemia, inhibition of platelet aggregation; 7 days.
- St. John's wort – induction of cytochrome P450 enzymes; 5 days.
- Others such as kava and valerian are sedatives, perhaps reducing the need for additional sedative agents – titrate!

Informed consent

Upto the 1950s, anesthesia claimed about one life for every 2000 anesthetics given. Particularly during the past 30 years, the frequency of anesthesia-related complications leading to morbidity and mortality has decreased markedly, but unfortunately not to zero. No one knows the actual incidence of preventable anesthetic deaths; currently quoted numbers range from 1 in 20 000 to 1 in 200 000 anesthetics, a reasonable estimate probably lying somewhere between these figures.

Anesthetic risks are usually smaller than the risks associated with surgical interventions, but they loom large when general anesthesia or heavy sedation is required for a non-invasive and essentially risk-free diagnostic examination. For example, when a small child needs anesthesia to hold still for a CT scan or MRI study, anesthesia essentially poses the only risks.

Many drugs used in general anesthesia interfere with ventilation – think of respiratory depression from narcotics, surgical anesthesia depressing reflexes and relaxing the muscles of the upper airway and, worst of all, the commonly used neuromuscular blocking agents, which spare the heart but paralyze the muscles of respiration. Recognition of these potential respiratory problems has led to the widespread use of endotracheal anesthesia, which requires the insertion of a tube into the trachea, sometimes a non-trivial matter. Unrecognized esophageal intubation and inability to gain control of the airway continue to claim lives. No wonder then that inadequate ventilation and hypoxemia have caused more grief than any other anesthetic complication. No organ depends more on continuous perfusion with oxygen-carrying blood than the brain. The consequences of brain hypoxia range from deterioration of intellectual function to death.

Anesthetics also affect the cardiovascular system by weakening the myocardium, by depressing autonomic control, and by a relaxing effect on vascular smooth muscle. Decreased preload, low cardiac output, and hypotension can result with potentially disastrous consequences.

Regional anesthesia carries the risks associated with potential local anesthetic toxicity, resulting in hypotension or convulsions. In addition, the injection of drugs into a nerve plexus, a nerve, or into the epidural or subarachnoid space, carries the risk of physical damage, bleeding, and infection. These complications occasionally cause permanent neurologic changes and even paralysis.

Few drugs are free of the potential for triggering an anaphylactic response, which can be difficult to diagnose in a patient under general anesthesia. Interestingly, of all the medications used during an anesthetic, the class of drugs most likely to cause an anaphylactic reaction is not antibiotics, but rather the paralytic muscle relaxants. The resulting severe hypotension and bronchospasm can then threaten the life of the patient.

Anesthetic morbidity is not easily defined but is certainly more common than mortality. Intraoperative hypotension and arrhythmias are common and, unless severe, are not even mentioned as complications. Within hours after general anesthesia, 25% of all patients may experience transient cognitive dysfunction; a similar percentage suffer from nausea and vomiting and/or sore throat, and a very small number have peripheral nerve impairment, which usually resolves within weeks. Occasionally, we chip a tooth during tracheal intubation, cause a hematoma with an i.v. catheter, or produce more significant complications with invasive monitors, for example a pneumothorax or catheter-related bloodstream infection with a central venous catheter.

In short, anesthesia does pose dangers. This raises the question of how to tell a patient about potential complications in anesthesia or other procedures. Should we pat the patient on the back and say, "Don't worry, I'll take care of you"? Or should we enumerate all possible complications? What does the patient need to understand, and what are we legally required to explain? The informed consent process should result in the active participation of an autonomous and competent patient choosing an anesthetic course based on the information and compassionate medical advice. Physicians have been criticized for being either overly paternalistic or aloof and impersonal. Frequent complaints concern failure to explain findings and/or treatment plans.

While it would be ideal for each patient to understand the details of his or her medical care and participate in all decisions, that level of true "informed consent" is unattainable. Patients will almost invariably be cared for by several experts. Even an expert physician in one field cannot fully appreciate the depth of knowledge an expert in another field brings to the table; how much less then can a medically naïve patient hope to understand all ramifications of diagnosis, prognosis, treatment options, and complications?

Informed consent should fulfill both ethical and legal obligations in the physician–patient relationship, including the pros and cons of the anesthetic options and certainly a description of complications with a 10% or greater risk of occurrence. In addition, rarer complications relevant to a particular operation, for example post-operative visual loss following a long complex spine procedure, should be discussed, especially if their disclosure might affect the patient's decision whether to proceed or seek alternative therapy. Otherwise, it is ethically preferable and legally sound to ask whether the patient wishes to hear about the less common but more serious risks before presenting a comprehensive and dizzying list. For example, enumerating risks of heart attack, stroke, and death from anesthesia need not further upset a patient who is undergoing a necessary operation. He already knows he could die from the operation itself or from refusing surgery.

When speaking with patients, before asking for their signature on a document entitled "Informed consent," we find ourselves confronted by a multi-horned dilemma. We wish to explain our findings and therapeutic options, realizing that the patient has a right to make decisions about his or her care. While we do not wish to be paternalistic, we have the obligation to offer our opinion as to the best treatment plan so that the patient has the benefit of our knowledge. Sometimes, our opinion can be colored by our personal skills and experiences; when two treatments are equivalent in all aspects, we should prefer the one with which we have more and better experience. The legally required "informed consent" process, therefore, calls for skillful and compassionate blending of information and guidance covering (i) risks, complications, and consequences of the proposed treatment, (ii) alternatives, and (iii) conflicts of interest.

Notes

1 www.anest.ufl.edu/EA.

2 From the *Hevea brasiliensis* tree.

3 This and other guidelines from the American Society of Anesthesiology are available from their website at www.asahq.org.

4 NPO stands for the Latin nil per os = nothing by mouth.

5 The American Society of Regional Anesthesia publishes updated guidelines regularly. See www.anest.ufl.edu/EA.

Airway management

We have made remarkable advances in techniques to secure a patent airway, and have developed new equipment and methods to monitor breathing. Yet, respiratory complications remain the leading cause of anesthesia-related deaths, with the majority related to failure to obtain control of the airway. Here we will discuss: (i) how to evaluate the airway of a patient; (ii) the impact of the planned procedure designed to protect the airway; and (iii) how to manage the airway. First, let us explain why all this matters.

Any time we anesthetize a patient, we must be prepared to take over his ventilation at a moment's (or less) notice because anesthesia can interfere with ventilation in so many ways. We may have weakened, with muscle relaxants, the patient's ability to breathe. We may have put him into a deep coma, anesthetizing his respiratory center and relaxing the muscles in his mouth and pharynx so that his air passage is obstructed. We might have suppressed his urge to breathe with hypnotics and narcotics during nothing more than a minor surgical procedure. Whatever the roots of the failure to breathe, we must be ready to support inadequate spontaneous effort or take full command of ventilating the patient's lungs, which means establishing or re-establishing a patent airway and, if necessary, breathing for the patient.

Therefore, before anesthetizing ANY patient, we examine the airway, looking for physical findings that can be reassuring or worrisome.

Examination of the airway

Direct laryngoscopy (see below) requires neck flexibility, a mouth that can open widely, and no excessive pharyngeal tissue or a large tongue to get in the way. These features cannot be measured directly, but the following steps help us to assess problems that might arise during laryngoscopy:

- Assess mouth opening: inter-incisor distance should exceed 4 cm in an adult.
- Determine the mentum–hyoid (>4 cm) or thyromental (>7 cm) distance: shorter distances suggest an "anterior" or very cephalad larynx, which would be difficult to visualize by conventional laryngoscopy.
- Investigate the posterior pharynx (modified Mallampati classification) by having the sitting patient fully extend his neck, maximally open his mouth, and stick out his tongue with or without phonation. Figure 2.1 shows how we classify the visible structures.
- Determine the ability to move lower in front of the upper incisors (prognath), which is a good sign. To accomplish this we ask our patients to bite their upper lip.
- Evaluate neck mobility: full extension through full flexion should exceed 90°. Patients who might require further evaluation or a special approach to minimize neck movement during intubation include:
  - (i) those with rheumatoid arthritis and/or Down's syndrome: the transverse ligament that secures the odontoid can become lax, introducing cervical instability and the potential for cervical cord trauma with direct laryngoscopy;
  - (ii) trauma patients who may have damaged their cervical spine (Table 2.1).
- Finally, patients with a history of difficult intubation and any obvious airway pathology (vocal cord tumor, neck radiation scar, congenital malformation, mediastinal mass, etc.) should be further investigated. Patients with a history of snoring and/or morbid obesity also cause us concern.

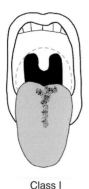
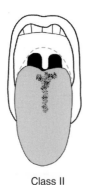
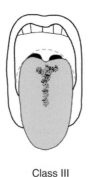
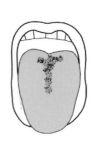

Fig. 2.1 Modified Mallampati classification: Class I: soft palate, fauces, uvula, pillars; Class II: soft palate, fauces, portion of uvula; Class III: soft palate, base of uvula; Class IV: hard palate only.

Class I   Class II   Class III   Class IV

Table 2.1. Trauma evaluation of the cervical spine: findings that may compel radiographic assessment

Midline cervical tenderness

Focal neurologic deficit

Decreased alertness

Intoxication

Painful, distracting injuries that might mask neck pain

From Hoffman, J. R., Mower, W. R., *et al.* Validity of a set of clinical criteria to rule out injury to the cervical spine in patients with blunt trauma. *N. Engl. J. Med.* 2000; **343**:94–9.

See www.anest.ufl.edu/EA for a thorough review of airway evaluation.

Airway management techniques

Mask–ventilation

Simple as it seems, the ability to mask–ventilate a patient is *the* essential airway management technique that needs to be practiced and learned by every health-care provider. Most important is the patient's head position: Do not let the patient's neck flex and thus potentially occlude the airway, which makes mask–ventilation difficult to impossible. Proper mask technique includes the following:

  (i) Select an appropriate size mask to fit over the patient's nose and mouth and provide an airtight seal without pressure on the eyes.

 (ii) Place the head in sniffing position (occiput elevated, neck extended) or directly supine, with the neck neutral to slightly extended.

(iii) Positioning yourself at the patient's head, apply the mask to the face with a pincer grip by thumb and index finger of the left hand. Place the third finger on the mentum and pull the chin upward.

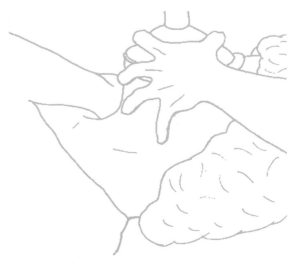

Fig. 2.2 Mask–ventilation technique.

The fourth finger remains on the mandible, not the soft tissue under the jaw where it might cause compression and obstruction. With the pinkie at the angle of the mandible, pull the jaw forward to open the posterior pharynx (a painful maneuver in an awake patient!) (Fig. 2.2).

(iv) Then, ventilate the patient's lungs with a self-inflating bag, Mapleson or anesthesia machine circle system. Keep inflation pressures to the minimum required to ventilate the lungs, in an effort to prevent inflation of the stomach (ideally no more than 20 cmH$_2$O pressure).

What to do when mask–ventilation proves to be difficult:

- Reposition. Make sure the mandible is being pulled anteriorly.
- Add a second person to try two-handed mask–ventilation. One person uses both hands to hold

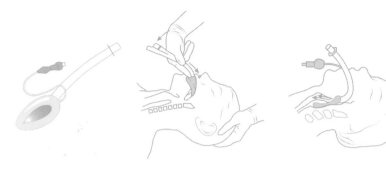

Fig. 2.3 Laryngeal mask airway. We advance the LMA along the roof of the mouth of the anesthetized patient, until it seats at the esophageal inlet. We inflate the cuff, which causes the LMA to rebound slightly. Finally, we confirm placement by the presence of end-tidal CO_2 on the capnograph. LMA: laryngeal mask airway.

the mask and pull the jaw anteriorly. The other compresses the breathing bag.

- Use an oral or nasal airway to establish a pathway past the pharyngeal tissue and tongue. This is not advisable in the awake patient (he would retch) nor under light anesthesia (he might develop a tight laryngospasm, which would make matters worse). A nasal trumpet can be inserted after lubrication, even if the patient is awake.
- If the patient has a beard, try placing an occlusive dressing (with a hole for the mouth) over the beard, or apply Vaseline® to the mask.
- The edentulous patient usually does better with his false teeth in place, but make sure they can be easily removed. If the patient is comatose, an oral airway may help.

Laryngeal mask airway

Developed in the 1980s, the laryngeal mask airway (LMA; Fig. 2.3) has supplanted tracheal intubation for many general anesthetics. The device is basically the progeny of a face mask mated with an endotracheal tube, allowing positioning of the mask just above the glottic opening. While there are available versions intended to protect the airway from gastric aspiration (e.g., LMA Proseal®), none can guarantee it. The major advantages of the LMA over tracheal intubation are the lower level of skill required for placement, decreased airway trauma (especially of the vocal cords), and reduced stimulation such that lightly anesthetized, spontaneously breathing patients can tolerate the device. Also, the properly positioned LMA places the laryngeal inlet in clear view for a fiberoptic scope, making tracheal intubation through the device an attractive technique in the management of the unexpected difficult airway.

To place the LMA, we induce anesthesia, usually without paralysis, then:

(i) place the patient's head in the sniffing position;
(ii) stabilize the occiput and slightly extend the neck with the right hand, allowing the jaw to fall open;
(iii) press the deflated LMA against the hard palate with the gloved index finger, and gently advance it until encountering the resistance of the upper esophageal sphincter.

There are many variations to this technique, including using a semi-inflated mask or the popular initial insertion upside-down, then rotation in the posterior pharynx (not recommended by the manufacturer). When difficulty arises, try moving to the front of the patient, placing the right hand on the top of the LMA and using the index finger to coax the tip of the LMA down toward the laryngeal inlet. Any restriction to mouth opening makes the latter technique impossible. When correctly positioned, the cuff comes to sit at the base of the hypopharynx at the esophageal verge. If viewed through a scope, the vocal cords (and many times the esophagus) will come into view within the LMA bowl. Thus, this airway does not protect against aspiration. While it can be used during controlled ventilation, we risk gastric distension if inflation pressure exceeds 20 cmH_2O and thus we would use pressure- not volume-controlled ventilation.[1]

We remove the LMA from the awakened patient, often without first deflating the device as it serves as a pharyngeal squeegee to pull secretions towards the teeth where they can be suctioned away. Because the LMA is less stimulating than an endotracheal tube, and unlikely to produce laryngospasm during its removal, in the spontaneously breathing patient the LMA can even be kept in place until removed in the PACU by nursing staff, thereby reducing

Table 2.2. Endotracheal tube sizes and approximate depths

Group	ETT size (mm ID)	ETT depth (cm from alveolar ridge)
Children	(4 + age)/4	(12 + age)/2
Adult women	7.0–8.0	20–22
Pregnant women	6.5–7.5	20–22
Adult men	8.0–9.0	22–24

ETT: endotracheal tube; ID: internal diameter.

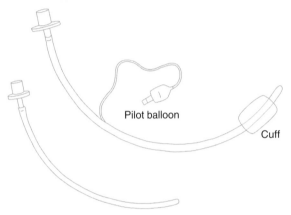

Fig. 2.4 Adult and pediatric endotracheal tubes. Note there is often no cuff on the pediatric tube.

Pilot balloon

Cuff

anesthetic wake-up time in the OR and improving OR throughput.

Endotracheal intubation

Oral intubation by direct laryngoscopy

We prefer to intubate the trachea when we need to have more control of the patient's airway, ventilate his lungs, and protect against aspiration of gastric contents. The use of a cuffed tracheal tube (Fig. 2.4) reduces the risk of aspiration in the adult.[2] Our first step is to confirm all necessary equipment is at hand:

- a properly checked anesthesia machine, or a self-inflating bag or Mapleson system with source of compressed oxygen, and a tight-fitting mask;
- endotracheal tubes (ETT) of appropriate sizes (see Table 2.2). Generally we like to have an extra tube a half size smaller than that anticipated ... just in case;
- a stylet that fits in the ETT – sometimes required to stiffen and shape the tube;
- a syringe to inflate the ETT cuff;
- an oral airway, in case intubation and mask–ventilation prove to be difficult;

- a laryngoscope handle and appropriate blades (Fig. 2.5), usually at least a curved (Macintosh) and straight (Miller), with confirmation that the light works!
- suction apparatus – for the inevitable oral secretions and potential regurgitation;
- induction drugs;
- an assistant schooled in application of cricoid pressure: manual pressure applied to the cricoid ring, compressing the hypopharynx against the vertebral body beneath, in hope of preventing passive regurgitation, and perhaps facilitating visualization of the glottic opening. Of note, cricoid pressure can at times complicate efforts at glottic visualization. The skilled laryngoscopist might reach over and adjust the assistant's hand to improve the view.

The smooth placement of an endotracheal tube requires skill and practice. We start with denitrogenating (pre-oxygenating) the patient's lungs before rendering the patient unconscious and immobile (including paralysis of the muscles of respiration) for the intubation. If the patient cannot breathe and we are unable to ventilate his lungs, his life is in danger. Fortunately, we can usually identify those patients in whom conventional endotracheal intubation will be difficult. It is vitally important to recognize them *before* administering medications that induce apnea. When possible, we assess denitrogenation by analyzing the content of exhaled gas. We seek an exhaled oxygen of >80%, ensuring the functional residual capacity (FRC, or volume of gas remaining in the lung following exhalation) contains overwhelmingly oxygen rather than nitrogen.

Intubation is typically performed with direct visualization of the larynx, that is, we like to *watch* the tube pass through the vocal cords. Unfortunately, without an instrument such as the laryngoscope, no direct line of sight exists through the open mouth to the larynx.

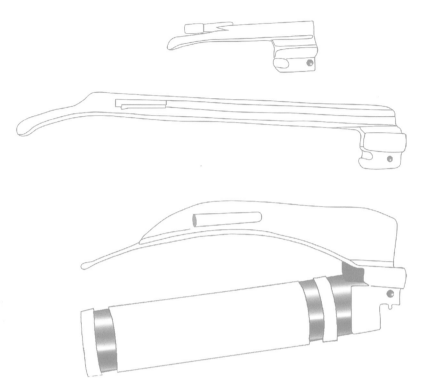

Fig. 2.5 Laryngoscope blades. The first two (Miller 0 and Miller 2) are classified as "straight" blades with which we lift the epiglottis to view the vocal cords. The last is the Macintosh 3 with handle. The tip of this blade is placed in front of the epiglottis, as shown in Figure 2.6.

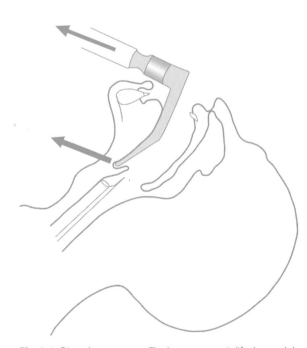

Fig. 2.6 Direct laryngoscopy. The laryngoscope is *lifted* toward the edge of the ceiling across the room, *not cranked* as that will damage the teeth and fail to provide the desired view.

Instead, we must find a way to bring the larynx into view – enter "direct laryngoscopy." Here we position the patient's head in the "sniffing position": flexed at the lower cervical spine and extended at the atlanto-occipital joint (see Fig. 2.6). We then advance a laryngoscope to the level of the epiglottis and use it to pull the lower jaw and tongue up and out of the way, opening up a line of sight to the larynx (usually). The exposure of the larynx varies and has been classified by Cormack and Lehane (Fig. 2.7). It is useful to note that the operator's view (Cormack–Lehane grade) can usually be improved by having an assistant apply a jaw thrust maneuver to the patient during the laryngoscopy.

Thus, to intubate a patient with a "normal airway," first position, denitrogenate (pre-oxygenate), and induce the patient as described above, then proceed as follows:

(i) Take the laryngoscope in your left hand; the right hand is responsible for everything else.

(ii) Place the right hand on top of the patient's head and accentuate neck extension. Note that some prefer to perform a scissor-like maneuver with the right thumb and index finger to open the patient's jaw.

Grade 1   Grade 2   Grade 3   Grade 4

Fig. 2.7 Cormack and Lehane classification of laryngeal view. Grade 1: full view of the glottis; Grade 2: only the posterior commissure is visible; Grade 3: only the epiglottis is seen; Grade 4: no epiglottis or glottis structure visible.

(iii) Advance the laryngoscope down the right side of the mouth to the level of the tonsillar pillars. Sweep the tongue to the left as you bring the laryngoscope to the midline. If the patient's tongue sneaks over the right margin of the blade try again as you can't see well through a tongue.

(iv) With a straight blade, lift the epiglottis; with a curved blade, place it in the vallecula (at the base of the epiglottis). As above, lift forward and upward (along the axis of the laryngoscope handle). Do not pry or crank with the laryngoscope! Teeth might be broken.

(v) When you can see the glottic opening clearly, grasp the endotracheal tube (hold it like a pencil – not a dagger) with the right hand (preferably without losing sight of the glottis), and advance the tip into the trachea just until the cuff disappears completely beyond the vocal cords.

(vi) Inflate the cuff only to the point of no air leakage, and *confirm tracheal position*.

This last point is *very* important. Patients do not die from esophageal intubation; they die when esophageal intubation is not recognized! You must be *absolutely* sure the tube is in the right place. A fiberoptic bronchoscope that finds the tip of the tube below the cords and above the carina would be ideal but is impractical as a clinical routine. A chest radiograph, both PA and lateral, confirming location in the trachea would also work, but is similarly impractical for OR applications. Instead, we must use clinical clues and technology.

(a) *Confirmation of exhaled CO_2* is the gold standard, either by quantitative capnography as in the operating room, or the more mobile colorimetric sensors typically used outside the operating room. Note, however, that this only guarantees ventilation of the lungs. It does not specifically identify the ETT as placed in the *trachea*. Pharyngeal position of the tube with ventilation (as with an LMA) may yield CO_2. Conversely, during cardiovascular collapse, with minimal or no pulmonary blood flow, little or no CO_2 will be returned to the lungs from the periphery, and end-tidal CO_2 might not be measurable. Place a sensor anyway because the return of detectable CO_2 will indicate effective resuscitative efforts and perfusion of the lungs.

(b) *Breath sounds*. While not definitive for tracheal placement, breath sounds should be present across the chest and absent over the stomach. We can rule out endobronchial intubation when we hear good breath sounds bilaterally (auscultating over each lateral chest wall). Emphasis on the *bilaterally*; listening close to one side of the sternum, we often mistake breath sounds transmitted from the other side.

(c) *Condensation*. While reassuring, "fogging" in the clear plastic ETT caused by condensation of the moisture from the humidified exhaled gas on the dry and cool ETT during exhalation is no ironclad guarantee. In fact, if lubrication is added to a stylet or scope to ease its removal from the ETT, condensation should *not* be expected.

(d) *Palpation of the ETT cuff*. Still not flawless, but when combined with the presence of exhaled CO_2, ballottement of the cuff in the suprasternal notch (notable by the bounce felt in a gently squeezed pilot balloon) does confirm tracheal position.

(e) *Chest excursion* should be symmetric.

While the above represents the standard intubation sequence, recent advances in technology present us with devices for indirect laryngoscopy via tiny cameras placed at the tips of blades of various designs. These provide superb alternatives when direct visualization proves impossible or is contraindicated. The wise clinician practices with these devices in routine airways as preparation for future emergencies.

"Can't intubate" situations

Here the hearts (of the caregivers) begin to pound … when the vocal cords cannot be visualized. If this problem arises after adequate pre-oxygenation, you will have

Table 2.3. Rescue techniques when intubation fails

Non-invasive

- Continued mask–ventilation
- Blind intubation (usually more successful via the nose)
- LMA; perhaps used as a conduit to intubation
- Combitube® or King Airway® (a blindly-placed double-lumen tube through which ventilation may be achieved regardless of its location: trachea or esophagus [provided the vocal cords are open])
- Lighted stylet (a lighted malleable stylet inside an ETT used to identify the trachea by a pretracheal glow in the neck)
- Fiberoptic intubation (with or without LMA as a conduit)
- Intubating stylet or airway exchange catheter (more malleable than an ETT and may include a lumen through which oxygen can be insufflated into the lungs while attempting to pass the ETT)
- Retrograde intubation (a wire placed via the cricothyroid membrane is advanced into the nose or mouth, then used as a guide for intubation) – not all that non-invasive and not routinely successful

Invasive

- Cricothyrotomy (with a needle and jet ventilation)
- Percutaneous tracheostomy (possible in a minute)
- Surgical tracheostomy (takes many minutes)

won valuable time before serious hypoxemia ensues. The first thing we try is to change the patient's position, the laryngoscope blade, and/or the laryngoscopist. If this does not help (and the patient is still apneic), then another technique must be attempted (Table 2.3).

The selection of rescue technique depends on the situation, experience of the physician, availability of equipment, and whether mask–ventilation is possible (Fig. 2.8). For example, "can't intubate, can't ventilate" scenarios necessitate rapid intervention, and thus, fiberoptic intubation would not be a likely choice for an inexperienced physician; placement of an LMA is much more likely to be successful. Failure to ventilate for more than a few minutes requires progression to an emergent surgical airway via either a cricothyroidotomy performed by the anesthetist, or a surgical tracheostomy. Contrast this with a "can't intubate, *can* ventilate" scenario, in which we may be able to mask–ventilate the patient's lungs between attempts with alternative devices, or until they awaken, at which

time we can perform an awake fiberoptic intubation. Remember that non-depolarizing muscle relaxants cannot be reversed (unless you are outside the USA where sugammadex is available [see Chapter 12]) until the patient regains at least one twitch on the train of four (ulnar stimulation), which may require 30 minutes or more depending on the muscle relaxant and dose administered. For this reason, we choose short-acting drugs, e.g., succinylcholine, when we anticipate difficulties: if intubation fails, the drug effect will wear off within a few minutes, and the patient can once again breathe spontaneously.

Awake fiberoptic intubation

Sometimes an indirect visualization technique becomes necessary, either during airway rescue, or when a preoperative examination suggests a likelihood of difficult intubation. In such cases, perhaps the most definitive technique is to secure the airway while the patient is still awake and breathing spontaneously. Awake fiberoptic intubation requires topical anesthesia for the patient's comfort, as well as to blunt the gag reflex that would prevent successful intubation of the trachea. All too frequently, secretions will smear the optics of the scope: an anti-sialogogue can be helpful.

Several nerves are involved in the sensation of the upper airway (Fig. 2.9). It is not much of a mnemonic, but try to remember a variant to TGIF (Thank God it's Friday) namely **TGIR**: "Thank God it's recurrent." It's lame, but perhaps just lame enough to be memorable! All but the first of these make up the gag reflex.

We anesthetize the posterior tongue and oro/nasopharynx by spraying 4% lidocaine, having the patient gargle viscous lidocaine, or applying the latter to a swab gradually advanced into the nose or against the base of the palatoglossal arches. Glossopharyngeal blocks also work well. We can continue to topicalize down to the base of the tongue or block the superior laryngeal nerves by injecting 1% lidocaine close to where the nerves penetrate the thyrohyoid membrane (Fig. 2.10). The transtracheal block is accomplished by injecting 2–4% lidocaine directly into the tracheal lumen through the cricothyroid membrane (after confirming needle location by easily aspirating air). Be sure to point the needle toward the carina. You are very close to the vocal cords, which you do not want to damage with a needle pointed cephalad!

This technique is better tolerated with sedation, though the risk:benefit of potential airway compromise

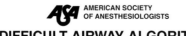

AMERICAN SOCIETY OF ANESTHESIOLOGISTS

DIFFICULT AIRWAY ALGORITHM

1. Assess the likelihood and clinical impact of basic management problems:
   - A. Difficult Ventilation
   - B. Difficult Intubation
   - C. Difficulty with Patient Cooperation or Consent
   - D. Difficult Tracheostomy

2. Actively pursue opportunities to deliver supplemental oxygen throughout the process of difficult airway management

3. Consider the relative merits and feasibility of basic management choices:

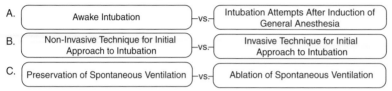

A. Awake Intubation –vs.– Intubation Attempts After Induction of General Anesthesia

B. Non-Invasive Technique for Initial Approach to Intubation –vs.– Invasive Technique for Initial Approach to Intubation

C. Preservation of Spontaneous Ventilation –vs.– Ablation of Spontaneous Ventilation

4. Develop primary and alternative strategies:

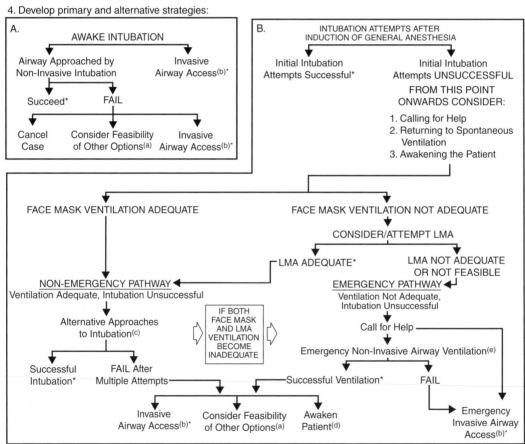

*Confirm ventilation, tracheal intubation, or LMA placement with exhaled CO_2

a. Other options include (but are not limited to): surgery utilizing face mask or LMA anesthesia, local anesthesia infiltration or regional nerve blockade. Pursuit of these options usually implies that mask ventilation will not be problematic. Therefore, these options may be of limited value if this step in the algorithm has been reached via the Emergency Pathway.

b. Invasive airway access includes surgical or percutaneous tracheostomy or cricothyrotomy.

c. Alternative non-invasive approaches to difficult intubation include (but are not limited to): use of different laryngoscope blades, LMA as an intubation conduit (with or without fiberoptic guidance), fiberoptic intubation, intubating stylet or tube changer, light wand, retrograde intubation, and blind oral or nasal intubation.

d. Consider re-preparation of the patient for awake intubation or canceling surgery.

e. Options for emergency non-invasive airway ventilation include (but are not limited to): rigid bronchoscope, esophageal-tracheal combitude ventilation, or transtracheal jet ventilation.

Fig. 2.8 ASA Difficult Airway Algorithm. Reprinted with permission.

Table 2.4. Airway device selection

	Mask	LMA	ETT
Procedure duration	Short	Short–Medium	Any
Protects against aspiration?	No	No	Yes
Positive pressure ventilation	PIP <20 cmH$_2$O	PIP <20 cmH$_2$O	Any
Stimulation by device	Low	Medium	High

PIP: Peak inspiratory pressure; pressures above 20 cmH$_2$O may distend the stomach.

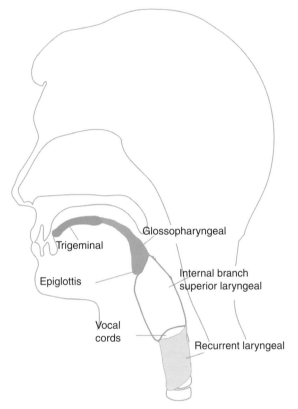

Fig. 2.9 Innervation of the airway. Anterior two-thirds of the tongue – **T**rigeminal nerve (V); posterior third of tongue to epiglottis – **G**lossopharyngeal nerve (IX); epiglottis to vocal cords – **I**nternal branch of superior laryngeal nerve (Vagus, X); trachea below vocal cords – **R**ecurrent laryngeal nerve (Vagus, X).

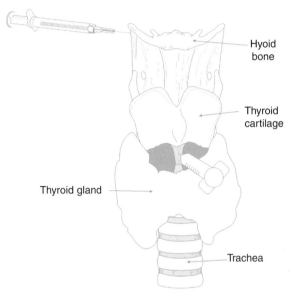

Fig. 2.10 Airway blocks for awake fiberoptic intubation. Location for superior laryngeal nerve block (top left) and transtracheal (center) injection of local anesthetics.

and aspiration – more likely with a numbed larynx – must always be taken into account.

Airway management plan

For many operative procedures requiring general anesthesia, any of these techniques (mask, LMA, ETT) may be appropriate, but there are times to prefer one over another. We take into account the planned procedure and the patient's status (Table 2.4). An emergency laparoscopic appendectomy should probably be performed with an ETT because of the high risk of aspiration (full stomach and increased intra-abdominal pressure from laparoscopy), while a professional singer undergoing a minor elective procedure might be better served with a mask or LMA.

Should Plan A prove unsuccessful, we always have Plans B–F waiting in the wings. First, depending on our level of concern, we always consider calling for help from colleagues who may have different airway management skills from our own. Then we turn to devices with which we have the most comfort and experience, such as the LMA. Next we select from the numerous other devices marketed for airway management, including optical laryngoscopes (a hybrid of a laryngoscope and fiberoptics) and devices designed for esophageal or supralaryngeal placement and supraglottic ventilation.

Our last resort is direct access to the trachea through the neck.

A word about the patient with a potentially unstable cervical spine: many times trauma patients arrive from the Emergency Department without a "cleared" cervical spine. Though radiographs can identify fractures and displacement, they fail to reveal torn or damaged ligaments, all pointing to instability of the cervical spine. If the patient has received painkillers, is intoxicated or comatose, and thus can give neither a useful history nor report cervical pain, we are in a quandary: the trauma patient's full stomach suggests the need for rapid-sequence intubation to minimize the risk of aspiration, while direct laryngoscopy may traumatize the spinal cord. The options become these:

(i) *An asleep airway technique.* One that does not require neck movement, such as intubating through an LMA, using a video-laryngoscope (Glidescope, AirTraq, and others), lighted stylet, or retrograde intubation. In skilled hands, these techniques may be performed with relative speed. A lengthy process increases the likelihood of aspiration.

(ii) *Awake fiberoptic intubation.* May be difficult and even dangerous to an at-risk cervical spinal cord in an intoxicated, uncooperative patient, and may take too long in the patient with multiple traumatic injuries.

(iii) *Blind nasal intubation.* Again, skilled hands dramatically increase the likelihood of success, but this technique is contraindicated in the presence of a base-of-skull fracture, e.g., with "raccoon eyes" or with cerebrospinal fluid dripping from the nose, as the endotracheal tube could enter the brain via the fracture site. Furthermore, if we incite a nosebleed, subsequent attempts at fiberoptic intubation may be visually compromised.

(iv) *Direct laryngoscopy with in-line stabilization.* A second person stabilizes the neck (without pulling on the head) in an effort to minimize neck extension. While probably inadequate in the patient with known cervical spine injury, this technique might be used for the patient with a low likelihood of trauma whose "clearance" was limited only by intoxication.

(v) *Awake tracheostomy.* Far more invasive than the other techniques, we reserve this primarily for patients with upper-airway trauma that will prevent other intubation techniques.

Regardless of the technique selected, the physician administering any general anesthetic must be prepared for failure of that plan and be ready to institute an alternative airway management technique. Finally, extra pairs of skilled hands are always useful. Call for help *early* when things are not going as planned!

Notes

1   With volume-controlled ventilation, a set tidal volume is delivered with little regard for the required inflation pressure, up to a set limit. Contrast with pressure-controlled ventilation, in which a set pressure is delivered for a period of time, without concern for the actual tidal volume.

2   Cuffed ETTs are not often used in infants because the cuff rests near the cricoid ring, the narrowest part of the baby's airway, and may cause laryngeal edema and possibly obstruction upon extubation. In fact, we want a leak around a child's ETT at about 20 cmH$_2$O airway pressure.

Vascular access and fluid management

We tend to forget that we humans (and many of our animal relatives) are mostly water. When we think about it, we must marvel how the body stores the bulk of this water in cells and the interstitial, extracellular fluid, where much of the water is tied up in gel. Suspended in this interstitial bog is the vascular compartment, comparatively puny in volume but most important because of its rapid transport of fluids, nutrients, and waste throughout the system, and its continuous and efficient exchange of water with the interstitial compartment (Fig. 3.1). Clinically, we can see dehydration in sunken eyeballs, tenting skin and dry lips, or the excess of fluids in edema and swollen eyes; we can even hear it should water collect in the alveoli.

Vascular access

During anesthesia, and whenever the oral route is unavailable, we give fluids parenterally. As long as we need to give only physiologic solutions, we can administer them subcutaneously; however, the uptake and distribution of such a depot of fluids take time. Much preferred and much faster is the intravenous route. Thus, vascular access assumes a critically important role in the peri-operative care of patients. The vascular bed also offers an ideal route for many drugs that need to be distributed throughout the body. Finally, intravascular pressures provide information on cardiovascular function. Thus, vascular access has become a skill, and fluid management a science, mastered by anesthesiologists.

Our skin is a wonderful organ (actually our largest). It wraps us securely into an elastic, fairly tough, self-repairing, protective envelope. When we break this envelope, we expose the patient to considerable risks. In addition to hazards associated with the actual placement of needles and catheters, infectious complications contribute significantly to morbidity and mortality of the hospitalized patient, particularly in the intensive care unit, where we frequently employ central venous access. Such catheter-related bloodstream infections (CRBSI) are now reported in CRBSI per 1000 catheter days with a goal of less than 2. Thus, we pay great attention to the details of central venous catheter placement and subsequent interaction with the catheter. In addition to CRBSI, infectious complications include local site infection, septic thrombophlebitis, endocarditis, and other metastatic infections such as osteomyelitis and abscesses of lung or brain.

Peripheral venous cannulation

Let's go through the steps involved:

(i) *Explain the need* for vascular access and obtain consent from the patient. Parents can be of great help in preparing a child for an i.v.

(ii) *Topicalize*. If there is sufficient time (30–45 minutes), a topical anesthetic such as EMLA (eutectic mixture of local anesthetics) can be applied to the intended site. This is most worthwhile for small children.

(iii) *Acquire equipment* (*Table 3.1*). We usually select the largest catheter appropriate for the selected vein and intended use. As an example, if we anticipate only minimal blood loss and a short-duration procedure, a small 22-gauge catheter, which will readily allow administration of over 30 mL/minute under gravity drip, is sufficient.

(iv) *Wash your hands*. Soap and water or a chlorhexidine-containing solution are both acceptable. Best to do this in front of the patient.

(v) *Don clean gloves*. They need not be sterile. From now on, you are dealing with the patient's blood, and you should expose neither yourself nor the patient to the possibility of infection.

(vi) *Select the site*. This involves more than just looking for the most visible vein. We often use the back of the hand because veins are both visible and easy to immobilize, and if you are unsuccessful you have an opportunity to try

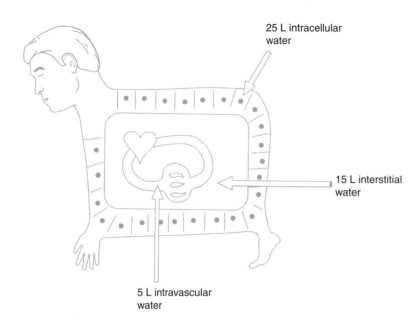

25 L intracellular water

15 L interstitial water

5 L intravascular water

Fig. 3.1 An uncharitable view (not to scale) of a 70 kg man as a tub filled with water (amounting to 60% of his total body weight [TBW]). This water is tucked away in cells (~65%, 40% TBW), caught in the extracellular space (~25%, 20% TBW), with a portion located in the interstitial gel (15% TBW) and the rest circulating in the intravascular compartment (~10%, 6–7% TBW).

Table 3.1. Equipment for peripheral intravenous access

Tourniquet

Gloves (that fit – you, not the patient)

Site prep, e.g., chlorhexidine

Local anesthetic (1% lidocaine plain ~0.5 mL and 25–27-g needle)

i.v. catheter (? gauge, ? length) ×2 in case of a miss

4×4 sponge (to clean up afterward)

Clear occlusive dressing

Pre-torn tape

i.v. fluids, primed and free of bubbles

again more proximally. Things to consider: use the non-dominant hand, avoid "creases" where kinking is likely, e.g., wrist, seek a relatively straight vein without venous valves that may hinder its cannulation; inserting at a venous fork is helpful as the vein tends to be better stabilized. Finally, we do not normally cannulate an arm that has been the target of an arteriovenous shunt (as for dialysis) or a lymph node dissection (as in a mastectomy).

(vii) *Apply a tourniquet.* Should be tight enough to obstruct venous return without restricting arterial flow. A working pulse oximeter confirms the tourniquet is not too tight. Do not actually tie a knot, just fold one side under the other to enable a very easy release.

(viii) *Prepare the site.* We prefer to use a bactericidal agent such as chlorhexidine in alcohol; next best would be an iodine-containing solution, e.g., betadine, which must be allowed to dry and should not be wiped off with alcohol. Finally, a patient allergic to both of the above can have the site washed with alcohol alone.

(ix) *Inject local anesthetic.* Awake patients benefit greatly if we take the time to first anesthetize their skin. It requires only a tiny volume (~0.1 mL) of local anesthetic injected immediately adjacent to (not over) the vein, minimizing the risk of obscuring visibility of the vein. While injection of lidocaine burns, we can reduce the discomfort by:

• Counter-irritation – with a free finger, scratch the patient's skin near the injection site, this "confuses" the nerve endings and reduces pain.

• Inject slowly since we are creating a fluid space that wasn't there before.

• Some argue that using local anesthesia insures two sticks instead of one, and that a "needle is a needle." We beg to differ: first, the local should be administered with a 25–27-g needle, which is barely felt by most patients; second, the i.v. does not always go in on the first try; and third, the pain of the i.v. catheter needle without local is worse than the local anesthetic injection (personal experiences).

(x) *Stabilize the vein* with traction below the puncture site.

(xi) *Puncture the skin* at a 30–45-degree angle (through the local anesthetic wheal!).

(xii) *Proceed into the vein* either directly from above or from the side; make sure you can see the clear plastic hub of the needle to observe the return of blood.

(xiii) *Advance catheter.* When you see a flash of blood, reduce your angle and advance a tiny amount (literally 1–2 mm) to get the catheter tip (not just the needle tip) into the vein, then fully advance the catheter off of the needle until the hub touches the skin. You cannot thread the flexible catheter without the stiff needle as a stylet, and the needle should not be reinserted as the catheter may be punctured.

(xiv) *Remove the tourniquet* (facilitated by proper placement in the first place). Note this occurs before pulling the needle out of the catheter.

(xv) *Apply gentle pressure* just proximal to the tip of the catheter, not over the catheter itself, to prevent a bloody mess and embarrassment.

(xvi) *Remove the needle* and dispose in a "Sharps" container.

(xvii) *Connect i.v. fluid administration set* that has been pre-primed (de-aired). Open the roller clamp to observe free flow, then slow down the administration as indicated by the patient's condition.

(xviii) *Observe the i.v. site* to confirm intravascular and not interstitial placement (not foolproof but helpful). Sometimes this can be difficult to judge and one's confidence may be initially low. Bleeding back into i.v. tubing that is open to air at a stopcock, or observing a slowed drip rate while applying firm circumferential compression of the arm well above the insertion site is a strong indicator of successful i.v. placement.

(xix) *Secure the i.v.* With due respect to those who consider this an art form, find a method that allows visibility of the entry site (to observe for infection) and the area over the tip of the catheter (to detect infiltration). Secure the i.v.

so that motion will not dislodge it. A loop in the tubing prevents a small amount of traction from pulling directly on the catheter. We avoid circumferential taping unless employing a very elastic material, to prevent a tourniquet effect should the catheter become dislodged over time.

The fluid administered depends on the goal of the infusion. In general, fluids should be administered through a programmable pump with adequate safety measures. That said, in anesthesia we usually control the rate of fluid administration through the i.v. tubing's roller clamp. In this case, *do not hang more fluid than the patient would tolerate as a bolus.* For an infant, do not hang a bag containing more than 20 mL/kg solution without a buretrol (a 150–200 mL reservoir attached between the i.v. fluid bag and the catheter). If the roller clamp is inadvertently left open, the patient will not be fluid overloaded. Use of an infusion set containing a microdrip chamber (60 drops per milliliter instead of 10 or 20 as with adult drip sets) also decreases the likelihood of fluid over-administration.

When we recognize the potential need for rapid fluid administration (read: major bloodletting), we plan our intravenous access accordingly. The maximum attainable flow rate depends on the resistance of the system, including the length and diameter of everything from the tubing to the vein itself. So, remove any small-diameter connectors and select a shorter, larger catheter (at least an 18-g in an adult).[1] Selecting a large vein for rapid flow is obvious, but the effect of cold fluids on a vein's caliber may be underestimated. Finally, two medium bore i.v.'s placed distally accommodate more fluid than a single large bore, in part because the downstream (towards the heart) resistance of the vein usually exceeds that of the i.v. catheter. Substantial flow increases can be achieved simply by elevating the infusion set. Using "pressure bags" may be necessary to achieve a desired flow, but allowing fluids to flow in passively is preferred. When i.v. catheters occasionally infiltrate, meaning the tip has migrated out of the vein, lower driving pressure results in less volume delivered into the interstitial tissue, reducing the chance for compartment syndrome or tissue sloughing.

Central venous catheterization

The complication rate of central venous catheterization (Table 3.2) is much higher than for peripheral i.v.'s, thus the first question should be whether central

Table 3.2. Complications of central venous catheterization and how to prevent them

Infectious complications:

- Use antimicrobial-impregnated catheters.
- Avoid the femoral route; subclavian (SC) has the lowest incidence, followed closely by internal jugular (IJ).
- Employ sterile technique (handwashing, removing jewelry, wearing mask, cap, gown, sterile gloves, full body drape). Simply treat it like a surgeon would an operation.
- Avoid antibiotic ointment at insertion site (this encourages resistant organisms and fungi) but use a chlorhexidine-impregnated disk.
- Disinfect catheter hubs when injecting or attaching tubing.
- Minimize duration of catheterization.

Mechanical complications: the most common are arterial puncture (femoral>IJ>SC), hematoma, and pneumothorax (SC>>IJ). For the IJ and femoral route these can be almost completely avoided by the use of ultrasound guidance during placement. It is not clear if its utility will be confirmed for SC catheterization.

- Optimize likelihood of success including proper positioning of the patient.
- Use a "finder needle" if ultrasound guidance is unavailable – this smaller gauge needle makes a much smaller hole if it ends up in the wrong place. The introducer needle is then advanced along the finder needle into the vein.
- If air is aspirated during any attempt, do not proceed to the contralateral side as bilateral pneumothoraces are extremely poorly tolerated (if you aspirated air during a femoral placement attempt you have bigger problems).

Thrombotic complications: most common with femoral site, and least for SC.

Table 3.3. Indications for central venous catheterization

- Need (anticipated or actual) to infuse fluids at a great rate.
- Administration of agents that require a central route (some vasoactive drugs, hyperalimentation, high concentrations of electrolytes).
- Need to transduce central pressures (pulmonary artery and occlusion pressures as well as cardiac output are available with a pulmonary artery catheter).
- Stable venous access in patients without other accessible sites, e.g., morbid obesity.

venous cannulation is truly necessary (Table 3.3). When placed emergently under suboptimal circumstances, for instance in a trauma patient, these catheters should be replaced within 48 hours to reduce the risk of infection, i.e., CRBSI.

The next question deals with access site. The three most common insertion sites are as follows:

- *Subclavian (SC)*. Once placed, this catheter location is probably the most comfortable for the patient and enjoys the lowest infection rate. Unfortunately, it carries a significant risk of pneumothorax (up to 3%), and the procedure can be very difficult when landmarks are obscured, as in obesity.
- *Internal jugular (IJ)*. Anesthesiologists favor this location because of accessibility (we're already at the head of the patient) and the extraordinarily low risk of pneumothorax. Incidentally, we prefer the right IJ over the left due to the "straightness" of the route to the heart, its generally larger diameter, and because we need not worry about injuring the left-sided thoracic duct.
- *Femoral*. Probably technically the easiest (remember "VanGogh" – vein, artery, nerve, gonads) and quickest, with the lowest rate of serious complications (though highest rate of minor complications). However, these catheters are more difficult to keep clean and therefore more likely to be a source of infection. The femoral route should be considered the third choice in most cases.

In addition to selecting a catheter size and length appropriate to the patient and indication, there are other features to consider (Table 3.4).

Table 3.4. Types of central venous catheters

- Antimicrobial-impregnated – this is important! It reduces CRBSI.
- Single vs. multi-lumen – depends on the intended use. If multiple drugs need to be infused at the same time, or we wish to simultaneously measure CVP while giving fluids and medications, a multi-lumen catheter should be selected. Importantly, fewer lumens lowers the likelihood of a subsequent CRBSI.
- Pulmonary artery (PA) catheter – if we want pulmonary artery or occlusion pressures, or cardiac output determination, a PA catheter (also known as a Swan–Ganz catheter) will do the trick. There are many types of these with variable capabilities (thermodilution cardiac output, continuous cardiac output, pacing port, continuous mixed venous oxygen saturation, etc.); make sure you check carefully before opening the (expensive) package.

Because the majority of catheters in anesthesia are placed in the IJ location in an anesthetized patient, we will describe this technique. In an awake patient, we would add a pre-procedure time-out, sedation, continual reassurance, and local anesthesia.

Internal jugular (IJ) catheter placement technique

Once we have confirmed the need for central venous catheterization, obtained the patient's consent, and collected all equipment, we work as follows:

(i) Optimally position the patient: Trendelenburg's position[2] (head-down, to increase the size of the vein and prevent air embolism), with the head turned no more than 45° to the opposite side. Continuous ECG rhythm monitoring will facilitate detection of guidewire-induced heart irritation.

(ii) Prepare: don cap and mask, remove watch and any wrist/hand jewelry, wash hands with chlorhexidine/alcohol gel, gown, put on sterile gloves, open catheter tray in easy reach. The patient should be fully covered with a large fenestrated drape. Ultrasound equipment for visualization is highly recommended and should also be prepared with a sterile sleeve over the transducer.

(iii) Prepare the site: currently recommended is a 30-second isopropyl alcohol chlorhexidine solution scrub, but an iodine solution can be substituted in case of allergy. The solution should be allowed to dry before continuing.

(iv) Identify the insertion point: while there are many possible sites along the vessel, for an IJ catheter we advocate a mid to high approach to minimize the possibility of pneumothorax. One technique: place the third finger of the left hand in the sternal notch, the thumb on the mastoid process, and then bisect the line with the index finger, adjusting to palpate the carotid at this level. Do not try to push the carotid out of the way, as both vessels lie in the same sheath and probing with your finger will shrink the readily compressible IJ. If the external jugular vein crosses at this location, move above or below it. The modern clinician heeds the advice of the experts and uses ultrasound imaging to view intended (IJ), and unintended (carotid), targets during the procedure.

(v) If not employing ultrasound guidance (because there is a total power failure in the hospital and you are performing the procedure with a flashlight carefully aimed by a junior medical student [who is also wearing a sterile gown, hat, and mask]), using a finder needle (22–23-g) attached to a syringe, begin about 1 cm lateral to the carotid pulse (that means a finger is continuously gently palpating the pulse until the IJ is located), aiming toward the ipsilateral nipple. Advance the needle through the skin, then gently aspirate on the plunger as you slowly advance the needle. In the average patient, the IJ should be no more than about 1.5 cm deep. If blood is not aspirated, slowly withdraw the needle and adjust the needle direction slightly. First check that the vein does not lie more lateral, then cautiously check more medially and caudally.

(vi) When blood is aspirated, gently transfer the finder needle/syringe to the left hand. With the right hand, carefully advance the needle through which the wire will be inserted along the finder needle and into the vessel until blood is easily aspirated.

(vii) Remove the finder needle and also the syringe from the needle that will receive the wire, and confirm intravenous location (see below). Keep your thumb (in a sterile glove!) over the hub of the needle when there is nothing attached to minimize blood loss and avoid a potentially catastrophic air embolism if the central venous pressure is low, or should the patient suddenly decrease it by taking a gasping breath.

(viii) Verify the vessel you have cannulated is in fact the IJ and not the carotid. While obvious with ultrasound visualization, the total power failure in which you are working requires 20th-century proof. Verify that the pressure in the accessed vessel is low by connecting a short piece of i.v. tubing to the needle. When you lower the tubing it should slowly fill with blood. Upon raising the tubing above the level of the heart (actually the central venous pressure to be more precise), the blood should flow back into the patient documenting a low vessel pressure.

(ix) Advance the wire through the needle. Here, we must monitor ECG to detect the extrasystoles that warn us if we have advanced the guidewire too far, i.e., into the heart. A series of atrial or ventricular extrasystoles prompts us to withdraw the wire a few centimeters.

(x) Remove the needle, make a small skin incision adjacent to the wire, then advance the dilator over the wire (often the dilator is already integrated into the introducer). Intended to both dilate soft tissues and allow easier advancement of the flimsy catheter it is unnecessary and potentially damaging to advance the stiff dilator entirely to its hub; it need only reach the vessel. If the dilator is separate, remove it and thread the catheter over the wire. If integrated, feed the catheter off the dilator as though it were an i.v. in the hand. Make sure to hold the wire while advancing or removing equipment over it, so as not to remove it, or (worse yet) fully insert it into the patient.

(xi) Remove the wire, cap off the ports, aspirate and flush each, and suture the catheter in place. We add a chlorhexidine-impregnated disk at the skin entry site and dress with a clear occlusive dressing. No antibiotic ointment should be used at the skin entry site.

(xii) At some point we must obtain a chest radiograph to confirm the catheter tip position. For an IJ catheter placed in the OR this is typically done immediately after the operation.

For a subclavian catheter with its higher placement-associated risk of pneumothorax this is often done sooner. The optimal location for a catheter placed via the IJ or SC route is just above the right atrium, where it will not perforate atrial tissue. On the X-ray the tip of the catheter is ideally positioned opposite the take-off of the right mainstem bronchus. The X-ray can also rule out pneumothorax and can suggest an extravascular location of the catheter.

Pulmonary artery catheterization

In addition to the risks of central venous catheterization listed above, pulmonary artery (PA) catheterization has caused catastrophic pulmonary artery rupture and comes with the increased risk of arrhythmias, complete heart block (particularly if the patient has a pre-existing left bundle branch block), pulmonary embolism, and cardiac valve damage. Thus, this invasive technique requires rigorous justification. Do you really need to have PA pressure, PA occlusion pressure (PAOP, also known as pulmonary capillary wedge pressure, PCWP), cardiac output, or access to mixed venous blood? How will it affect your management?

After placing an introducer (a special large-bore central venous catheter) via the central venous access technique above, a pulmonary artery catheter (PAC) is sterilely inserted through a hemostatic valve in the introducer. We are still gowned, gloved, etc., as above.

(i) Prepare the catheter: flush the PAC ports. Test the balloon for symmetric inflation (with 1.5 mL air) and passive deflation on removal of the syringe. Connect the PA (distal) port to a pressure transducer with the waveform on the monitor in view. Cover the catheter with the clear plastic sheath[3] that maintains internal sterility for subsequent manipulation of catheter depth (be careful you put the catheter in the proper end of the sterility sheath).

(ii) Advance the catheter through the introducer to 20 cm and confirm the central venous pressure (CVP) waveform from the distal lumen on the monitor (see below). Instruct an assistant to inflate the balloon.

(iii) Advance the catheter while keeping track of its depth as well as the waveform transduced from its tip (Fig. 3.2). From a right IJ access point the

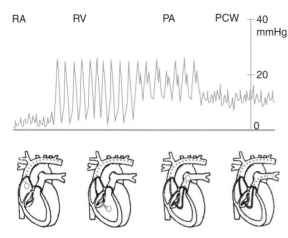

Fig. 3.2 Pressure tracings during placement of a pulmonary artery catheter. RA: right atrium; RV: right ventricle; PA: pulmonary artery; PCW: pulmonary capillary wedge. (Reproduced with permission from Dizon, C. T. and Barash, P. G. The value of monitoring pulmonary artery pressure in clinical practice. *Conn. Med.* **41**(10):623, 1977.)

RV tracing should appear before the catheter has been advanced about 30 cm, the PA waveform within 10 cm after that, and the PAOP around 50 cm. If they do not, deflate the balloon, pull back the catheter until you again see a CVP or RV waveform, reinflate the balloon and try again. Over-insertion can cause arrhythmias, pulmonary infarction, PA rupture or even a catheter knot, necessitating a vascular procedure to remove the catheter.

(iv) Once the PAOP tracing is obtained, deflate the balloon and confirm reappearance of the PA trace. If this does not occur, withdraw the catheter a few centimeters until it does. Continue manipulation until the PA trace with the balloon deflated becomes the PAOP (or wedge) trace on inflation. Always inflate the balloon to just barely occlude the PA pressure in order to avoid rupturing the vessel. Always watch the waveform during any catheter manipulation or balloon inflation. And remember … *balloon up on catheter advancement, balloon down on withdrawal.* Also know that as the catheter warms to body temperature it will always migrate distally a bit. Anticipate that it may re-wedge after the balloon has been deflated and withdrawing it a few centimeters may become necessary.

(v) Aspirate to confirm intravascular location, and flush all ports. Obtain a chest radiograph when

Table 3.5. Blood volume estimates

Population	Blood volume (mL/kg body weight)
Premature neonates	95
Infants	80
Adult men	70
Adult women	60

convenient, to confirm proper location. The tip should be within the mediastinal shadow.

Fluid management

As mentioned at the start of this chapter, we are mostly water, actually salt water with some other chemicals thrown in for good measure. The intravascular compartment, replete with cells and proteins, differs from the rest of the body. In fact the blood volume also differs with age and gender (Table 3.5). We may lose fluid in a number of ways, from the obvious – hemorrhage, urine, vomiting – to the less obvious – sweat, evaporation from exposed viscera or trachea, transudation between compartments. While fluid escapes from anywhere, replacement occurs only via the intravascular compartment.

Fluid types

Many types of fluid are available for intravascular administration (Table 3.6).

- *Crystalloid.*

  - *Hypotonic solutions.* With an osmolality less than that of serum (275–295 mOsm/kg), these are rarely used in anesthesia (except pediatrics), because the "extra" water finds itself going to where the salt is. Hence, very little of the infused fluid remains intravascular (<10% of D_5W), electrolytes are diluted, and cells swell.

  - *Isotonic solutions.* Preferred, though still only about 25% of the infused crystalloid volume remains intravascular, with the rest seeping into the interstitial space (apparent in the puffiness you see in patients who have received several liters); the most common representative is 0.9% sodium chloride (also known as normal saline).[4] Another nearly isotonic solution is lactated Ringer's

39

Table 3.6. Composition of common intravenous fluids

	Na$^+$ (mEq/L)	Cl$^-$ (mEq/L)	K$^+$ (mEq/L)	Ca^{2+} (mEq/L)	Other	Approximate pH	Calculated mOsm/L
D$_5$W					Dextrose 5 g/L	5.0	253
Normal saline	154	154				4.2	308
Ringer's lactate	130	109	4.0	3.0	Lactate 28 mEq/L	6.5	273
Hespan	154	154			Hydroxyethyl starch, 6 g/dL	5.5	310
3% NaCl	513	513				5.0	1027
In normal serum	136–145	98–106	3.5–5.1	4.2–5.3		7.35–7.45	275–295[a]

[a] Serum osmolarity is estimated as $2 \times [Na^+] + glucose/18 + BUN/2.8$.

(which also contains lactate, potassium, and calcium). Its measured osmolarity of about 260 mOsm/L is a bit below its 273 mOsm/L *calculated* tonicity so technically it is actually slightly hypotonic.

- *Hypertonic solutions.* Available in solutions from 1.8% to 10% NaCl; 3% is the most common. While almost 65% of the infused volume remains intravascular, these solutions may cause cellular dehydration, hypernatremia, and hyperchloremic metabolic acidosis.
- *Colloid.* Containing large molecules, these solutions tend to remain intravascular (assuming capillary integrity).
  - *Hetastarch (hydroxyethyl starch; Hespan®, Hextend®).* Associated with coagulation abnormalities with infusion of volumes exceeding 20 mL/kg.
  - *Pentastarch.* Hetastarch's younger brother, allegedly with less effect on coagulation.
  - *Albumin.* Very expensive; often refused by Jehovah's Witnesses.
- *Blood or blood components.* Associated with many risks and expense (see below).
- *Blood substitutes.* We need solutions capable of carrying oxygen, without the risks and expense of blood transfusions. Unfortunately, as of this writing, these solutions – including perfluorochemical emulsions, stroma-free hemoglobin, and synthetic hemoglobin – still remain in clinical trials.

Fluid requirements

We have for many years calculated the intra-operative fluid requirement as follows:

(i) *Maintenance.* The 4–2–1 rule (Table 3.7) was used to guide basic hourly isotonic fluid requirements.

For a 70 kg man, this would amount to 40 + 20 + 50 = 110 mL/h.

Recently this rule has come into question and likely overestimates fluid requirements.

(ii) *Fasting replacement.* We applied the 4–2–1 rule for the duration of fasting and replaced 50% over the first hour, then 25% over each of the next two hours. The current recommendation assumes ~80 mL/fasting hour.

(iii) *Insensible losses.* Perspiration and airway fluid losses amount to only about 1 mL/kg/h. Evaporative losses depend on the degree of exposed tissue, and particularly viscera, and range from 2 mL/h for simple cases, up to 30 mL/h for exteriorized viscera. Note however this is not weight-dependent. Previous recommendations resulted in higher insensible loss estimates.

(iv) *Urine output.* Replaced mL for mL.

(v) *"Third space" losses.* Transfer of fluid to this sequestered, extravascular space occurs with surgical trauma, and is replaced with isotonic solution in the short term: 4–10 mL/kg/h depending on the degree of surgical trauma, e.g., peripheral operation vs. open abdomen.

Table 3.7. The 4–2–1 rule for calculation of maintenance fluid requirements

Body weight	Fluid administration
For the first 10 kg	4 mL/kg/h
For the next 10 kg	Add 2 mL/kg/h
For each kg above 20 kg	Add 1 mL/kg/h

   Replacement rate decreases with subsequent hours of surgery.

(vi) *Blood loss.* We replace small amounts with crystalloid (3 mL per mL blood lost); in larger resuscitations, colloid and/or blood is administered 1:1 with blood loss.

Intra-operatively, we gauge fluid status by tracking vital signs, surgical progress, urine output (an inexact measure), and volume replacement. If the status is unclear, we may opt for invasive monitors such as central venous pressure monitoring (see Chapters 7 and 9), or trans-esophageal echocardiography, which enables visualization of ventricular volume. A less invasive approach is to transduce the peripheral venous pressure from an i.v. (assumes no constriction around the arm and that we can see a nice phasic pressure waveform – just like from a central venous catheter).

Evolving fluid replacement strategy

Giving excess fluid risks harm and challenges the cardiovascular system, the lungs, wound healing, and recovery of gastrointestinal function post-operatively. This topic has engendered passionate arguments for decades and opinion varies across a wide spectrum. Currently the pendulum has swung back in favor of a more conservative approach to fluid, and especially crystalloid, administration. The approach now advocated by many ignores pre-operative NPO deficits. Fluid administration begins with colloid in the form of a 6% synthetic starch solution given to replace blood loss at a 1:1 ratio. If blood loss exceeds 1.5 L then crystalloid is added. The net effect is a much smaller intra-operative weight gain, on the order of 2 kg less. Given that each kilogram represents one liter of fluid that has to go somewhere in the body and then later has to be eliminated, this is a non-trivial difference. This strategy continues to evolve, but seems to be gaining ground. In the face of hypotension and suspected hypovolemia, however, the correct strategy is of course to correct the hypovolemia.

Blood loss

When we anticipate a large blood loss, we might calculate the "allowable blood loss" (ABL) – not the amount we "allow" the surgeon to lose, but rather the tolerable blood loss volume after which we would likely need to transfuse.

$$ABL = \frac{\left(Hct_{initial} - Hct_{allowed}\right)}{\left(Hct_{initial} + Hct_{allowed}\right)/2} \times EBV$$

where we use the initial and minimum acceptable hematocrits ("allowed"), and the estimated blood volume (EBV) (Table 3.5). Unfortunately, we struggle to determine when we have reached the ABL. We report the estimated blood loss by looking at the surgical field, checking the volume in the suction canisters (subtracting any irrigation used), and examining the surgical sponges (a soaked 4×4 holds about 15 mL blood, a soaked lap sponge, 150 mL). More accurate, but generally impractical, measures include weighing the sponges or washing them out and checking the color of the effluent. In lieu of an accurate measure, we use hemodynamic clues as well as serial hemoglobin determinations.

This brings up the common misconception that we can assess blood loss by checking the hematocrit or hemoglobin concentration. Unless the patient has been carefully hydrated back to "euvolemia" (normal total blood volume), this is *not true*! Only if an equal volume of some other fluid is added (either from the interstitial space, or by us) does the hematocrit fall. If left to nature's device, it may take up to 2 days to reach steady state. Depending on the fluid, often much more than the actual volume of blood lost must be given to account for the small percentage that actually remains intravascular. The volume that escapes is not lost though; it replenishes the interstitial space that so generously donated fluid to the bloodstream before treatment could be instituted. This replenishment is vital for the transport of oxygen between the blood and tissues. Massive hemorrhage and hypotension compromise oxygen delivery to tissues; to maintain cellular integrity, these cells resort to anaerobic metabolism, with a by-product of lactic acid. We often gauge our resuscitation by the severity of and then recovery from lactic acidosis. Unfortunately, too great a contribution of fluids to this interstitial space can result in

Table 3.8. Blood types and their frequencies in the population

Type	Frequency	Antibodies	PRBC	FFP, cryo, platelets
A	45%	Anti-B	A or O	A, AB
B	8%	Anti-A	B or O	B, AB
AB	4%		Any	AB
O	43%	Anti-A and anti-B	O	Any
Rh+	90%		Any	Any
Rh−	10%	± Anti-Rh+	Rh−	Any

For platelets, as long as they are "packed" and therefore containing a low antibody titer, any type can be transfused in any patient, though we prefer to use Rh− in women. When transfusing platelets of an incompatible blood type, the packs must be red cell free.

impressive swelling and discomfort for the patient post-operatively. Accurate estimation of volume status and management of hydration remains a target of much research in anesthesia.

Blood replacement

As reviewed elsewhere (see section on the blood in Chapter 11), the trigger for red cell transfusion is based not on a single laboratory value, but rather on an assessment of the adequacy of oxygen delivery. When we deem replacement necessary – after considering the risk:benefit ratio and the wishes of the patient, e.g., Jehovah's Witness – we must decide what products to order.

Blood transfusions need to be ABO compatible. There are four major types, plus the rhesus factor (Table 3.8). In an emergency, when type-specific blood is not available, O− ("negative") blood can serve as a "universal donor." Because only about 7% of the population has this blood type (and not all happen to be blood donors), and 90% of the population is Rh+, it is usually safe to use O+ blood in an emergency, at least in men. A problem arises for Rh− women who might someday carry an Rh+ fetus. Maternal anti-Rh antibodies will cross the placenta, causing potentially fatal erythroblastosis fetalis.

For nearly all transfusions, we administer packed cells (rather than whole blood, which enables us to collect and use plasma for separate infusion). For type O transfusions, this minimizes the administration of type O serum with its anti-A and anti-B antibodies. Once we have given more than four units of type O packed cells, however, we are obliged to continue with type O transfusions because of the administered antibody load. Lacking antibodies to A, B, and Rh makes type AB+ patients the universal recipient. A pity that they are a distinct minority (3%)!

Pre-operatively, the expected need for blood transfusions covers the spectrum from: the patient will certainly not require a transfusion (no need to determine the patient's blood type) to: we know that without several transfusions the patient cannot survive (we must prepare several units of blood for this patient). To negotiate the area between these extremes, we can do the following:

(a) "Type and screen": The patient's blood is ABO and Rh typed and screened for common antibodies (indirect Coombs test). This quick (minutes) and inexpensive test (if there is anything in today's hospital that can be called inexpensive) misses only about the 1% of uncommon antibodies and is therefore usually sufficient, unless the patient has had multiple transfusions in the past and has developed many unusual antibodies.

(b) "Type and crossmatch": The patient's blood is typed and the type-matched (potential) donor's cells are exposed to the patient's serum. This is more involved than type and screen, costs more money and takes at least an hour, but readies donor blood for an immediate transfusion. We request a specific number of units to be typed and crossmatched if experience tells us to expect a large blood loss.

When we call the blood bank and ask for blood to transfuse, they always crossmatch it first, significantly delaying its arrival at the bedside. The ordering of type-specific blood is an option, though there are risks of incompatibility. Thus the time to call the blood bank is EARLY, when the situation appears to be going awry.

Table 3.9. Transfusion guidelines

Packed red blood cells (PRBCs):

- Rarely transfuse if Hgb >10 g/dL; almost always if Hgb <6 g/dL
- If Hgb is 6–10 g/dL, base decision on patient's risk for complications of inadequate oxygen delivery and risk for additional blood loss. In a typical 70 kg patient one unit PRBC transfusion is expected to increase Hgb by 1 g/dL and hematocrit by 3%
- Consider pre-operative autologous blood donation, cell saver (intra-operative blood recovery and re-infusion), acute normovolemic hemodilution

Platelets:

- Prophylactic transfusion for surgery usually indicated if <50 000/microL; or <100 000/microL and high risk of bleeding; not indicated for states of increased destruction, e.g., ITP
- Indicated for microvascular bleeding with <50 000/microL; or <100 000/microL and risk for increased bleeding
- May be indicated despite adequate platelet count if there is known platelet dysfunction and microvascular bleeding
- Transfuse 1 u/10 kg. In a 70 kg patient each unit will increase the platelet count by approximately 10 000/microL
- 1 single donor pheresis unit ≅ 6 random donor units

Fresh frozen plasma (FFP):

- Urgent reversal of warfarin therapy (5–8 mL/kg)
- Correction of known coagulation factor deficiencies for which specific concentrates are unavailable
- Correction of microvascular bleeding with elevated (>2 times normal) INR or aPTT, or when suspected factor depletion as after transfusion of more than one blood volume
- Treatment of heparin resistance (e.g., antithrombin III deficiency) in a patient requiring heparin
- Give enough to achieve at least 30% of normal plasma factor concentration (10–15 mL/kg)
- Platelets for transfusion also contain plasma: 4–5 u platelets or 1 single-donor unit contains factors equal to about 1 u FFP
- Often given 1:1 with PRBCs in trauma resuscitation

Cryoprecipitate:

- Prophylactic use in peri-operative or peripartum patients with congenital fibrinogen deficiencies or von Willebrand's disease unresponsive to desmopressin (DDAVP, 1-deamino-8-D-arginine vasopressin)
- Bleeding in patients with von Willebrand's disease if specific concentrates are unavailable
- Patients with a fibrinogen level <80–100 mg/dL (normal 150–450 mg/dL)
- Correction of microvascular bleeding in massively transfused patients with an unknown fibrinogen

Drugs for excessive bleeding:

- Desmopressin and topical hemostatics (e.g., fibrin glue and thrombin gel) should be considered
- Recombinant activated factor VII: consider when all above have failed

ITP: idiopathic thrombocytopenic purpura; INR: international normalized ratio; aPTT: activated partial thromboplastin time. Guidelines published in *Anesthesiology* 2006; **105**:198–208.

Table 3.9 provides some basic transfusion guidelines, though we encourage you to check for updates regularly. Table 3.8 describes which products may be transfused, based on the patient's blood type.

Depending on the storage medium employed, packed red blood cells (PRBC) come to us with a hematocrit of 50–80%, the latter a very viscous suspension that does not infuse well. We often dilute the PRBC unit with as much as 250 mL of normal saline (addition of hypotonic solutions will cause cell lysis, while calcium-containing fluids, e.g., Ringer's lactate, can initiate *in-vitro* coagulation in contact with

Table 3.10. Transfusion reactions

Transfusion reaction	Incidence	Comments
Non-hemolytic reaction	1:100–5:100	Fever, chills, urticaria
Hemolytic reaction	1:25 000	Hypotension, tachycardia, hemoglobinuria, microvascular bleeding, DIC; fatal ~1:500 000
Infectious diseases	Rare (<1:100 000)	Hepatitis A, B, C; HIV
	Significant (1:2)	CMV (immunocompromised patients should receive CMV-negative units)
	Unknown	West Nile and other viruses, prions
Bacterial infection	Rare	Limit by transfusing over less than 4 hours
TRALI (transfusion-related acute lung injury)	1:5000–1:10 000	Transfused serum vs. recipient white cells; increased capillary permeability → non-cardiogenic pulmonary edema and ARDS-type picture. The number one cause of mortality after transfusion
Other		Dilutional thrombocytopenia, citrate toxicity → acute hypocalcemia with infusion of >1 u/5 min Immunodulation: Transfused blood decreases the immune response and worsens long-term outcome after cancer surgery. Incidence unknown

These figures are frequently updated as new screening tests become available.

citrated blood). Blood is stored at 1–6°C and should be infused through a warmer. We use special infusion sets that contain a filter (≤170-micron) to trap clots or other debris.

Risks

Blood transfusions are inherently dangerous (Table 3.10). In addition to the frequent non-hemolytic reactions, ABO incompatibility threatens the potential of a hemolytic reaction with hypotension, hematuria, and fever. The diagnosis can be made more readily if the patient is awake since the symptoms of nausea, vomiting, flank or back pain, and dizziness frequently accompany a transfusion reaction. Therapy includes stopping the infusion immediately (we return both the remaining banked blood and a sample from the patient for testing), treating mild symptoms with antihistamines and acetaminophen to reduce fever, and perhaps adding corticosteroids to reduce the immune response. We worry most about the potential for shock, kidney failure, and disseminated intravascular coagulation (DIC). In this last nasty syndrome, the antigen/antibody reaction can trigger factor XII (Hageman), which kicks the kinin system into action leading to the generation of bradykinin and, through it, damage to endothelium (oozing), hypotension, and thrombosis via the release of endogenous tissue thromboplastin. Human error plays a large part in transfusion reactions, which account for more than half of transfusion-related deaths … translation: *double check all blood (patient and donor blood types) before transfusing!*

Unfortunately, there are several types of transfusion reaction, and some can manifest even several days after the transfusion.

As we are largely water, maintenance of the patient's fluid status represents one of anesthesiology's greatest challenges. Using vigilance, anticipation, appropriate monitors, and vascular access, we manage fluids, blood, and blood products to maintain stability and perfusion of vital organs.

Notes

1   The traditional units of measure can be very confusing. Larger catheters are measured in "French" (or Charrière), with 3 Fr to the millimeter. In contrast "gauge," an inverse unit of measure, defines needles and intravenous catheters. Each successive increase in "gauge" represents a decrease in diameter of about

10%. Thus a 21-g i.v. catheter is only about 50% the size of a 16-g.

2   Named for Friedrich Trendelenburg (the emphasis is actually on the "Trend," not the "del," as still pronounced by his family) – 1844–1924; his original description was a 45° head-down angle (we do much less as even at 20° head down the patient will want to slide down the table) with the legs and feet hanging off the bed (actually draped over the shoulders of an assistant).

3   Locally called a Swandom.

4   Interestingly the calculated osmolarity of this solution (308 mOsm/L based on 154 mEq/L each of Na^+ and Cl^-) would lead one to think that it is actually hypertonic. However, not all of the ions are dissociated in solution, with the undissociated NaCl only exerting 1 mOsm/L effect. Thus, when the osmolarity is actually measured instead of simply calculated, it is found to be isotonic.

Regional anesthesia

We can imagine future clinicians prescribing treatments that would exclusively affect a single cell type or a specific organ without spillover effects. That type of explicit therapy would be the opposite to general anesthesia, the name of which implies generalized effects of the anesthetic drugs. Indeed, anesthetics delivered via the lungs or by intravenous injection flood all organs in the body, causing numerous undesired effects. How much better to pinpoint the effect with regional anesthesia. Here, we deliver the drug selectively to the innervation of the surgical site. We are closer to the ideal but not quite in heaven. We lack the specificity of drugs that would block only one type of fiber (e.g., pain) and spare all others (e.g., motor) or that restrict their activity solely to the surgical site. We also have to contend with side effects that arise when the anesthetic drug gains access to the circulation, and performs mischief far from its intended site of action. Nevertheless, regional anesthesia provides a tool that can be used to great advantage for many patients.

Four distinct processes lead to the sensation of pain (Fig. 4.1):

(i) *Transduction*. Noxious stimulation of a peripheral receptor releases local inflammatory mediators that cause changes in the activity and sensitivity of sensory neurons. *Pre-incisional* infiltration of local anesthetics effectively blocks transduction.

(ii) *Transmission*. Once the noxious stimulus has been transduced, the impulses travel via (unimaginatively named) A-delta and C fibers to the dorsal horn of the spinal column where they synapse. The dorsal horn cells may be subject to "wind-up" or enhanced excitability and sensitization. Like a bandit cutting telegraph lines in an old (really old) Western, regional anesthesia can cut transmission of these signals.

(iii) *Perception*. Afferent fibers from the dorsal horn travel to higher CNS centers, mostly via the spinothalamic tracts. Activation of the reticular formation probably increases arousal and contributes the emotional component of pain. Central-acting agents such as opioids alter perception.

(iv) *Modulation*. Efferent pathways including inhibitory neurotransmitters modulate the afferent nociceptive information.

The complexity of pain perception goes beyond this quick anatomic/physiologic summary. Strong emotional stimuli, endogenous endorphins, and distraction can completely block pain perception, as is often true for injuries sustained in battle (or when being eaten by a lion). Thus, in addition to the described processes of getting the signal from injured tissue to the brain, psychological factors influence the pain experience.

While we can interfere with the impulses traveling up the nervous pathways at any stage, mounting evidence suggests that multi-modal and pre-emptive (before incision) therapy can both improve immediate post-operative pain control and reduce the risk of a subsequent chronic pain syndrome.

Transduction of superficial noxious stimuli can be inhibited with pre-incisional local infiltration. As the name implies, regional anesthesia involves anesthetizing a specific portion of the body, thereby preventing transmission. Because pain sensation travels via nerves (A-delta and C fibers to be specific) from the site of the injury to the spinal cord (dorsal columns) and then up to the brain, the nerve impulse can be interrupted at numerous sites. Consider an operation on the big toe. Local anesthetic infiltration suffices for only the most superficial of procedures. For anything deeper, we make use of our knowledge of the area's innervation and the anatomic course of the nerves through the body. Sensory impulses can be interrupted in several locations including the ankle, popliteal fossa, sciatic notch, or at the spinal cord level. The first three would be considered peripheral nerve blocks because they block the transmission of the "pain message" before it reaches the central nervous system. We can also block

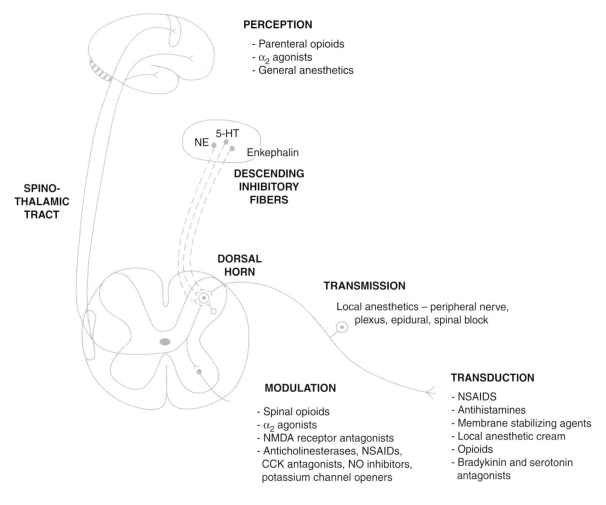

PERCEPTION

- Parenteral opioids
- α_2 agonists
- General anesthetics

NE 5-HT Enkephalin

DESCENDING INHIBITORY FIBERS

SPINO-THALAMIC TRACT

DORSAL HORN

TRANSMISSION

Local anesthetics – peripheral nerve, plexus, epidural, spinal block

MODULATION

- Spinal opioids
- α_2 agonists
- NMDA receptor antagonists
- Anticholinesterases, NSAIDs, CCK antagonists, NO inhibitors, potassium channel openers

TRANSDUCTION

- NSAIDS
- Antihistamines
- Membrane stabilizing agents
- Local anesthetic cream
- Opioids
- Bradykinin and serotonin antagonists

Fig. 4.1 Pain processes. See text for explanation. NE: norepinephrine; 5-HT: serotonin; NMDA: *N*-methyl-D-aspartate; NSAID: non-steroidal anti-inflammatory drug; CCK: cholecystokinin; NO: nitric oxide. (Reproduced with permission from Kelly, D. J. *et al.* Preemptive analgesia I: physiological pathways and pharmacological modalities. *Can. J. Anesth.* **48**(10): 1001, 2001.)

the message at the level of the central nervous system with an epidural anesthetic (which could be a caudal block), or a spinal (properly called a subarachnoid) block. Together, these last approaches are called neuraxial anesthesia. And all can be effective for big toe surgery.

When used for operative anesthesia, we typically supplement a regional block with sedation; the patient need not be aware for most procedures. A balance must be struck between the patient's comfort and the side effects of sedation, primarily respiratory depression. Also, all our sedatives, even midazolam (Versed®), linger and produce a hangover effect. Therefore, the patient will not be fully functional following the procedure, or even for the remainder of the day. Some patients do not wish, or cannot afford, to be out of action for an entire day and would prefer the reassuring conversation of a caring anesthesiologist over drug-induced anxiolysis.

We may be tempted to choose regional anesthesia for patients with cardiovascular or pulmonary problems, arguing that a properly conducted regional technique stresses these systems less than does a general anesthetic. Be careful! If the regional block is unsuccessful, if there are complications, or if the block wears off during the operation, the patient may require emergency general anesthesia and possibly also tracheal intubation. Similarly, regional anesthesia must be used with caution in patients with a recognized "difficult airway."

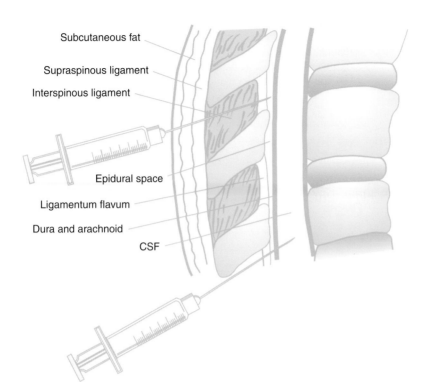

Subcutaneous fat

Supraspinous ligament

Interspinous ligament

Epidural space

Ligamentum flavum

Dura and arachnoid

CSF

Fig. 4.2 Layers of the back for neuraxial anesthesia. The upper needle demonstrates the location of the epidural space. Usually a catheter would be threaded for continuous epidural infusion of local anesthetic ± opioids. The lower needle is in the intrathecal space, where CSF would be readily aspirated. We place intrathecal needles below the lowest extent of the spinal cord (L1–2 in adults) to minimize the risk of damage to the spinal cord.

Table 4.1. Classification of nerves

Class	Size	Function
Aα (myelinated)	Large	Proprioception, motor
β		Touch and pressure
γ		Motor
δ	Small	Temperature, sharp pain
B (myelinated)	Small	Sympathetic preganglionic
C (unmyelinated)	Small	Dull pain, temperature, sympathetic postganglionic

If we fear difficulty managing the patient's airway, we would be ill-advised to perform a regional anesthetic to "avoid the airway" without adequate preparation (additional airway equipment, etc.).

Neuraxial anesthesia

Neuraxial anesthesia involves the placement of a variety of agents (local anesthetics, opioids, alpha$_2$-receptor agonists, and other adjuncts) into the intrathecal (subarachnoid) or epidural space (Fig. 4.2), either by a single injection or by a continuous-infusion catheter technique. The medications act directly on the spinal cord and, for epidurals, also on the spinal roots. This results in decreased transmission of impulses through the various nerves (Table 4.1).

Some local anesthetics have differential effects on various nerve types. For analgesic applications we would prefer to block only the pain impulses, but no agent is quite that specific. Bupivacaine and its relatives (levo-bupivacaine and ropivacaine) block sensory more than motor fibers and are the agents of choice for labor analgesia, where we desire maintenance of maternal mobility ("Push! Push!").

The dermatomal level (Fig. 4.3) achieved depends on several factors (Table 4.2). Consider a cesarean delivery, for which we require a T4 sensory level to minimize discomfort with uterine manipulation. For an epidural, we select a local anesthetic and concentration (e.g., 2% lidocaine with epinephrine), then administer it in ~5 mL boluses until we achieve the desired level (or we reach the maximum dose allowed).

For a spinal we administer a calculated dose and then might use gravity to influence the level of the

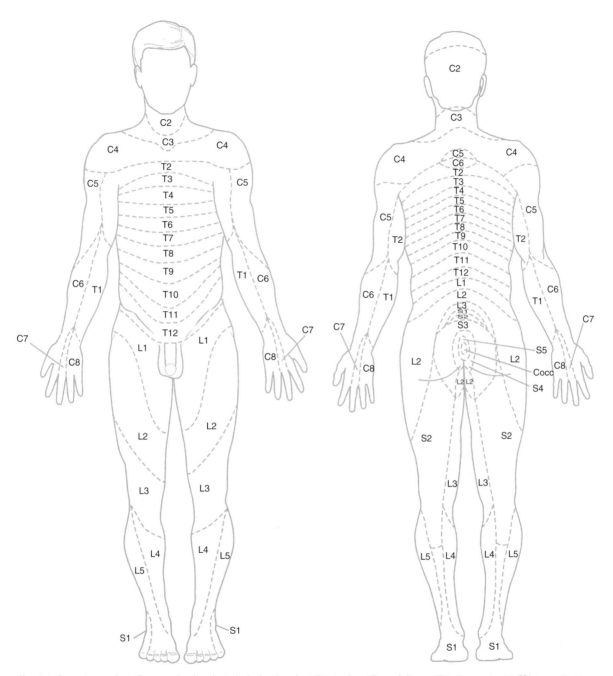

Fig. 4.3 Dermatome chart. Common landmarks include the thumb at C6; nipples at T4; umbilicus at T10; iliac crest at L1; fifth toe at S1. Note that the perineum is innervated by S2–4.

block. Normal cerebrospinal fluid (CSF) has a specific gravity (density relative to water) of 1.0006 ± 0.0003 (as a ratio, it's a dimensionless unit). Any agent of a different density, injected into the CSF, will distribute according to gravity. That is, a hyperbaric drug will "sink," and hypobaric will "float." We can affect the resulting anesthetic level by tilting the patient.[1] The level required depends on the surgical procedure (Table 4.3). To achieve a T4 level for our cesarean delivery, we inject hyperbaric local anesthetic (e.g., 12 mg

Table 4.2. Factors determining the spread of neuraxial anesthesia

	Spinal	Epidural
Dose	Mass of drug only	Mass of drug and volume
Level of injection	Yes	Yes
Age	Yes	Yes
Patient position	Yes relative to agent baricity[a]	Minor effect
Obesity	Minor effect	Minor effect

[a] Baricity is the density (specific gravity) of the injected agent, relative to spinal fluid (see text).

Table 4.3. Dermatomal level requirements for a selection of operations

- T4–5: upper abdominal surgery
- T6–8: intestinal, gynecologic or renal surgery
- T10: transurethral resection of the prostate, hip or inguinal hernia surgery
- T12: lower extremity surgery with a thigh tourniquet
- L1: Knee surgery
- L2–3: Foot surgery
- S2–5 (saddle block): perineal surgery, hemorrhoidectomy

of 0.75% bupivacaine with dextrose) intrathecally at a level below where the spinal cord ends (~L1–2). When the patient assumes a supine position, the local anesthetic "sinks" to the thoracic kyphosis (Fig. 4.4). If, after a few minutes, the level of the block remains too low, we can carefully lower the patient's head; as the drug, which we made "heavy" with dextrose, follows gravity, the level will rise. After some minutes (the actual time depending on the agent selected), the drug will be "fixed" and no further manipulation of its level can be achieved by altering the patient's position.

Hemodynamic effects

Unfortunately, autonomic nerves (sympathetic here) are the easiest to block and cannot be independently spared. The sympathetic block usually extends at least two dermatome levels higher than the somatic sensory block. Basal sympathetic tone causes vasoconstriction peripherally, thus its elimination results in vasodilation (venous and arterial). Up to about a T4 level (nipple line), hypotension results primarily from decreased preload secondary to vasodilation proportionate to the sympathetic level (the higher the block, the more of the peripheral vasculature escapes from nervous control, relaxing vascular tone). The baroreflex response will attempt to maintain cardiac output. While its efforts to vasoconstrict the blocked area are thwarted, vasoconstriction in the unblocked area works overtime. Sympathetic stimulation reaches the heart via the "cardiac accelerators," which travel in T1–4 nerves; thus a higher block may inhibit sympathetic stimulation of the heart, resulting in bradycardia and a greater decrease in cardiac output and blood pressure. Epinephrine, rather than atropine, resuscitates severe bradycardia following neuraxial block.

Pulmonary effects

If the neuraxial anesthesia level covers the thorax, intercostal muscle function will be impaired. While not a problem for most patients, those who recruit accessory muscles for normal breathing may have difficulty. Fortunately, the diaphragm receives its innervation from C3–5, and therefore the neck should ideally never be affected by neuraxial anesthesia. If it *is*, the block is *much* too high and the patient will complain (if he still can) of dyspnea. Manual ventilation with bag and mask will be required. While a head-up position can encourage a hyperbaric spinal block to recede, often tracheal intubation for maintenance of the airway will become necessary, especially in an obstetric patient at high risk for pulmonary aspiration of gastric contents. Occasionally respiratory depression accompanies neuraxial anesthesia not from blockade of motor impulses, but from hypotension-induced ischemia of the respiratory center in the brain. These patients are often somnolent as well. The alert clinician should not require a declining pulse oximeter to recognize this problem. We converse with our patient both for its distractive capacity (for the patient, not us – ideally), and as a monitor of her mental status. Frankly, we can learn

Table 4.4. Risks and complications of neuraxial anesthesia

- Hypotension – common, often heralded by nausea (treat by increasing preload, cardiac output, and blood pressure with volume loading; phenylephrine also finds use)
- Hypoventilation due to opioids, blockade of accessory muscles of ventilation or medulla hypoperfusion from high spinal
- High spinal – with resultant hypotension/hypoventilation (avoid by careful and fractionated dosing of epidural catheters – for fear they have migrated intrathecally)
- Bradycardia/asystole – *rare* but requires aggressive treatment with epinephrine
- Post-dural puncture headache – probably from leaking CSF
- Local anesthetic toxicity (minimized by careful and fractionated dosing, and testing the catheter to ensure extravascular placement)
- Neurologic damage – epidural hematoma, cauda equina syndrome or trauma by needle – RARE
- Infection – meningitis, arachnoiditis, or epidural abscess – RARE
- Transient neurologic symptoms – usually mild buttocks/leg pain for ~1 week after spinal anesthetic. Incidence 10–20%, more frequent and more severe with lidocaine
- Backache – usually transient
- Minor effects – urinary retention, pruritus, shivering

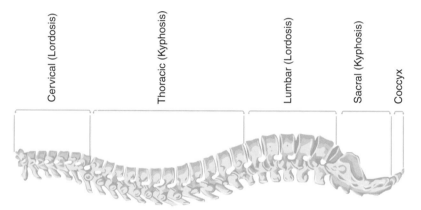

Cervical (Lordosis)   Thoracic (Kyphosis)   Lumbar (Lordosis)   Sacral (Kyphosis)   Coccyx

Fig. 4.4 Shape of the spine. Note that in the supine patient, hyperbaric intrathecal medications will "sink" to the thoracic kyphosis. An interactive simulation of this is available at the VAM website from our link www.anest.ufl.edu/ea.

much from our patients about innumerable topics. A high spinal obviously interferes with small talk. More commonly, patients become dyspneic, even with only a mid-thoracic level of anesthesia, and usually without any decrease in their oxyhemoglobin saturation. We attribute this to loss of chest wall proprioception, which removes a feedback loop that reassures the patient's brain that ventilation is maintained.

If the patient complains of shortness of breath, first confirm that the level of anesthesia is not too high. For example, test their grip strength bilaterally. If reassured on that point, let the patient put a hand in front of her mouth so that she can feel her exhaled breath. This may restore the feedback loop and the patient's sense of well-being. If necessary, apply supplemental oxygen but continue to monitor for hypoventilation.

Complications

Of the potential complications to neuraxial blockade (Table 4.4), we fear formation of an epidural hematoma most. Because the spinal cord runs in the spinal canal, a closed space, anything that abnormally takes up room causes compression of other structures. Should an epidural blood vessel get nicked on insertion of a needle or catheter (common), and that vessel fail to clot normally, the resulting hematoma can cause increased pressure and ischemic damage to the spinal cord. For

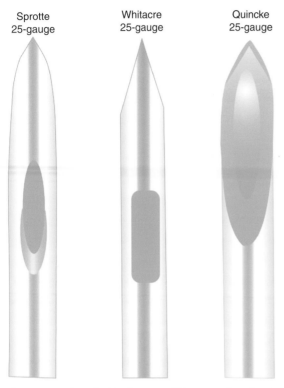

Sprotte
25-gauge

Whitacre
25-gauge

Quincke
25-gauge

Fig. 4.5 Spinal needles. The Sprotte and Whitacre are "pencil-point" needles, which are thought to *spread* the dural fibers rather than cutting them, as a hypodermic-like pointed Quincke needle might, thereby reducing the incidence of post-dural puncture headache.

this reason, patients who are anticoagulated or thrombocytopenic are rarely considered candidates for neuraxial blocks. This risk of epidural hematoma is present both at insertion *and* removal of the catheter.

Post-dural puncture headache, another complication, deserves special mention: the patient develops pounding headaches when sitting up and finds great relief by lying down. A hole in the *dura mater* does not seal immediately. The size and shape of that hole has implications for the future development of a post-dural puncture (spinal) headache. We can minimize the risk of this headache by using "pencil point" needles (Fig. 4.5) in the smallest diameter practical, e.g., 25–27-g. As you might imagine, post-dural puncture headaches are particularly bad when we inadvertently nick the dura with the large epidural needle[2] during an attempt to place an epidural catheter. This so-called "wet tap" has a high incidence of headache, particularly in the pregnant patient. Treatment includes bedrest, hydration, analgesics, caffeine, and an epidural

blood patch in which the patient's own blood is sterilely injected into the epidural space, providing usually immediate relief.

Technique

Neuraxial block placement requires both skill and the patient's cooperation. Table 4.5 lists the steps for placing either a spinal or an epidural anesthetic. A combined spinal–epidural (CSE) begins as an epidural, but after identification of the epidural space with the epidural needle (Fig. 4.6), a thin spinal needle is passed through that needle and into the intrathecal space for injection of drug. The spinal needle is withdrawn, and the epidural catheter threaded as above.

Indications

Many factors must be considered including location of operation and, therefore, anesthetic level required, duration of surgery, and implications for cardiovascular and respiratory function. For example, we would not use spinal anesthesia in a patient in hemorrhagic shock or with significant aortic stenosis who would not tolerate a drop in preload and afterload (Table 4.6).

Peripheral nerve blocks

With neuraxial anesthesia, it is difficult to block only the area of interest. Almost by definition, surgical anesthesia at the desired level includes everything "south" as well; this is particularly true with spinals. Peripheral nerve blocks provide an alternative, interrupting nerve impulses at specific points in their course, rather than the entire spinal cord. Table 4.7 lists some of the blocks we perform.

While local anesthetics can diffuse a small distance, depositing the drug in close proximity to the desired nerve increases the likelihood of a successful block. Therefore, knowledge of anatomy is paramount. Sometimes anatomic landmarks suffice; for example, we can deposit local anesthetic in the axillary sheath by traversing its artery. For most blocks, however, in order to ensure the needle tip lies within millimeters of the intended nerve (and not *in* the nerve), we use one of three common techniques:

(i)   Paresthesia technique, in which placement of a needle in close proximity to a nerve causes a "pins and needles" sensation in the nerve's peripheral sensory distribution. Depending

Table 4.5. Neuraxial blockade placement

Position patient with back flexed, sitting up or lying on the side

Identify a palpable interspace (if possible) at the desired level[a]

Remove hand/wrist jewelry and watch

Put on a hat, mask and sterile gloves

Sterilely prepare with chlorhexidine alcohol scrub[b] and drape a wide area

Infiltrate skin and deeper planes with local anesthetic (1% lidocaine)

Spinal	Epidural
Insert guide needle, if <23-g spinal needle; smaller needles are not stiff enough to penetrate the skin	Insert epidural needle through skin (see Fig. 4.6)
Advance needle through layers: subcutaneous tissue, supraspinous ligament, interspinous ligament. If the needle is midline, there should be little pain. Redirect if bone is contacted. Ask the patient whether they feel the needle pressure left, right or middle	
Increased resistance may be noted in the ligamentum flavum, then a "pop" as the dura is punctured. CSF returns through the needle when the stylet is removed	Apply a glass syringe with 2–3 mL saline and a small air bubble. Ballottement of the syringe causes compression of the bubble. Slowly advance the needle with continuous gentle pressure until there is a "loss of resistance," where the saline is easily injected into the epidural space, really a potential space that experiences negative pressure when the dura is pressed upon by the needle. (CAREFUL! DO NOT aspirate at this point.) Thread a catheter through the needle 3–5 cm into the epidural space
Apply syringe with medication, aspirate and watch for "swirl" if the densities of the CSF and local anesthetic are sufficiently different	Attach syringe to catheter and aspirate. If you aspirate blood, the catheter tip is probably in an epidural vein. If you aspirate clear liquid, the tip may be in the subarachnoid space. But even if you cannot aspirate anything, the next step will make doubly sure
Administer medications through the needle	"Test dose" catheter with epinephrine-containing local anesthetic (e.g. 1.5% lidocaine with epinephrine 1:200 000) to confirm catheter is not intravascular (epinephrine-induced tachycardia) or intrathecal (rapid numbness/weakness)
Position patient for gravity-dependent spread (hyperbaric spiral)	Secure catheter. Position patient. Administer medications through catheter. Start with conservative dose, wait to give it a chance to work and then, if necessary, repeat injections until desired anesthetic level is achieved

[a] Spinals should be placed below where the spinal cord ends (usually L1–2 in an adult, lower in a child); epidural location depends on the region to be anesthetized.
[b] While this counters the product's labeling, ample evidence and our societies recommend its use.

on the area of the intended block, specific paresthesias can be sought with manipulation of the needle. This technique can be uncomfortable for the patient, yet requires the patient to be sufficiently awake to respond. We need to watch the patient while gauging the pressure we apply to the plunger of the syringe. The patient will let us know if he feels an "electric shock" or pain – signs we associate with the intraneural placement of the needle, at which point we do not proceed to inject drug under high pressure, which would compress the nerve in its sheath, causing nerve ischemia and injury.

(ii) Nerve stimulator technique, in which we apply a small electrical current to an insulated needle, causing stimulation when near a motor nerve. We adjust the needle position to achieve the maximal motor response in the desired distribution. This technique enables us to exploit anatomical cues to direct needle movement. For example, stimulation of the phrenic nerve (the patient will hiccup) when performing an

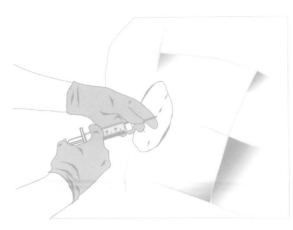

Fig. 4.6 Technique of neuraxial block placement. In this case the epidural space is sought with a "loss of resistance to saline" technique, noting when the fluid in the syringe is suddenly easily injected.

Table 4.6. Indications and contraindications for neuraxial anesthesia

Indications

Surgical anesthesia, particularly below the umbilicus, and especially where consciousness is desired, e.g., obstetrics

Post-operative pain management

Labor analgesia

Chronic pain management

Contraindications

Patient refusal/inability to cooperate

Elevated intracranial pressure (risk of herniation)

Infection at site

Inadequate volume status

Critical aortic stenosis or other lesion that does not tolerate swings in preload/afterload

Coagulopathy[a]

[a] For recommendations on management of patients taking anticoagulants see www.anest.ufl.edu/EA.

interscalene block tells us the brachial plexus lies just a centimeter posterior in the neck. This technique is less uncomfortable for the patient than the paresthesia technique, and sedation may be used.

(iii) Ultrasound-guided technique (Fig. 4.7), in which needle insertion into nerve sheaths or around vessels is guided by ultrasound-enabled visualization of those structures (much like looking at a child in its mother's womb). This technique eliminates much of the needle probing necessary using landmarks, paresthesias or electrical stimulation alone to locate nerves whose anatomical course can differ between individuals. Use of ultrasound increases success, shortens onset time, and reduces complications of regional anesthesia.

Indications

Peripheral nerve blocks may be performed for operative procedures, as well as for post-operative pain management. Through blockade of nerve impulses, pre-emptive analgesia may be obtained. Furthermore, catheter techniques enable post-operative pain management with continuous infusions of local anesthetic and/or opioids. Such infusions can improve perfusion to the operative extremity, reduce pain with movement, speed recovery, and improve quality of life even weeks after the operation when the infusion has long been discontinued.

Intravenous regional anesthesia (IVRA)

Also called a Bier[3] block, this is perhaps the simplest, safest, most foolproof regional anesthetic technique. We replace the blood in the venous system of an extremity with local anesthetic (large volume, low concentration, e.g., 0.5% lidocaine WITHOUT epinephrine) by first exsanguinating the extremity (usually arm), applying a tourniquet, then infusing the local anesthetic distal to the tourniquet. We obtain excellent anesthesia within minutes. It will last until the tourniquet is deflated. The local anesthetic will flow retrograde through the venous system into the vasa nervorum that bathe each nerve fiber. Unfortunately, not infrequently the patient will be troubled by tourniquet pain. Therefore, this technique is best suited for operations lasting less than an hour. The procedure is safe as long as the tourniquet holds tight, preventing the local anesthetic from gaining access to the central circulation and causing systemic toxicity. If the local anesthetic has been in the extremity for at least 20–30 minutes when the operation is complete, the tourniquet can be safely deflated without toxic effects. The safest practice, however, is to "cycle" the tourniquet a few times by briefly deflating it and then immediately reinflating it, thereby allowing only a small amount of unbound local anesthetic into the circulation at a time.

Table 4.7. Indications for peripheral nerve blocks

Peripheral nerve block	Indication
Cervical plexus	Carotid endarterectomy
Stellate ganglion	Complex regional pain syndrome (CRPS) of the upper extremity (also called reflex sympathetic dystrophy, RSD)
Upper extremity	
Brachial plexus	Shoulder, arm, wrist, hand procedures
Distal nerves (median, radial, ulnar)	Forearm, hand procedures
Digital nerves	Fingers – do not use epinephrine-containing local anesthetics in finger and toe blocks. Vasoconstriction of digital arteries can lead to distal necrosis
Intercostals	Rib fractures or chest tube placement
TAP (transverses abdominus plane)	Abdominal surgery below the umbilicus
Celiac plexus	Chronic pain in abdomen, especially pancreatic cancer
Lower extremity	
Femoral, obturator, lateral femoral cutaneous	Procedures of the thigh and knee
Sciatic and saphenous	Lower leg, calf, ankle, foot procedures
Ankle	Foot procedures

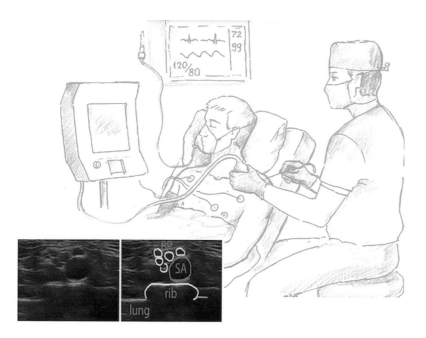

Fig. 4.7 Supraclavicular ultrasound-guided block of the brachial plexus. Note the patient is sedated, perhaps with a small amount of supplemental oxygen, and fully monitored during the procedure. The ultrasound picture insert demonstrates a typical supraclavicular image and a schematic illustration of the anatomic structures (SA: subclavian artery; BP: brachial plexus). The left side of the image corresponds to the lateral side of the patient. Illustration by B. Ihnatsenka, MD.

Local anesthetic toxicity

Local anesthetics exhibit dose-related toxicity. Therefore, concerns about potential toxicity grow with increasing doses of local anesthetic (see also Chapter 12). Typical volumes of local anesthetics used for various blocks follow (we use lidocaine 1.5% as an example):

Subarachnoid block	5 mL
Epidural block (with epinephrine)	20 mL
Brachial plexus block (with epinephrine)	30 mL
Intercostal block (multiple levels)	20 mL
Finger block (*without* epinephrine)	3 mL

Of these, intercostal nerve blocks lead to the highest local anesthetic blood levels and therefore are most likely to cause toxicity. In order to reduce the rate of absorption we often use a solution that is premixed with 1:200 000 epinephrine (5 mcg/mL), which not only reduces the absorption of the drug and thus the chance of toxicity, but also prolongs the anesthetic effect.

An added advantage of the epinephrine: should the injection be inadvertently intravascular (as into an epidural vein), the prompt development of epinephrine-induced heart rate increase will give a clear signal, the injection aborted, and attention paid to the vital signs and mental status.

Either an inadvertent intravascular injection or rapid absorption of properly placed local anesthetic can trigger toxic manifestations. We reduce this risk by dividing the dose, if it is a larger volume, into multiple smaller boluses, looking for signs of toxicity in-between. Early typical symptoms include a metallic taste, ringing in the ears, and tingling around the mouth. Sleepiness or mental status changes often accompany these symptoms. Central nervous system toxicity progresses to seizures (treated with *small* intravenous doses of midazolam or propofol) and eventual coma. Cardiovascular effects include hypotension due to vasodilation and myocardial depression, but may progress to complete cardiovascular collapse. This is particularly true with bupivacaine, whose slow unbinding from sodium receptors causes stubborn ventricular arrhythmias.

As with all emergencies, the treatment includes the common sense steps, such as to stop injecting and then to follow the standard ABCs of basic life support. "A" (airway) and "B" (breathing with oxygen) are particularly important since hypoxia and acidosis worsen the toxicity. In addition, removal of local anesthetic (and other drugs at toxic levels) from the circulation can be facilitated by the administration of intralipid (see Chapter 12). It sounds obvious, but do not use lidocaine to treat local anesthetic-induced ventricular arrhythmias! Use amiodarone (start with 1 mg/kg slowly i.v.) instead. Early evidence suggests that epinephrine, at least in high doses, may actually reduce survival in this setting.

Anesthesiologists skilled in both regional and general techniques offer patients a broad range of options for their operation. Regional anesthesia occupies a niche in outpatient surgery, where rapid awakening and minimal nausea/vomiting are sought. In many procedures, regional with light general anesthesia provides good operative conditions for the surgeon and excellent post-operative analgesia. Regional anesthesia plays a growing role in post-operative pain.

Notes

1 At www.anest.ufl.edu/EA resides a link to an interactive subarachnoid block/spinal anesthesia simulator which allows the student to manipulate baricity, patient position, and drug binding to help clarify the interactions.

2 There are many needles used for insertion of an epidural catheter; they tend to be large (to accommodate a 20-g or larger catheter), slightly blunt (to reduce the risk of dural puncture), and with a curved tip (to encourage the catheter to pass into the epidural space). Common designs include the Tuohy (introduced by Edward Boyce Tuohy [pronounced "Too-ee"] around 1945) and the Weiss (designed by Jess Bernard Weiss around 1961). The latter is basically a Tuohy needle with wings at the hub.

3 August Karl Gustav Bier (1861–1949), a German surgeon, introduced intravenous regional anesthesia in 1908. He also administered and received the first spinal anesthetics in 1898 (and experienced one of the first post-dural puncture headaches the next day).

General anesthesia

General anesthesia requires many preparatory steps. These include the pre-operative evaluation of the patient and the procurement and preparation of all equipment to be used (as well as emergency alternatives we hope not to need), drugs to be given, intravenous cannulae to be inserted for the infusion of the necessary fluids, monitors, and the tools and techniques needed for the establishment of an open airway. Elsewhere in this book you will find all of these topics addressed. Here, we will limit ourselves to a discussion of how to induce and maintain general anesthesia and how to ease the patient out of the drug-induced coma before transfer to the post-anesthesia care unit (PACU).

Pre-operative holding

Once the preparations for general anesthesia are complete, the patient's history and physical examination are reviewed, consent is verified, and the machine and equipment are set up and tested (we need to be sure they will work as expected), we are ready to bring the patient to the operating room. We return to our patient in the pre-operative holding area, check the i.v. and offer a sedative for anxiety, which most patients willingly accept. A few might also benefit from analgesia for acute pain. Recall that opioids and sedatives act synergistically to depress ventilation, so choose the one the patient needs most, and continue to monitor if they must be combined. Additionally we have by now considered our plan for post-operative pain and might consider a pre-emptive analgesic such as a non-steroidal anti-inflammatory, acetaminophen, or gabapentin (see Chapter 12 for a more detailed review of each of these). Gastrointestinal optimization might be indicated, with H_2 blockers, pro-kinetic agents (e.g., metoclopramide), and/or a non-particulate oral antacid.

Induction, maintenance, and emergence

Once the patient moves to the operating table, we apply monitors and check pre-induction vital signs. Now we are ready to send the patient on one of the strangest journeys of his life: general anesthesia. We will administer drugs by injection and inhalation that will effectively disengage his brain, removing conscious thought, and interfering with some unconscious activities as well. If we use neuromuscular blocking agents, ventilation will cease, and he will be unable to move. In short, without intervention to maintain these systems, particularly ventilation, the patient will most certainly die.

To appreciate the enormity of this statement, consider the extreme of this condition: once general anesthesia has been established for some cardiac procedures, we might lower the patient's temperature to the point where all currently monitored variables cease to show evidence of life. There will be no heartbeat, no electrocardiogram, no spontaneous breathing, no blood flow, the patient's temperature will be about 18°C (a bit cooler than room temperature) and the electroencephalogram will show no deflection. There will be no reflex, no motion, and no reaction to any intervention. If, at this point, you were to bring in an observer, unaware of what had been done, he might well pronounce the patient dead. In the operating room we call this DHCA, short for deep hypothermic circulatory arrest. And yet, if we restore blood flow and gas exchange, and raise the temperature, the patient's neurologic, cardiac, and respiratory functions will slowly resume their own life and, once the temperature approaches normal and the effects of drugs wear off, the patient will wake up. We cannot imagine a more profound responsibility than that of the anesthesiologist taking a patient to such an extreme approximation to death while guarding his life.

In routine general anesthesia we do not drive the system to the extreme just described. Yet, a defenseless patient under general anesthesia will expect the anesthesiologist to stand in for him and his dignity and attend to him with focused attention and great skill.

During general anesthesia, we must provide the patient with sleep, amnesia, and analgesia; we must

57

monitor his vital signs and keep them within physiologically reasonable limits, and we must facilitate the surgeon's work as much as possible so she, too, can do her best for the patient.

Pre-oxygenation

The establishment of a patent airway is our most important safety concern. Disaster overtakes the patient within a matter of minutes if he cannot breathe for himself (because we eliminated desire and/or ability to breathe with sedatives or paralytics), and we cannot ventilate his lungs (because his airway is obstructed by soft tissue and because we cannot intubate his trachea for any number of reasons). Then minutes, even seconds, count. If, before inducing apnea, we replace the nitrogen in his lungs with oxygen, we can gain 3–6 minutes (more with a large functional residual capacity [FRC]) before arterial hypoxemia occurs. Therefore, we routinely pre-oxygenate (i.e., "denitrogenate") patients before inducing anesthesia. This procedure is simple: we apply a face mask that seals around the nose and mouth well enough to prevent entraining nitrogen-containing room air from around the mask, and select a flow of oxygen high enough to prevent the patient from inhaling his exhaled gas. The latter is vented and, after one minute of deep breathing or several minutes of quiet breathing, the patient's FRC will contain very little nitrogen, much oxygen, and the usual amount of water vapor and carbon dioxide.

Induction

We now introduce hypnotic, analgesic, and anesthetic drugs into the body either by intravenous injection or via the lungs (in the past intramuscularly or even rectally). While inhalation anesthesia can be induced without the help of intravenous drugs, the most common approach is to inject a fast-acting drug such as propofol (1–3 mg/kg), often with the addition of an opioid to blunt the response to manipulation of the larynx. Within a couple of minutes, these drugs will reach their peak effect, at which time intubation of the trachea becomes feasible, usually with the help of muscle relaxants. Propofol offers sufficient relaxation of the muscles that oppose laryngoscopy that we can often intubate without adding a muscle relaxant, especially in children.

Instead of intubating the trachea, we have the option of inserting a laryngeal mask airway (LMA), which does not require the use of a muscle relaxant

and is particularly welcome when the patient need not be intubated at all and is breathing spontaneously throughout the operation (see Chapter 2).

Once we have placed the endotracheal tube or LMA and have confirmed its proper location by auscultation and continual end-tidal CO_2, we maintain the level of anesthesia by inhalation, intravenous (TIVA, total intravenous anesthesia) or a combination anesthetic. A number of halogenated drugs are available (halothane, isoflurane, desflurane, sevoflurane), but we use only one at a time (though we may use more than one during a case, especially with children). Each is delivered with oxygen-enriched air. Sometimes we combine the halogenated agent with oxygen and 50–70% nitrous oxide. The latter provides modest analgesic background (equivalent to about 10 mg morphine) without much cardiovascular depression. Surgical anesthesia (the patient will not respond to the incision) can be obtained within a matter of minutes so that the induction of anesthesia need not delay the incision.

Propofol is the poster child agent for TIVA. Purported advantages of this technique are shortened wake-up and PACU times, and reduced risk of postoperative nausea and vomiting. Rather than halogenated agents, patients for outpatient surgery might receive a propofol infusion (for sedation and sleep) with nitrous oxide (to provide a modicum of analgesia and ensure amnesia), supplemented with small amounts of analgesics.

The rapid sequence induction

Patients who need general anesthesia, even though they have a full stomach (having recently eaten or having a condition that interferes with gastric emptying such as trauma or pregnancy), require a special technique, the so-called rapid-sequence induction (Table 5.1). With a full stomach, the specter of regurgitation and aspiration arises. The technique calls for a thorough denitrogenation, followed by the administration of propofol or thiopental and succinylcholine or rocuronium in rapid succession while we maintain pressure on the cricoid ring (the so-called Sellick maneuver[1]). Remember, the cricoid is the only ring of the trachea that does not have a membrane posteriorly and, instead, is cartilaginous throughout its circumference. So, pushing on it compresses the distal hypopharynx (not the esophagus, as believed for many years). How hard should one push on the cricoid while doing this? 20–30 newtons.[2] You can feel the cricoid ring under the skin of the front of the

Table 5.1. Steps in a rapid-sequence induction

Once you have started a rapid-sequence induction, you have lost the opportunity to check or obtain missing equipment. Thorough preparation, therefore, is mandatory.

Preparation

1. Prepare and check for function:
   - suction on, audible and next to the patient's head
   - intubation equipment:
     - tubes – one too large, one just right, one too small – check cuffs
     - laryngoscope – two different blades (usually straight and curved) – check lights
     - Stylet or intubating bougie
   - machine and backup self-inflating resuscitation bag
   - emergency airway equipment immediately available including LMA and cricothyrotomy set
2. Have available a helper skilled in applying cricoid pressure and to assist as necessary
3. Prepare patient:
   - give antacid if circumstance permits
   - obtain vital signs, print ECG strip

Induction

1. Pre-oxygenate/denitrogenate to an end-tidal oxygen of ideally at least 80%
2. Tell the patient he will feel pressure on his neck as he falls asleep; meanwhile the assistant gently locates the cricoid ring
3. In rapid succession, administer an intubating dose of propofol (or thiopental) followed by an intubating dose of succinylcholine, while the assistant begins to apply cricoid pressure (20–30 newtons,[2] 2–3 kg)
4. As the patient falls asleep, the assistant increases cricoid pressure (40 newtons)
5. Sixty seconds after the succinylcholine entered the vein (or when apnea and relaxation coincide), intubate the trachea under direct laryngoscopy
6. Inflate the cuff of the endotracheal tube and connect to the breathing circuit, then inflate the lungs
7. Confirm endotracheal position of tube by:
   - watching chest rise – bilaterally
   - observing for appearance of condensation (fog) in the ETT
   - listening over the stomach for absence of breath sounds
   - observing the capnogram for appearance of carbon dioxide for 6 breaths
8. Then tell assistant to release cricoid pressure after confirming correct position of the tube
9. Secure tube and begin anesthesia

neck just under the larynx. Only once we have inflated the cuff and confirmed the proper position of the endotracheal tube can we stop the Sellick maneuver.

Positioning

For many operations, the patient can lie on his back. Others require positions that may take an hour or more to be accomplished (e.g., some neurosurgical operations). We need to understand what position favors access for the surgeon and what positions present dangers for the patient (interference with ventilation,

compression of nerves, extreme flexion or extension of joints or simply are not tolerated because of arthritis or contracture). Thus, the positioning is a joint surgical/anesthesia task during which a lot of foam padding finds application between patient and hard surfaces. The most common post-operative nerve palsy affects the ulnar nerve, which is exposed to pressure at the ulnar groove of the elbow. The nerve runs superficially through the cubital tunnel at the elbow, between the medial epicondyle and the olecranon. When struck it elicits tingling in the hand and hence is commonly, if not oddly, referred to as the "funny bone." Pronation of the forearm (rolling the hand palm downward) flattens the groove and increases the risk for pressure injury. Simultaneous stretch on the nerve compounds the risk so we keep the patient's arms supinated when placed out to his sides, and well-padded with elbows bent to about 90° if the patient is positioned prone with the arms up in "surrender" position.

Depth of anesthesia and monitoring

Once the patient is positioned, we must keep the anesthetic level so that the patient will neither feel pain nor remember the operation. Yet this "anesthetic depth" must be balanced against the hemodynamic consequences (hypotension) of excess anesthetic, as well as the potential for delayed wake-up. If the patient is not paralyzed, there will be little doubt that he will move, alerting us if he feels pain, though isolated cases report intra-operative awareness and recall even in this setting. We need to gauge the depth of anesthesia clinically and with the help of instruments. The clinical assessment includes monitoring heart rate and blood pressure, which should be neither high from sympathetic response to noxious stimulation, nor low from overdose with anesthetics. In recent years processed EEG signals have become available that help gauge the depth of anesthesia by generating a score linked to EEG activity, which becomes depressed as anesthesia deepens. In addition to these signals we keep track of the intravenous drugs the patient has had, of their effects and duration, and of the concentration of expired anesthetics, which reflect blood and finally brain levels. Thus, the conduct of general anesthesia calls for continual attention to a number of parameters and variables.

At the same time, we monitor pulse oximetry, blood pressure, heart rate, ECG, tidal volume, respiratory rate and peak inspiratory pressure, inspired oxygen, the concentration of respired gases and vapors, and the capnogram. Should blood loss, deep anesthesia, surgical activity (for example compressing the vena cava), an embolism (e.g., air aspirated into an open vein), or a process originating in the patient (such as anaphylaxis or coronary insufficiency) cause a problem, we should be able to discover the effects as early as possible so that we can take corrective actions. Alteration of the ST segment may herald myocardial ischemia requiring optimization of the myocardial oxygen supply:demand ratio, and possibly even a change in the surgical plan

for emergent cardiovascular intervention. However, the degree, or even presence, of such depression may be altered merely by changing the monitoring mode of the ECG device, for example to limit the interference of electrocautery on the signal, or adjusting its amplification. The astute clinician considers all details, from pre-existing patient risk, to intra-operative events, through nuances of monitoring, in assessing and reacting to all findings.

We also assess the degree of muscle relaxation with the help of a nerve stimulator (twitch monitor) and by watching the operation and gauging muscle tone, which might impede the surgeon's work. Thus, we cannot be satisfied with just watching the monitors; we need to keep an eye on the patient, his face, his position, and the surgeon's progress.

A tedious aspect of our work is the obligation to keep a record of all these events and of our activities, such as the administration of drugs and fluids, adjustment of ventilator settings, and even of surgical events ("aorta clamped at 9:24 a.m.!"). Automated record-keeping systems are becoming increasingly sophisticated.

Emergence

Well before the surgeon puts in the last stitch, we begin preparation for having the patient wake up. This might call for the reversal of a non-depolarizing neuromuscular blocking drug and the scaling back of inspired anesthetic concentrations. Furthermore, our goal is to have the patient awaken quickly and without pain, but only **after** the operation concludes; therefore, we titrate opioids or our regional anesthetic to anticipate the pain level without unacceptable respiratory depression, while also considering the risk for postoperative nausea and vomiting. It is a fine art to gauge the surgical process and the patient's requirements so that the patient opens his eyes when the dressing goes on. "Hello," we say, and, after confirming the patient is strong, able to protect his airway (cough or gag reflex), breathing and following commands, we suction his airway and say, "All done! Let me take out that tube," when we pull the endotracheal tube or the LMA. While the patient is not likely to remember such words, they provide a fitting ending to a perfect anesthetic!

We then accompany the patient to the PACU, where we go through a formal process of turning the care of the patient over to a specialized PACU nurse, unless the patient is fit for early discharge home or needs to be admitted to the intensive care unit.

Table 5.2. Likely initial direction of trends of commonly monitored signals in patients under general anesthesia with mechanical ventilation[a]

Problem	BP	HR	SpO$_2$	ETCO$_2$	PIP	Breath sounds	Example of a cause
Breathing system obstruction	Up	Up	Down	Down	Up	Abnormal	Kinked ETT
Transfusion reaction	Down	Up	Down	Down	Up	Abnormal	Patient ID error
Anaphylaxis	Down	Up	Down	Down	Up	Abnormal	Allergic reaction to muscle relaxant
Pulmonary edema	Down	Up	Down	Down	Up	Abnormal	Heart failure from fluid overload
Aspiration		Up	Down	Down	Up	Abnormal	Full stomach with regurgitation
Asthma		Up	Down	Down	Up	Abnormal	Reaction to ETT with light anesthesia
Myocardial infarction	Down	Up		Down		Abnormal with edema	Coronary artery plaque rupture
Cardiac tamponade	Down	Up		Down		Normal	Central venous catheter perforation
Pulmonary embolism	Down	Up	Down	Down		Normal	Fat embolism from femur fracture
Hemorrhage	Down	Up		Down		Normal	Torn vena cava
Esophageal intubation	Up	Up	Down	Absent		Abnormal	Difficult intubation
Light anesthesia	Up	Up			Up	Normal	Increased surgical stimulus
Malignant hyperthermia	Up	Up		Up		Normal	Muscular dystrophy
Disconnect		Up	Down	Absent	Down	Abnormal	Table turned
Endobronchial intubation	Up		Down		Up	Abnormal	ETT advanced too far
Pneumothorax	Down	Up	Down		Up	Abnormal	Left nephrectomy
Addison crisis	Down	Up		Down		Normal	Following chronic steroid therapy without supplementation

[a] These may vary with severity, duration, and the patient's condition.
BP: blood pressure; HR: heart rate; SpO$_2$: oxyhemoglobin saturation; ETCO$_2$: end-tidal carbon dioxide; PIP: peak inspiratory pressure; ETT: endotracheal tube; ID: identification.

Problems

Things don't always run smoothly. If critical incidents occur, they must be discovered and corrected in time, lest they lead to disasters. To catch early trends, however, presents more difficulties than one might think, because most signals we monitor are rather non-specific. Thus, a low SpO_2 could be the result of a mainstem intubation, i.e., past the carina and thus only ventilating one lung, an asthma attack, or faulty hospital gas piping; low blood pressure might be the consequence of bleeding, deep anesthesia, or a measuring artifact. Therefore, with any deviation from normal, we need to think holistically about the patient and the anesthesia system with all of its components.

In Table 5.2 we have listed trends in various monitored parameters as they often appear during certain problems. Observe two points:

(i) Usually we cannot arrive at a diagnosis by simply looking at the monitors. We need additional information, which we must urgently collect when trends herald trouble.

(ii) Breath and heart sounds turn out to be very helpful. Always listen to heart and lungs (wheezing, crackling, uneven breath sounds or – importantly – normal breath sounds) to include or exclude certain items from a differential diagnosis. Equally important is the peak inspiratory pressure.

To complicate matters even further, not all patients react in an identical manner. Coexisting diseases or previous pharmacologic interventions can obscure changes or reverse the direction of an expected change. Finally, trends can reverse direction, depending on how long the problem existed and how grave the incident. For example, hypercarbia and hypoxemia secondary to inadequate ventilation because of obstruction in the endotracheal tube can first cause sympathetic stimulation and a rise in blood pressure and heart rate. However, if the problem persists, pressure will decline and, with severe hypoxemia, extreme bradycardia can supervene.

A particular problem virtually unique to anesthesia deserves special mention: *malignant hyperthermia*. Patients with this rare ($\approx$1:20 000) inherited defect in intracellular calcium control are asymptomatic until given succinylcholine or anesthetic vapors, which can trigger a violent increase in metabolism with skyrocketing O_2 consumption and CO_2 production. The condition may be heralded by masseter muscle rigidity (difficulty opening the patient's mouth). Tachycardia and rapidly rising end-tidal carbon dioxide ($ETCO_2$) precede by many minutes a murderous (literally) fever. Later high creatine kinase levels and red colored urine reflect extensive muscle damage. Immediate cooling and i.v. dantrolene have greatly improved the prognosis. Hydration, diuretics, and bicarbonate administration prevent myoglobinuria-induced renal failure. Hyperkalemia is expected and treated aggressively. Triggering agents must be eliminated and subsequently always avoided. Patients diagnosed with this condition should be registered with MHAUS (Malignant Hyperthermia Association of the US) and wear a Medic Alert bracelet. Furthermore, with autosomal dominant inheritance, family members should consider being screened either by a muscle biopsy or genetic testing for a ryanodine receptor mutation.

Notes

1 Brian A. Sellick (1918–1996), a British anesthetist who made numerous contributions in cardiothoracic anesthesia, is best known for a seminal paper describing cricoid pressure to prevent gastric reflux and distension from mask–ventilation.

2 A "newton" is not, as one may guess, the force of one apple falling from a tree, but rather is equivalent to 0.225 pounds.

Post-operative care

The post-operative care of the patient can be divided into an early and a continued phase. The early phase lasts from the moment the patient leaves the operating room until he is discharged from the post-anesthesia care unit (PACU) or its equivalent. For all but the most minor of outpatient procedures, the care is then continued, a phase that can extend for days or even weeks.

Early post-operative care

Based on his medical condition and the planned operative procedure, we will have classified the patient as ambulatory (also known as outpatient), as "post-operative admit" (the patient comes to the hospital on the day of the operation and is admitted to the hospital after his operation), or as an inpatient (the patient is already in the hospital, or will be admitted for pre-operative preparation, and will stay there post-operatively). Two categories of patient might bypass the PACU (formerly called the recovery room): (i) ambulatory patients who had a minor procedure and are expected to be ready for discharge in a matter of minutes and (ii) patients requiring intensive care because of serious pre-operative medical problems or major operations with potential complications. The latter are admitted directly to the intensive care unit (ICU) upon completion of the operation.

For patients coming to the PACU we consider three factors: the patient's pre-operative condition; the effects of the just completed therapeutic (surgical, radiological, obstetrical, electroconvulsive) or diagnostic procedure; and the effects of the anesthetic. As we turn the patient's care over to the PACU staff, we provide a formal "report" of his condition including the following:

- pre-existing medical conditions with particular emphasis on pre-existing respiratory, cardiac, and chronic pain issues;
- surgical disease, operative and anesthetic course, and any problems encountered;

- fluid status including what was administered, estimated blood loss, and urine output;
- medications administered in the operating room. We mention antagonists given to counteract lingering neuromuscular weakness or respiratory depression or nausea and vomiting. Should the patient need more such medication, the PACU physician can either continue the already initiated treatment or, if the patient does not respond, switch to another drug;
- concerns regarding the procedure or the patient, including the plan for post-operative pain management;
- issues requiring follow-up such as pending laboratory evaluations, a chest radiograph to confirm central venous catheter placement, when the next dose of antibiotics is due, etc.

Because handoff communication is one of the root causes in a majority of adverse events, this handoff should be formal and thorough, with time for questions, and even a "read-back" to ensure the major issues were understood. Finally, we make certain the patient is stable, record a first set of post-operative vital signs, and ensure that all documentation is complete and correct.

In the PACU, we first worry about safety. We consider waning anesthetic drug effects as they relate to adequacy of oxygenation, which in turn requires an alert respiratory center (is there a hangover effect from CNS depressants or opioids?) and the muscle power to breathe (is there a hangover effect from muscle relaxants or a regional anesthetic?), an open airway (is there obstruction of the upper airway?), and no encumbrance to breathing from dressing, position, or the surgical procedure. Adequacy of oxygenation also requires adequate circulation (is the blood pressure normal and the ECG unchanged from its pre-operative state?). The pulse oximeter will speak volumes to these questions. If the patient is *breathing room air* and his oxygenation (as measured by pulse oximetry located peripherally) is normal, we can be assured of adequate breathing.

We assess the central nervous system, recognizing that the patient usually will have had a number of drugs with CNS effects. With modern anesthetic techniques and drugs, we expect the patient to rally from the depressant effects of the drugs fairly rapidly and to become responsive, if not immediately oriented. Up to 25% of elderly patients will be delirious after a general anesthetic for a major surgical procedure. Once a patient is not only responsive but also oriented, we know that his brain is perfused and oxygenated.

Most patients will arrive with an intravenous infusion. It is very often difficult to ensure the patient is in a neutral fluid balance (blood pressure and urine output can be affected by surgical stress and medications). If his insensible losses (about 800 mL/day) and intra-operative losses (from evaporation from exposed surfaces, e.g., intestines, bleeding and from edema caused by the surgical trauma) have been replaced, fluid therapy will simply continue to replace insensible losses.

Often enough, however, some bleeding continues – usually invisibly – into the traumatized tissue. Fluid therapy will need to be adjusted to meet the patient's requirements as judged by cardiovascular signs and urine production. A balanced salt solution such as normal saline or Ringer's lactate will serve as long as there is no need to worry about electrolytes, red blood cells, and plasma proteins.

While we worry about altered mental status, hemodynamic derangements, excessive pain, and other serious signs of imminent danger, our patients often have very different concerns. When expecting to survive, patients worry almost three times as much about being nauseated, gagging, and vomiting as they do about their next biggest concern: post-operative pain. We might have expected such a result based on the number of common words for vomiting (barf, puke, retch, hurl, blow, spew, regurgitate, reversal, up-chuck).[1]

Approximately 20–30% of all, and up to 80% of high-risk untreated surgical patients, will experience post-operative nausea and vomiting (PONV). In adults, female gender, non-smoking, use of post-operative opioids, and a prior history of PONV or motion sickness each increases risk by approximately 20%. Surgery longer than 30 minutes and certain operations (e.g., strabismus, breast, gynecologic, laparoscopic or ophthalmologic, or posterior fossa craniotomies) increase the risk of PONV even further. Thus a non-smoking female with a history of motion sickness having a

laparoscopic hysterectomy can be predicted to benefit greatly from prophylactic anti-nausea medication.

Nausea and vomiting represent very complex responses involving at least the chemoreceptor trigger zone (CTZ) and the vomiting center. Chemically, numerous neurotransmitters (dopamine, serotonin, histamine, acetylcholine via muscarinic receptors) and chemical irritants (narcotics, chemotherapy agents) can be involved. Additionally, the brain processes afferent inputs from the vestibular system, the gastrointestinal (GI) tract, and even the respiratory center, superimposing these on any emotional effects associated with provocative smells, tastes, and sights. Certain combinations of stimulants are a recipe for PONV.

Treatment guidelines, thankfully, are quite simple. Prophylaxis is recommended for all patients at moderate or high risk for PONV, typically administered before the end of surgery, and usually involving a 5-hydroxytryptamine (5-HT$_3$, serotonin) receptor antagonist. Unfortunately, prophylaxis offers only about a 50% reduction of risk. In patients thought to be very high risk, we employ a multi-modal approach, adding a second agent (to reduce remaining risk another 50%) with a different mechanism of action (think of dexamethasone, or a dopamine receptor antagonist like droperidol, a histamine blocker like diphenhydramine, or a "dirty" drug that has a little action at many receptor sites, like promethazine). If relief of PONV lasts at least 6 hours before recurring, we repeat the therapy (though we do not re-dose long-acting drugs like dexamethasone and scopolamine). If the original therapy failed to provide at least 6 hours relief we would instead reconsider possible triggers for PONV, and try agents with a different mechanism of action.

Of course, this won't help one whit if you are on a plane and a passenger behind you starts retching (or the nurse can't go immediately to check out the ordered drug). But one can still offer help. Many find relief from steady and firm (to the point of inducing mild discomfort) pressure at the P6 (Neiguan) acupuncture point (Fig. 6.1). Alternatively, presumably because of the respiratory center's influence, rhythmic "sniffing" of peppermint or, to make it seem more medicinal, an alcohol swab from the first-aid kit, has been shown to help (but any smell should work).

Early post-operative pain

As we reassure ourselves as to the patient's safety, we begin to consider his pain. Three points need

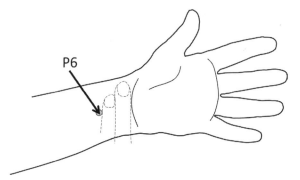

Fig. 6.1 Schematic of the P6 acupuncture point where pressure is applied to reduce nausea. The point is two fingerbreadths proximal to the ulnar crease between the palmaris longus and flexor radialis tendons.

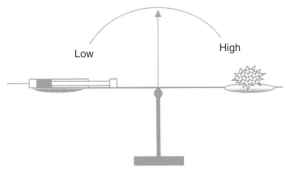

Minute ventilation

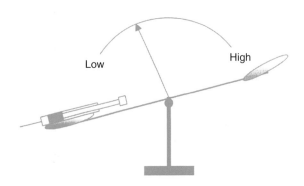

Minute ventilation

Fig. 6.2 Ventilatory response to $PaCO_2$. The first diagram shows that noxious stimulation (spiked beasty on the right) can counteract the respiratory depressant effect of narcotics (syringe), maintaining a normal ventilatory response to $PaCO_2$. In the lower diagram the pain has vanished and the respiratory depressant effect of the narcotic becomes unmasked; minute ventilation is low. Such depression can even result in apnea.

attention: (i) surgical incisional pain will decrease over time, (ii) analgesic effects left over from the anesthetic will wane over less time, and (iii) pain counteracts the CNS depressant (respiratory) effects of narcotic analgesics (Fig. 6.2). Thus, pain management in the PACU must seek a balance of three shifting slopes of which we do not know the rate of change. This translates into: *watch the patient* and titrate drugs to balance adequate analgesia and avoid respiratory depression, meanwhile considering the onset time and duration of each drug administered. As long as the patient cannot take oral medication, a practical approach for the acute phase of pain management in the PACU can make use of intravenous morphine in 2.0 mg increments for the average adult. It takes about 5 minutes for such a dose to show any effect, and closer to 30 minutes for actual equilibration. Therefore, wait at least 5 minutes before giving the next dose. Many factors influence the patient's response to such treatment. A patient on chronic narcotic therapy will require more, a frail elderly person less. Titrate! Titrate! Titrate! There are also non-narcotic medications to be considered such as acetaminophen and ketorolac in appropriate patients.

After minor surgical procedures, many patients will not require opioids at all, and most can take oral medication. Chapter 12 gives drugs and dosages.

Complications

There would be no need for a PACU if it were not for the occasional complications that require early recognition and prompt treatment. Here is a quick review of potential problems encountered in the PACU.

Desaturation

Differential diagnosis

- *Hypoventilation. Always first assist ventilation to establish normal SpO_2 and $PaCO_2$!* Then consider causes and their treatment.

  - *Residual neuromuscular blockade.* Suspected when the patient shows an abnormal respiratory pattern, particularly the tracheal tug, i.e., downward motion of the larynx with inspiration, or rocking respirations where the chest caves in and the abdomen expands with inspiration. Test by asking the patient if he can hold his head off the bed for 5 full seconds. Treat with reversal agents if less than a full dose was administered in the OR. Continue to support ventilation until strength returns. Patients at high risk for pulmonary

65

aspiration of gastric contents may benefit from airway control via repeat intubation.

- *Residual sedation.* Consider dose of benzodiazepines (can be reversed with flumazenil).
- *Narcosis with carbon dioxide retention.* Typically a slow, deep respiratory pattern; consider asking him to take breaths every few seconds for a minute or so. If this restores the saturation then be suspicious the patient is retaining enough carbon dioxide to tip the alveolar gas equation towards hypoxemia. Also consider cautious reversal of opioids with naloxone diluted to 40 or 80 mcg/mL solution.
- *Bronchospasm (wheezing).* Intubation is a strong stimulant for bronchospasm; treat with bronchodilators.
- *Laryngospasm (stridor).* If related to the operation, e.g., neck operation with possible hematoma formation, it becomes a surgical emergency. Otherwise try continuous positive airway pressure, letting the patient exhale against resistance (5–10 cmH$_2$O) and maintaining that pressure throughout the respiratory cycle. If there is no air movement, a tiny dose of succinylcholine can break the spasm.
- *Pain.* Particularly with a subcostal incision where deep breathing is painful.

- *Ventilation/Perfusion mismatch*
  - *Atelectasis.* Probably the most common cause of post-operative hypoxemia. Ask the patient to take a single deep breath and hold it for as long as he can. If the saturation recovers then you've made the diagnosis of atelectasis from shallow breathing.
  - *Aspiration of gastric contents.* Particularly in high-risk patients, or if intubation required multiple attempts.
  - *Pneumothorax.* Especially after subclavian central venous access. Obtain a chest radiograph, but be prepared to relieve the pneumothorax by puncture (second intercostal space, mid-clavicular line) should a tension pneumothorax develop in the meantime.
  - *Pulmonary embolism.* Thromboembolism is the most common. May need $\dot{V}/\dot{Q}$ (ventilation/

perfusion) or CT scanning. Most surgical patients require some form of prophylaxis against deep vein thrombosis (DVT).
  - *Pneumonia.*
  - *Mainstem intubation.*
- *Diffusion block*
  - *Pulmonary edema.*
- *Inadequate FiO$_2$*
- *Other*
  - *Hypoglycemia* or other electrolyte abnormalities.
  - *Caffeine withdrawal* for multi-cup coffee drinkers.
  - *CNS event.*

Management

(i) Airway

- Chin lift, neck extension; continuous positive airway pressure (CPAP) often helps. For this, use a bag and mask system (Mapleson – see Chapter 8) with a high flow (15 L/min) of oxygen. Apply the face mask tightly, letting the patient exhale against resistance (5–10 cmH$_2$O) and maintain that pressure throughout the respiratory cycle.

(ii) Breathing

- Supplemental oxygen (make sure it is flowing).
  - Via nasal cannula, but with oxygen flows of 2 L/min the inspired O$_2$ only increases by about 6%.
  - Via standard tent face mask for an inspired O$_2$ of up to 50%.
  - Via partial rebreathing face mask for an inspired O$_2$ of up to 80%.
  - Via non-rebreathing face mask for an inspired O$_2$ of up to 95%.
- Encouragement – "take a breath and then another and another!", often effective with narcotic depression.
- Bag–Mask – use with self-inflating bag or Mapleson.
- Check ventilator settings, O$_2$ concentration and end-tidal CO$_2$ if the patient is intubated.

(iii) Studies to consider

- Chest radiograph if abnormal breath sounds (pneumonia, atelectasis, pneumothorax, ± aspiration). Keep in mind, however, that a portable film may not provide the highest quality and consolidation takes some time to manifest radiographically.

- Arterial blood gas.
- Twitch monitor if patient appears still to be weak.

Hypotension

Differential diagnosis

- Inadequate preload
  - Inadequate fluid resuscitation
  - Continued hemorrhage
  - Venodilation due to medications or sympathetic blockade (e.g., neuraxial anesthetic or analgesic)
  - Pulmonary embolism
  - Increased intra-abdominal pressure, e.g., big uterus pressing on vena cava
  - Increased intra-thoracic pressure, e.g., tension pneumothorax
  - Pericardial tamponade, especially if central venous access was obtained
- Poor myocardial contractility
  - Residual anesthetics
  - Myocardial ischemia
  - Fluid overload ("far-side" of the Starling curve)
  - Pre-existing cardiac dysfunction
  - Electrolyte disturbance
  - Hypothermia
- Inadequate afterload
  - Sepsis
  - Vasodilation due to medications (e.g., residual antihypertensives) or sympathetic blockade, e.g., neuraxial anesthetic or analgesic
  - Anaphylaxis
- Arrhythmias
  - Bradycardia
  - Loss of atrial kick
    · Atrial fibrillation/flutter
    · AV dissociation
  - Electrolyte disturbance

Management

- Physical examination (especially chest auscultation).
- ECG (at least 5-lead strip) to detect arrhythmias and ischemia.

- Advanced cardiac life support (ACLS) protocol if abnormal rhythm.
- Hemoglobin level.
- Intravascular fluid resuscitation ± blood transfusion.
- Supplemental oxygen.
- Elevate legs to enhance venous return.
- Consider transthoracic echocardiogram.
- Consider chest radiograph.
- Consider invasive monitoring.
- Check electrolytes, especially Ca^{2+} for inotropy and K^+, Mg^{2+} for arrhythmias.

Hypertension

Differential diagnosis

- Pain
- Pre-existing hypertension
- Bladder distension
- Rebound hypertension (especially with missing dose of chronic clonidine)
- Endocrine problem (thyroid storm, pheochromocytoma)
- Malignant hyperthermia, neuroleptic malignant syndrome
- Delirium tremens
- Increased intracranial pressure

Management

- Treat pain or anxiety if present.
- Review for pre-existing hypertension and reinstitute antihypertensive therapy where appropriate.
- Check ECG.
- Look for additional signs of malignant hyperthermia.
- Check for high bladder dome or ultrasound the bladder to verify it is not full. If Foley catheter in place, check patency and remove any fluid-filled loops in the tubing, or perform in-and-out catheterization.

We hope that none of these problems arose or that they have been dealt with successfully, at which point we are ready to discharge the patient from the PACU.

PACU discharge

A frequently used checklist is the Aldrete Recovery Score (see Table 6.1). If the sum of points reaches 9 or

Table 6.1. Aldrete score for post-anesthesia recovery[a]

System	Description	Score
Activity	Able to move four extremities voluntarily or on command	2
	Able to move two extremities voluntarily or on command	1
	Unable to move voluntarily or on command	0
Respiration	Able to breathe deeply and cough freely	2
	Dyspnea or limited breathing	1
	Apneic	0
Circulation	Blood pressure ±20% of pre-anesthetic values	2
	Blood pressure ±20–49% of pre-anesthetic values	1
	Blood pressure ±50% of pre-anesthetic values	0
Consciousness	Fully awake	2
	Arousable on calling	1
	Non-responsive	0
Oxygenation	Able to maintain saturation >90% on room air	2
	Needs oxygen to maintain saturation >90%	1
	Saturation <90% even with oxygen	0

[a] A score of 9 or 10 suggests the patient is stable for discharge from the PACU.
Aldrete J. A. The post-anesthesia recovery score revisited (letter). *J. Clin. Anesth.* 1995; **7**:89.

10, we can discharge the patient from the PACU. The Modified Aldrete Score reaches a total score of 14 with the addition of up to 2 points each for pain and nausea/vomiting. Discharge is often acceptable with scores of 11 or more.

Outpatients

After outpatient procedures under local or peripheral nerve block anesthesia, perhaps with parenterally administered CNS depressants, e.g., midazolam (Versed®), propofol or opioids, the patient may bypass the PACU unless a medical condition would call for observation. It may be necessary to prescribe an oral analgesic that might include a mild opioid.

If no CNS depressant drug was used during the procedure and if the peripheral nerve block is behaving as expected (surgical anesthesia wearing off, but perhaps analgesia continuing), the patient can be discharged. We still insist that a relative or friend accompany him home because he will have been exposed to the stress of an operation – however minor – and will have been fasting and thus be at risk of swooning or even fainting and not being at the height of his reflex responses.

For those patients who required CNS depressants for a short operative procedure in which no severe post-operative pain is expected, e.g., a sigmoidoscopy under propofol sedation or a cataract removal under topical or local anesthesia preceded by a small (0.5–0.75 mg/kg) dose of methohexital (Brevital®) to minimize the discomfort of the retrobulbar block, the recovery process can be completed in a matter of minutes to an hour, at which point the patient can be discharged into the care of a relative or friend for transportation home. We always assume that drug effects and hormonal disturbances will linger for a matter of several hours to a day, so that upon discharge, the patient cannot be considered ready to drive an automobile or ride a bicycle or even cross the street by himself.

For those patients who remain in the hospital following their operation, PACU discharge signals the phase of continued post-operative care.

Continued post-operative care

The patient will go through important changes in response to a major operation with anesthesia. The stress of the inflicted surgical trauma will trigger a release of adrenocorticotropic hormones, cortisol, and catecholamines. Catabolism will overpower anabolism; the patient will be in a negative nitrogen balance. Coagulation changes might further thrombosis. Incisional pain and narcotic analgesics can reduce pulmonary gas exchange. Where the endotracheal tube contacted the tracheal wall, it will have impaired the mucociliary elevator. Together with narcotic inhibition of the cough reflex, already reduced in the elderly, patients may retain bronchial secretions, potentially leading to atelectasis and pneumonitis. Large fluid loads given during the operation need to be mobilized, yet antidiuretic hormone secretion will favor water and salt retention. An ileus after intra-abdominal procedures often takes days to resolve; nasogastric suction may deflate the stomach, but not without also removing electrolytes. In short, many major operations will leave the patient in a greatly debilitated state that can take several days or more to resolve.

If these processes are superimposed on extensive surgical operations, for example those affecting heart, lung, or brain, the patient will be admitted to the ICU. This will also be true for post-operative patients who come with pre-existing disease processes involving the cardiovascular (congestive heart failure, recent myocardial infarction), or respiratory (obstructive lung disease) systems, the central nervous system (stroke, tumor), metabolism (diabetes), hepatic or renal systems, or infection. The available frequency of observation, extent of monitoring, and immediacy of care in the ICU do not match what is available in the operating room, but greatly exceed whatever can be offered on the post-surgical ward.

When we visit the patient on the post-surgical ward, we will not only consult his chart to see the trends in vital signs (cardiovascular, respiratory, and temperature) but also assess fluid status and medications prescribed and given. We then talk to the patient to gauge his mental status (up to 25% of elderly patients can take up to a week to become fully oriented, and some 10% have cognitive impairment lasting for months) and to ask about his comfort. We might have to explain that hoarseness (from an endotracheal tube) or sore throat (from a rough laryngoscopy or residual irritation from an LMA or endotracheal tube) is likely to improve in a day or two. We continue to worry about pulmonary complications, e.g., atelectasis and pneumonitis, which are most likely in elderly men, in smokers, and after operations that involve the upper abdomen and the chest. Being aware that myocardial infarctions are far more likely to occur – many of them silently – on the second post-operative day than in the operating room, we pay special attention to the cardiovascular system. Hypotension, hypertension (often pre-existing), and

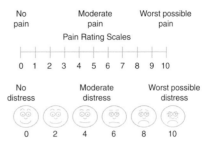

Pain assessment guide
Tell me about your pain

VAS = Pain intensity (0–10), patient report

If 0 is no pain and 10 is the worst pain imaginable, what is your pain now? ...in the last 24 hours?

Fig. 6.3 VAS pain assessment guide. Adult patients will be asked to select a number on the visual analog scale (VAS), while children can point to one of the faces to describe their pain.

arrhythmias are not uncommon. We document this post-operative visit, and bring concerns to the attention of the surgical team as needed.

Pain management

As anesthesiologists, we are particularly attentive to the patient's pain and its management. We now use a widely employed standardized method of assessing pain in adults and children (Fig. 6.3). In children incapable of relating their pain, physical signs can help (Table 6.2). The treatment of pain will be influenced by its severity.

If the patient is unable to take oral medication, we can institute patient-controlled intravenous opioid administration (PCA), a system that enables the patient to trigger an intravenous injection of a prescribed amount of a narcotic. The PCA pumps can be programmed to deliver a specific volume, then to lock the system for a predetermined period. When the patient pushes a button, a typical program might deliver (into a running intravenous drip) a 1 mg bolus of morphine. The pump then goes into a lockout mode, making an additional injection impossible for a pre-programmed period of, for example, 5 minutes. The pump can be programmed to limit the hourly injection to, for example, no more than 10 mg/h. Even that amount will be excessive if the patient self-administers the maximum, hour after hour. The dose and the lockout period have to be tailored for the individual patient

Table 6.2. Pain assessment guide in children; FLACC scale (face, legs, activity, cry, consolability)

	Behavioral/distress score (0–10, Caregiver)		
	0	1	2
Face	No particular expression or smile	Occasional grimace or frown, withdrawn, uninterested	Frequent to constant frown, clenched jaw, quivering chin
Legs	Normal position or relaxed	Uneasy, restless, tense	Kicking or legs drawn up
Activity	Lying quietly, normal position, moves easily	Squirming, shifting back/forth, tense	Arched, rigid or jerking
Cry	No cry asleep or awake	Moans or whimpers, occasional complaint	Crying steadily, screams or sobs, frequent complaints
Consolability	Content, relaxed	Reassured by occasional touching, hugging, or "talking to," distractible	Difficult to console or comfort

and with the caveat that ONLY the patient himself is ever allowed to push the button that makes the PCA deliver the next dose. While morphine is the standard, several drugs are available, among them hydromorphone (Dilaudid®) and fentanyl. In addition, for patients who pre-operatively have become tolerant to opioids, a background infusion, known as a "basal rate," of the narcotic may be required.

Depending on the operation (some cause much more severe and protracted pain than others; some limit oral intake for a longer period) and the patient (some are much more sensitive than others), a PCA pump might be available to the patient for a day or a week or more. Once narcotics are no longer needed, or the patient can tolerate p.o. intake, oral medications take over. A great variety of drugs are available (see Chapter 12).

Some patients will still have an epidural catheter in place that had served the anesthetic management during a thoracic, abdominal, or lower extremity operation and can now be used for pain management. Typically, we infuse a low concentration of local anesthetic combined with a narcotic through the catheter. By combining these drugs, we minimize the amount of motor block (paralysis) from the local anesthetic while limiting narcotic side effects (nausea, itching, and urinary retention) associated with larger doses of opioids. Once we establish a level of analgesia with a bolus injection, an infusion is begun and the patient might regulate the administration of additional drug with a PCA pump (PCEA: patient-controlled epidural analgesia). Dose and concentration of local anesthetic and lockout period will have to be adjusted for the individual patient and drugs infused. A typical arrangement might deliver 5 mL of 0.125% bupivacaine with 2 mcg/mL of fentanyl, with a lockout period of 20 minutes. Other approaches use a continuous epidural infusion alone.

The post-operative recovery will progress slowly. Every day, if all is going well, we can see improvements. Indeed, we can often see the moment when the patient "turns the corner" from negative to positive nitrogen balance. He will start shaving, she will do her hair and even put on lipstick. The patient will begin to eat, and we can switch from parenteral to oral medication. Many patients will be discharged from the hospital with prescriptions for oral analgesics. See Chapter 12 for a list of commonly used drugs, dosages, and duration of effect.

Chronic pain

Anesthesiologists have assumed an ever-increasing role in the treatment of patients with pain that ranges from the acute pain in the PACU, to the persisting (days rather than hours) post-operative pain, to the truly chronic (weeks and months rather than days) pain. The latter often does not arise from a surgical trauma but instead from tumors and degenerative diseases. The armamentarium of the chronic pain physician also differs from that of the acute care anesthesiologist. Gone are invasive monitors and moment-to-moment control of vital signs. Still very much in evidence are regional anesthesia procedures and a vast array of medications, most of them to be taken by mouth. Many patients with chronic pain suffer greatly from conditions for which we cannot find an anatomic explanation, conditions the treatment of which requires as much skill and compassion as should be expected by a patient with traumatic pain. Thus, for all patients with chronic pain, we emphasize a dual approach that includes not only pharmacologic treatment, but also non-pharmacologic treatment such as therapeutic exercise, distraction techniques and massage, which calls for the skills of nurses, physical therapists, and psychologists.

In the management of chronic pain, a number of different nerve blocks have been used. More common among them are stellate ganglion and paravertebral sympathetic blocks, e.g., for complex regional pain syndrome (CRPS), formerly called reflex sympathetic dystrophy (RSD), lumbar facet blocks or epidural steroid injection for back pain, and celiac plexus block, e.g., for pain from pancreatic cancer. Nerve blocks are often repeated to tide the patient over a condition that can be expected to improve. If that is not the case, neurolytic (destructive) nerve blocks can be considered. For these, alcohol or phenol has been used. Such blocks are employed most often for terminally ill cancer patients, not only because of the potential for serious side effects but also because axons often regrow with recurrence of pain in two or three months, and some patients develop a central denervation dysesthesia, which is very difficult to treat. Despite this, these blocks find use in some forms of severe chronic non-lethal pain (trigeminal neuralgia, shingles, severe CRPS), as well as sweating disorders (hyperhidrosis).

The first step will always be to assess the severity of pain, if for no other reason than to gauge the effectiveness of the treatment. A guideline for treatment might suggest the following:

- *For mild pain* (*VAS 4 or below*). Oral medication with acetaminophen such as tramadol/acetaminophen (Ultracet®) is often sufficient. If necessary, we might consider low-dose narcotics, such as oxycodone or hydrocodone.
- *For moderate to severe pain* (*VAS up to 7*). We would rely more on narcotics such as morphine or hydromorphone (Dilaudid®). Depending on the circumstances, centrally acting muscle relaxants, antidepressants, and anxiolytics can be added.
- *For the most severe or chronic pain*. Higher doses of narcotics, or narcotic-containing skin patches that steadily deliver drug transdermally, continuous infusions through implanted catheters, e.g., intrathecal or epidural pumps, and in patients who find no relief in pharmacologic approaches, neurolytic nerve blocks come into consideration.

In the past, many patients suffered greatly because physicians feared that opiate medication would lead to addiction. Such concerns must be tempered by the obligation to alleviate pain and will be abandoned when dealing with a terminally ill patient.

Note

1   A much-debated portion of the Sapir–Whorf hypothesis in linguistic relativity theory proposed that cultures develop more terms for ideas or objects of significant interest, for example "snow" in some Eskimo languages. In fact whole books have been written about this topic which we find impressive, surprising, intriguing, astonishing, amazing, a wee bit odd …

Monitoring

7

Introduction

Imagine stepping into an operating room. You see a patient draped for the operation, the surgical team, the anesthesiologist, an anesthesia machine, a ventilator, one or more infusion pumps, bags with intravenous fluids, and monitors with screens full of curves and numbers. But the picture is not static. The people move, the bellows of the ventilator go up and down, the drip chambers of the infusion sets show drops of fluids, and on the monitors the ECG, blood pressure, SpO_2, and capnographic patterns run across the screen. You behold this scene that presents an enormous amount of continuously changing data. You also hear the surgeon asking for an instrument, the scrub nurse saying something to the circulator, the anesthesiologist conveying to the surgeon information from the patient's medical record, the ventilator puffing, and a monitor beeping. Depending on your experience, you will know how to interpret what your senses absorb. You can imagine the scene with calm professionals at work at a routine task or one with frantic activity during an emergency punctuated by the urgently sounding alarms.

In this scene, *you* are the monitor. You absorb an abundance of signals that present data, which in your mind turn into information. You turn this information into knowledge, depending on what you know about the patient, the operation, and the clinical team. This knowledge depends on information about the patient's history and, ideally, acquaintance with the patient himself. If you were to record all the facts that you can comprehend, you would wind up with a very, very long list. On paper, it would take hours to synthesize, from such a comprehensive list of facts and ever changing trends, the current status of the patient. Such knowledge would enable you to make certain statements about this moment in time and projections into the immediate future.

When you think about monitoring, please remember that the physical diagnosis – still part of monitoring

in anesthesia – and the elaborate electronic monitors present only a minute fraction of the data that *you*, the clinical monitor, require and absorb in order to understand what is going on with your patient. The electronic monitors simply report; synthesis of the data is your job. They supplement in a modest way what the clinician perceives.

Let us now look at the small fraction of information generated by physical examination and by electronic and mechanical monitors.

Assume that the patient undergoes an operation under epidural anesthesia and light sedation. In addition to all the data described above, you will observe that the patient is breathing spontaneously. That means he has a heartbeat and a blood pressure sufficient to perfuse his respiratory center. If the patient responds appropriately to a question, we know his brain is adequately oxygenated. Now, that is a lot of information picked up without instruments!

Now assume the patient to be under general anesthesia and paralyzed, and that a ventilator mechanically breathes for him. Without getting a little closer, you cannot know if the patient has a heartbeat, a blood pressure, a perfused brain, or enough oxygen to keep the brain out of trouble. Enter focused monitoring …

Focused monitoring

Our goals in monitoring the patient under anesthesia are driven by two considerations:

(i) Are we ventilating the patient's lungs optimally and giving just the right amount of drugs and fluids? In other words, we monitor so that we can titrate our ministrations to a conceptual optimum.

(ii) Do the data we gather from the patient and the equipment indicate potential danger or trends that require our intervention? In other words, for safety's sake, we monitor variables that can indicate threatening problems, be they the consequence of anesthetic or surgical actions or based on the patient's disease.

Many signals we monitor subserve both titration and safety. For example, during anesthesia, we observe the patient's response to electrical stimulation of a motor nerve (the "twitch monitor") in order to *titrate* the administration of neuromuscular blocking drugs (muscle relaxants). At the end of anesthesia, we observe the same response in order to make sure that the patient has adequate muscle power to breathe without assistance – an important *safety concern*! Many, perhaps even most, other signals fall only into the safety category. For example, we typically monitor the ECG, oxygen saturation, and temperature for safety's sake, not for titration.

All monitoring builds on old-fashioned inspection, auscultation, and palpation. Indeed, instruments do not tell all, and at times may even fail. The clinician must still be able to assess the patient and the system without recourse to instruments. Rarely will the instruments alone make a diagnosis for you. More often than not, you will have to take into consideration facts not captured by instruments. First comes inspection.

Inspection

More than any other monitoring activity in the operating room, inspection must be practiced and honed. In anesthesia, the pattern of spontaneous breathing gives more important information than any other observation.

Spontaneous ventilation

During spontaneous breathing, the patient's chest should rise smoothly, with chest and abdomen moving in harmony. We speak of "rocking the boat" or paradoxical breathing when the abdomen rises during inspiration and the upper chest lags behind; opposite of what is normally observed, and a sign of respiratory impairment from upper airway obstruction, partial muscle paralysis, or pulmonary disease such as emphysema. The next glance should be directed at the larynx, which should be quiescent during breathing. With beginning respiratory insufficiency, the larynx moves downward a little with every inspiration, the so-called tracheal tug. The greater the respiratory impairment, the greater the laryngeal excursions with breathing, culminating in the agonal breathing pattern where larynx, floor of mouth, and tongue move with every

desperate inspiration. Particularly in children, flaring nostrils indicate respiratory weakness, often enough leading to respiratory failure when small children can no longer muster the effort to overcome weakness or obstruction.

The eyes

Don't forget to check the pupils. When the patient lies face-down or the surgeon works in the face, we must tape the eyes shut to guard against corneal abrasions. At other times, a look at the eyes can be helpful. During general anesthesia, the eyes should be still, the pupils constricted – or at least not dilated – and left should equal right (unless of course the patient has had cataract surgery in one eye). Light reflexes disappear under surgical anesthesia. Widely dilated pupils – if not the result of mydriatic drugs – indicate grave danger (the "open window to eternity"). The sclera may be injected under light anesthesia, as is also true for sleep. And while you are at it, take a look at the palpebral conjunctiva of the lower lid. The conjunctiva should be pink (not pale with anemia or bluish with hypoxemia or engorged by venous obstruction).

Head lift test

At the end of an anesthetic in which muscle relaxants were used, we make sure that the patient has the muscle power to maintain normal ventilation. While the nerve stimulator (see below) is helpful, a simple clinical test is even better: ask the patient to lift his head off the pillow and keep it up for 5 seconds. If he can do that, no more than 25% of his neuromuscular junctions remain blocked by muscle relaxants and you are reasonably assured that he will be able to maintain normal ventilation following extubation. When the operative site (neck, upper chest) makes a head lift test impossible, we assess not only the response to the nerve stimulator but also the pattern of breathing and SpO_2 relative to inspired oxygen.

Auscultation

Cool clinicians wear a stethoscope slung around their necks. Even cooler clinicians actually use the instrument to listen, for example, over the upper trachea: is air escaping at the end of mechanical inspiration? We welcome this sign in small children in whom we avoid compression of the tracheal mucosa with uncuffed endotracheal tubes. In adults we like to inflate the cuff of the endotracheal tube (ETT) so that a little gas will escape only when we exceed, by a few cmH_2O, the chosen peak inspiratory pressure. Inflating the cuff to a "minimal leak" pressure has two advantages. For one, it assures us that the cuff is not compressing the delicate, tracheal ciliated mucous membrane more than necessary. For another, it provides an emergency escape valve should excessive pressure build up in the breathing circuit. Though rare this has occurred when safety relief valves failed.

After intubation of the trachea, we listen over both lung fields for breath sounds and check the epigastrium to make sure that we are not delivering gas into the stomach during manual inspiration.

The lowly stethoscope (cheap, non-electronic, sturdy, time-honored) often makes diagnoses for us. Unless you are very clever with ultrasound, no electronic instrument identifies a pneumothorax. Enter the stethoscope and physical exam: breath sounds on one side and not the other, and chest rise more on one side than the other screams unilateral ventilation. It does not, however, scream "Insert chest tube now!", as this finding is also present with an overly aggressive ETT insertion that passes the carina. Withdrawing the tube a few centimeters is effective here. Also, consider a patient who becomes tachycardic, hypoxemic, and hypotensive, and assume that pneumothorax ranks high on your list of differential diagnoses. If breath sounds over the left chest equal those over the right and both sides of the chest move equally, a significant pneumothorax moves to the bottom of the differential diagnosis, and pulmonary embolism and cardiac tamponade move up. Don't abandon the stethoscope.

Remember to listen to heart sounds, either through the chest wall or with an esophageally placed stethoscope. With cardiovascular depression from deep anesthesia, the sounds become muffled. Cardiac tamponade will do the same. In either case, blood pressure will be low and heart rate high. Air embolism may cause the infamous mill wheel murmur produced by blood being beaten into foam in the heart. That is a late sign of air embolism, usually too late to be helpful. Therefore, when worried about the possibility of air embolism, we resort to more technical monitoring and watch the end-tidal CO_2 (it decreases with any kind of pulmonary embolism as loss of perfusion to a portion of the lung creates deadspace ventilation), and we monitor for air with a precordial Doppler instrument or with a transesophageal echocardiograph.

Palpation

How old-fashioned can you get? Putting a hand on the patient will give you all sorts of information. More than just the presence of a pulse, we may assess its quality. Is the patient warm, or cold and clammy? (The latter with sympathetic activity causing vasoconstriction and sweating.) Are his muscles fasciculating? (With shivering or after the administration of succinylcholine.) Put the palms of your hands on the clavicles, letting your fingers rest on the upper chest. Does the upper chest rise during spontaneous inspiration? (See above for "rocking the boat.") What is the muscle tone? In spontaneously breathing infants, the intercostal spaces should not retract during inspiration. Infants will also have flaccid fingers with muscle paralysis or deep anesthesia.

Instruments that supplement clinical monitoring

As we begin to focus on instruments to aid us in our monitoring task, we also need to ask for justification for their use. Does this monitor offer benefits that justify the cost (amortization of the instrument and cost of consumable supplies and, don't forget, time needed for application) and the potential hazards inherent with the use of the monitor? Several instruments have been identified as essential minimal monitors *always* to be used. With others, the clinician must decide whether a cost–benefit assessment justifies its use. Many monitors will be used routinely, others only with special indications. We must also point out that, over time, clinical practice changes with changing assessment of the value of this or that monitor.

The American Society of Anesthesiologists has published Minimal Monitoring Standards for patients undergoing general anesthesia.[1] In brief, these standards call for the monitoring of the patient's oxygenation (inspired gas and saturation of arterial blood [SpO_2]), ventilation (capnography and clinical assessment), circulation (ECG, arterial blood pressure), and temperature.

Non-invasive instruments

Some instruments put numbers on observations (feel a thready pulse and assume arterial hypotension; take a blood pressure and put numbers on the hypotension). Others provide information that our senses fail to detect (ECG and capnography, for example).

Blood pressure

The reference point for blood pressure recordings is the heart. An interactive simulation may clarify this.[1] In short, when upright your blood pressure just above the ankle will be much higher than in your upper arm – by the weight of the column of blood between ankle and heart.[2] Conversely, if you worry about cerebral perfusion pressure, remember that the pressure in the upper arm will be higher than that in the head if the patient stands or sits upright. Interestingly, while the mean blood pressure is affected by the column of blood between the heart and monitoring site, additional factors affect the actual peak (systolic) and trough (diastolic) readings. In a horizontal and recumbent patient, systolic pressure measured at the wrist exceeds that at the upper arm, and measurement at the ankle is higher still. How can blood flow toward a higher pressure? The pressure wave generated by the heart reflects off vascular bifurcations and arteriolar constrictions creating a "sloshing" much as children in a hot tub half-full of water can still create waves sufficiently high to spill over. Of course if the peaks of the waves lap at the lip of the tub, the troughs must be lower than the calm water line (mean). And so it is with arterial blood pressure as well. The systolic (peak) pressures rise as more reflected pressure waves are encountered, while the diastolic (trough) pressures decrease to a similar degree. Because energy is lost as blood moves forward, the MEAN pressure, the best measure of energy in the blood, decreases steadily from its left ventricular departure until it finally reaches the right atrium. You can monitor mean blood pressure in the upper or lower arm or just above the ankle (the best place if you have to use the lower extremity) and obtain reasonably accurate readings as long as the cuff is at the level of the heart (play with the interactive blood pressure cuff placement simulation[1]).

You should be able to take a blood pressure by cuff (with an integrated pressure manometer) and stethoscope listening for the Korotkoff sounds. You can also feel a pulse distal to the cuff and register systolic pressure when the distal pulse disappears. Instead of feeling the pulse, you can use a pulse oximeter probe placed distal to the cuff. Use it while inflating the cuff rather than during deflation. The pulse oximeter averages incoming data and thus takes a little time before reporting a signal, but it stops working rapidly when suddenly deprived of a pulsatile signal, as happens during inflation of the cuff. Disappearance of the waveform occurs at the systolic pressure.

The world (at least the Western world) has now taken to automatic electronic blood pressure devices that work as oscillometric sphygmomanometers. The concept is fairly simple. The unit inflates a cuff around the arm (or just above the ankle) and monitors the pressure in the cuff. Well above systolic pressure, the tight cuff transmits no pulsations to the unit. However, as the cuff pressure approaches systolic pressure, the pulsations of the artery begin to cause some oscillation of pressure in the cuff. When the cuff pressure falls just below systolic, the oscillations gain in amplitude, and the clever unit registers systolic pressure. Soon the cuff pressure drops to mean arterial pressure, at which point the oscillations reach their peak amplitude. You can imagine that now the oscillations become smaller and smaller and eventually disappear altogether as the cuff pressure drops to and below diastolic pressure. Identifying diastolic pressure presents the algorithm in the unit with the greatest challenge; hence diastolic pressures are more likely to be inaccurate, mean arterial pressure most likely to be accurate, and systolic pressure reasonably accurate. Oscillometric blood pressure recordings have become generally adopted in anesthesia where accuracy within ±10% is clinically quite acceptable. The measurements may become unreliable when arrhythmias, extremely slow heart rates, or a surgeon or tech leaning against the cuff on a tucked arm fools the algorithms that govern the systems.

Pulse and cerebral oximetry

An old saying goes: *The lack of oxygen not only stops the machinery, it wrecks it.* Hypoxia of the brain first causes confusion, then coma, and eventually irreversible brain damage. Other organs follow that pattern, even though most can survive hypoxia longer than the brain. Thus, knowing whether arterial blood carries oxygen to the organs assumes great importance. Because oxyhemoglobin is red and reduced hemoglobin bluish, this color difference can be exploited to assess the oxygenation of blood. Clinically, we recognize cyanosis, but we cannot well grade the degree of bluishness. In fact color alone equates poorly with saturation. The presence of at least 5 g/dL of deoxygenated "blue" blood is required for the color to be reliably seen by the unaided eye. Thus visible "cyanosis" means very different things in the anemic and polycythemic patient. An anemic patient with a hemoglobin of 8 g/dL would not develop visible cyanosis until his saturation approached 37.5% ([8−5]/8 × 100%), while a person with polycythemia and 20 g/dL of hemoglobin gets the blues at a saturation of 75%.

Enter pulse oximetry. The concept is what you might call "elegant." A probe sends light impulses into a finger, ideally one of the middle ones (or earlobe or nose or toe) and then collects the light that has passed through the tissue. The light comprises two wavelengths: one (infrared) more likely to be absorbed by oxyhemoglobin, the other (red) by reduced hemoglobin. By rapidly (too rapid for the eye to recognize) alternating the two wavelengths with no light at all, the unit is able to estimate the proportion of oxyhemoglobin to reduced hemoglobin. This is called "functional saturation." Some instruments include the other species of hemoglobin in blood (methemoglobin, carboxyhemoglobin) in their calculations and compare the oxyhemoglobin as a percentage of the sum of all known hemoglobins. This is called "fractional saturation," which will be a little lower than functional saturation.

We want to know the percentage of hemoglobin saturation with oxygen in arterial blood (rather than in the tissue or in arterial plus venous blood); therefore we need to catch the saturation reading in the artery, rather than in the whole finger. To accomplish this, the unit functions as a plethysmograph extrapolating only the light signal that varies (from arterial pulsation), and disregarding the rest of the signal (veins, fat, ambient lighting). The saturation is reported as SpO_2, the **p** referring to the fact that the measurement is based on pulse oximetry rather than on a direct *in-vitro* measurement of oxygen saturation from an **a**rterial blood sample, which would be SaO_2. A healthy person breathing room air at sea level (at least not at Mount Everest) should have an SpO_2 of about 98% ±2%. The device is remarkably accurate. Above an SpO_2 of 85%, the error is just ±2%, and increases only to ±3% for SpO_2 75–85%. With modern schools ending the practice of using medical students as research subjects, appropriate studies on volunteers induced to an SpO_2 below 75% are, not surprisingly, lacking. Here is a rough correlation of SpO_2 to arterial partial pressure of oxygen (PaO_2):

SpO_2	PaO_2
100%	100 mmHg or higher
90%	60 mmHg
60%	30 mmHg

In patients with normal lungs and nothing more than a small physiologic shunt (2–4%), the PaO_2 should be about 5 times the % oxygen. If it is substantially different, a shunt and/or hypercarbia likely exists. For your interacting pleasure there is a very nice web-based simulation that lets you manipulate the variables in the alveolar gas equation to demonstrate this point.[1]

As a plethysmograph, the pulse oximeter also reveals heart rate, rhythm, and a sense of pulse volume, which complements well our other monitors. Consider what we deduce from an ECG with a rate of 85 complexes per minute but a flat-line pulse oximeter. Presuming no technicalities (pulse ox probe disconnect, inflated cuff proximal to the probe), this defines pulseless electrical activity (PEA) and will be seen in dire situations of extreme hypovolemia, cardiac tamponade, tension pneumothorax, and severe electrolyte disturbances. A glance at the capnogram will show severely reduced $ETCO_2$ despite "adequate" ventilation. Only taken together do these monitors provide sufficient information for a definitive diagnosis.

There is also non-pulsatile oximetry; this oximetry bounces red and infrared light pulses off of tissue deep to the sensor, then analyzes the returning light. The most common application is over the forehead (cerebral oximetry) to gain insight into regional cerebral tissue oxygen saturation (RSO_2). By transilluminating the tissue (brain) several centimeters deep to the probe, we determine the saturation at the level of the venules, arterioles, and capillaries. This monitoring is of particular interest in cases where cardiac bypass is used and when treating severe brain injuries. A typical normal value is around 60% and we would be increasingly concerned if it decreased below 40%.

There is obviously much more to pulse and cerebral oximetry than outlined here. But we will not dwell on issues of other dyes interfering with the measurements, on the amount of pulsation required, on the influence of venous pulsation, or on the confounding effects of external light. For all of these issues we refer you to one of many exhaustive texts on monitoring or pulse oximetry.

The electrocardiogram

Intra-operative electrocardiography does not draw on the full power of this sophisticated monitor. Instead of 12 leads we usually settle for just three or five electrodes. With five electrodes we place green on the "gas pedal" (right leg, or at least south of the heart), red on the "stop pedal," "snow on the grass" (white to right shoulder over green), and "smoke over fire" (black to left shoulder over red). Add a brown electrode at the V5 position (over the fifth rib in the anterior axillary line) and we cover the heart nicely.

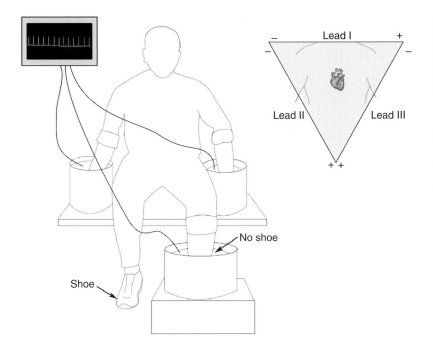

Shoe

No shoe

Lead I

−   +

Lead II   Lead III

+   +

Fig. 7.1 Einthoven's triangle. Willem Einthoven (1860–1927), the Nobel prize-winning Dutch physician and inventor, is best known for recording the electrocardiogram by using salt solutions to enable electrical conduction between the body and a recording galvanometer. The triangle is described by connecting three imaginary lines drawn between the arms and the left leg. The original device weighed over 500 pounds. Modern ones are obviously much smaller but rely on the same principle (the saltwater buckets have been replaced with conducting adhesive pads).

The electrical potential difference between any two electrodes represents an ECG "lead." The pair must have a positive and negative as defined by convention. Think of the positive lead as the exploring sensor (Fig. 7.1).

With the five-electrode ECG, the brown electrode serves as the exploring, positive electrode overlying the left ventricle; all the others become background. To detect myocardial ischemia, the precordial (V) leads are most useful, especially V3, V4, and V5. A precordial lead can be monitored even if you only have three electrodes. Simply choose a lead on the monitor, then take the positive lead from that configuration, e.g., the red electrode from lead II, and put it over the V3, V4, or V5 position. This yields a lead more sensitive for ischemia than any of the limb leads.

Many ECG monitors for the operating room offer a "monitoring mode," which is heavily filtered in order to reduce the artifacts induced by motion or electrical noise, e.g., the infamous electrocautery system. While the monitoring mode usually provides clean and stable tracings, the filtering can obscure diagnostic changes or it can mimic changes that will not be seen in a diagnostic 12-lead ECG. Thus, when observing ST segment depression in the monitoring mode, consider the clinical context and switch to diagnostic mode for confirmation before treating the patient. Similarly, when anesthetizing a patient at high risk for myocardial ischemia, use diagnostic mode and at least one precordial lead.

In the operating room we are primarily concerned with rhythm and ST segment elevation (impending infarct?) or depression (ischemia?). The best leads to detect such changes are leads II and V3–5. Lead II shows the best P waves and thus enables us to observe the cardiac rhythm, such as the nodal rhythm occasionally observed in the anesthetized patient. Cardiac output and arterial pressure fall a little when the ventricle is deprived of the 20% augmentation to filling provided by the "atrial kick." Leads V3–5 look at the left ventricle, the part of the myocardium most likely to suffer ischemia.

The ECG earns its keep in patients with heart disease and in the rare event of a cardiac arrest and resuscitation. When premature ventricular contractions arise in a patient who did not have them before, we are alerted and begin to search for an explanation. Hypercarbia is a common culprit. Think of ventricular hypoxia when ST segments begin to change (>1.5 mm ST depression or elevation; most ominous is a downward sloping, depressed ST segment), T waves flip, and particularly when the rhythm switches to ventricular tachycardia.

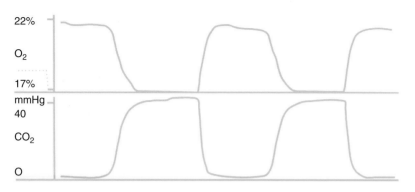

Fig. 7.2 Tracings from a gas monitor that show oxygen (top) and carbon dioxide (bottom) concentrations collected close to the mouth of a healthy volunteer breathing room air. As the person exhales, the oxygen concentration falls while carbon dioxide appears in the collected gas. During inhalation the oxygen analyzer registers room air (about 21% oxygen and no detectable carbon dioxide).

Monitoring respired gases

Capnography

The delivery of carbon dioxide to the lungs from the periphery depends first on the metabolic production of carbon dioxide. Capnography, therefore, says something about metabolism, which may be depressed by cold or fired up during hyperthermia. Capnography depends on blood flow to the lungs. It therefore says something about circulation, specifically regarding pulmonary blood flow. The delivery of carbon dioxide to the expired gas requires ventilation of alveoli and transport of alveolar gas to the outside. Capnography therefore says something about ventilation. Because the ambient air is free of carbon dioxide (well, not completely free with about 0.03% in air), the appearance of carbon dioxide in the inspired gas must mean that carbon dioxide is being added to the gas or that the patient is re-inhaling the carbon dioxide he just exhaled, for example from a breathing circuit with a defective valve that causes the deadspace in the circuit to increase. Thus, capnography, the measurement of carbon dioxide in the respired gas, really offers rich information that is easily acquired.

The respired gases can be sampled for analysis by aspirating gas from the breathing circuit – or from the nose of a non-intubated patient – and then delivering it to an analyzer. This is called "side-stream" sampling. We can also clamp an analyzing cuvette directly on the breathing tube so that all the respired gas passes through a system measuring the carbon dioxide, the so-called "on-airway" or "main stream" capnography. These methods use infrared spectroscopy to generate a continuous tracing of the changing carbon dioxide concentration in the respired gases. A capnogram results (Fig. 7.2).

If we wish only to detect the *presence* of carbon dioxide, as to document intubation of the trachea (as opposed to the esophagus) outside the operating room, the much less technology-dependent chemical method suffices. Though slow, the color change of a pH-sensitive indicator connected into the exhaled gas stream can display approximate ranges of carbon dioxide proving ventilation of the lungs is occurring. Recall, however, that lack of color change means only that no CO_2 is reaching the detector; you must determine whether this is from lack of pulmonary ventilation, or lack of pulmonary perfusion as in a cardiac arrest.

One clever method of analysis, the volume-based capnogram, plots carbon dioxide over the volume of gas exhaled (Fig. 7.3). It not only lets us estimate the end-tidal concentration of carbon dioxide but it also provides an estimate of deadspace.

Oxygen

When we connect a patient to an atmosphere other than room air, we assume full responsibility for the patient's oxygen supply. The patient might require only 21% oxygen at ambient pressure at sea level, or he might need much more, depending on clinical circumstances. Uncounted patients have died because that seemingly simple requirement was not met either because gases were mixed such that less than 21% oxygen was present in the inspired gas or because a gas other than oxygen came out of the cylinder or pipeline, as happens when cylinders are mis-filled or pipes delivering gases are switched by mistake. Monitoring oxygen in the inspired gas, therefore, has become mandatory when patients depend on us to prepare their respired gases.

Several methods are available. Ideally we would have a rapidly responding analyzer that generates "oxygrams" as shown in Figure 7.2. The technology for that relies on paramagnetic devices. Many current anesthesia machines incorporate a fairly slowly responding fuel cell. However, even an instrument with a response time of many seconds suffices.

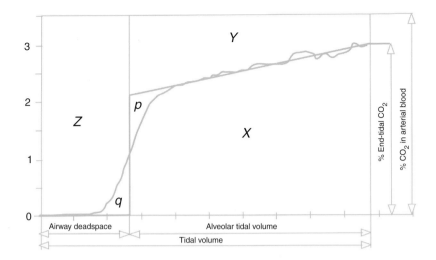

Fig. 7.3 Volume-based capnogram. Area Z (its top line is at the level of % CO_2 in arterial blood) represents the deadspace volume of the airway (V_D). Its right border is obtained by drawing a vertical line so that areas p and q are equal. X plus p represents the volume of exhaled carbon dioxide. Y represents wasted ventilation from alveolar deadspace.

Anesthetic gases

With side-stream gas monitors, it becomes possible to use the technology incorporated into capnography to analyze nitrous oxide and the halogenated inhalation anesthetics. The response time of these analyzers enables us to monitor both inspired and expired gas concentrations. We can thus watch what concentration the patient inhales in relation to what he exhales, and do so breath by breath. This frequently differs from the concentration set at the vaporizer which delivers gas to the breathing circuit, where the fresh gases are diluted by those the patient re-inhales (see Chapter 8).

Temperature

The body of an adult patient can absorb many calories before becoming noticeably warmer or, conversely, will cool only relatively slowly when losing heat by radiation (which accounts for most of the heat loss), evaporation (next in importance), convection, and conduction (least important).[3] However, monitoring the temperature, regardless of how slowly it changes, becomes important in babies and small children and in patients exposed to large heat losses as occurs with lengthy intra-abdominal or intrathoracic operations. In patients whose temperature drifts down to 35°C, wound infections may be more common. Other side effects of hypothermia include reduced enzyme activity, diminished blood clotting ability, and shivering (which increases oxygen consumption potentially contributing to myocardial ischemia), as well as patient discomfort.

Central blood in the pulmonary artery gives the most representative "core temperature." Tympanic membrane (really, these are ear canal thermometers), esophagus, bladder, nasopharynx, skin, and temporal artery offer other sites and have all but eliminated measurements made from the mouth and rectum. During endotracheal anesthesia, nasopharyngeal or esophageal temperatures can be measured easily with the help of a disposable thermocouple.

Skin temperature can be measured in the axilla and on the forehead. For the latter site, temperature-sensing adhesives are available that change color with changing temperature. Their accuracy is limited not only by the fact that ambient temperatures affect skin temperature but also because the temperature-sensitive liquid crystals do not offer good resolution. Temporal artery thermometry, where a scanner is touched to the forehead and pulled lightly across the skin overlying the temporal artery, has been shown to accurately measure core temperature and is steadily replacing other bedside thermometers.

Neuromuscular function

Because we use neuromuscular blocking agents (muscle relaxants, for short) so frequently, we need to monitor the degree of relaxation. Clinical judgment goes a long way, but instruments can gauge the degree of relaxation and provide numerical assessment. For this purpose, we use a nerve stimulator that delivers short pulses of a direct current. We use two electrodes placed fairly close together (Fig. 7.4) over the course of a nerve (usually the ulnar nerve near the wrist), and select one of several patterns of stimuli. Ideally the current is well below the level needed to stimulate the muscle

Table 7.1. Neuromuscular blockade monitor pattern descriptions

	Frequency	Pattern	Comments
Train of four (TOF)	2 Hz	Four twitches 0.5 s apart	Repeats every 12 s
Tetanus	50–100 Hz	For 5 s	Painful if awake
Post-tetanic stimulation	Single stimulus at 1 Hz		Follows a 5 s tetanus
Double burst	2 Hz	Three twitches, a 750 ms pause, followed by two more twitches	

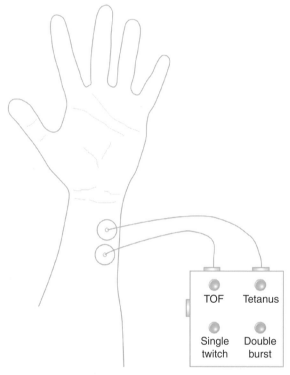

Fig. 7.4 Neuromuscular blockade (twitch) monitoring. Electrodes placed over the course of the ulnar nerve.

directly, as a healthy muscle will respond to strong, direct stimulation even in the presence of neuromuscular blocking agents. Thus, we are looking for maximal stimulation of the nerve only. Submaximal stimulation of the nerve can induce variability of response and thus make it impossible to tell whether an observed depression must be attributed to neuromuscular blockade or inadequate stimulation.

The most commonly used patterns of stimulation are shown in Table 7.1, with the typical patterns of response depicted in Figure 7.5. In addition to the response to nerve stimulation, we like to check the patient's muscle power if possible. Full return of muscle power can be assumed if the patient can lift his head off the pillow for 5 seconds, or bite on a tongue depressor so that you cannot withdraw it. If we suspect residual neuromuscular blockade in the PACU, we ask if the patient has double vision, or difficulty lifting his head, lifting an arm, squeezing a fist, or swallowing.

Doppler and ultrasound

The Doppler principle[4] has been applied to monitoring in anesthesia. We can place a Doppler pencil probe over a vessel to identify its location and blood flow or, with a broader emitter/receiver head, place it over the chest to detect the blood flow in the right atrium. When air appears in the blood flowing into the heart, it changes the reflective characteristics of the blood, transforming the Doppler signal into an easily recognized swooshing noise.

While ultrasound has been used for many years to spy on babies still in the womb and to view the functioning heart through the chest wall, more recently the equipment has been miniaturized into a finger-sized probe that views the heart from behind, through the wall of the esophagus (Fig. 7.6). This advance gives us a hands-free, relatively stable (and relatively non-invasive) view of the heart that does not impinge on the operative field. The technology continues to advance but currently allows views from multiple angles and Doppler analysis of flow (enabling estimation of pressures) across the cardiac valves for the experienced ultrasonographer. While invasive pressure monitoring offers indirect insights into cardiac physiology, with transesophageal echocardiography (TEE) we can actually *see* the heart doing its work. We can assess preload (how full is the left ventricle?), contractility (how much are the walls thickening?), and ischemia (are there sections of the ventricular walls that lag behind?). During cardiac surgery, we can evaluate valve repairs and septal defect closures. TEE is also a great way to detect air emboli and cardiac tamponade.

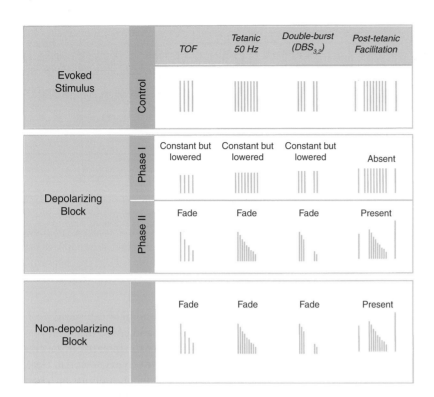

		TOF	Tetanic 50 Hz	Double-burst (DBS$_{3,2}$)	Post-tetanic Facilitation
Evoked Stimulus	Control				
Depolarizing Block	Phase I	Constant but lowered	Constant but lowered	Constant but lowered	Absent
	Phase II	Fade	Fade	Fade	Present
Non-depolarizing Block		Fade	Fade	Fade	Present

Fig. 7.5 Neuromuscular blockade monitor patterns. The figure shows the response we expect to see in a normal muscle before giving any muscle relaxants (control); after the administration of succinylcholine (Phase I), a depolarizing muscle relaxant which, after continued administration, assumes the pattern of a so-called Phase II block; and finally following the administration of a non-depolarizing muscle relaxant, resulting in a pattern resembling the Phase II block from succinylcholine. (Reproduced with permission from Kalli, I. S. in Kirby *et al. Clinical Anesthesia Practice*, W. B. Saunders, p. 446, 2002.)

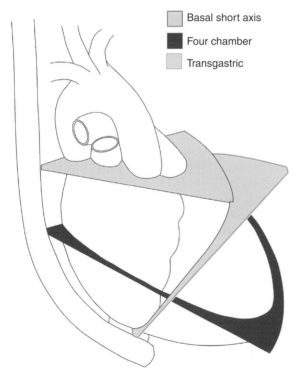

■ Basal short axis

■ Four chamber

■ Transgastric

Fig. 7.6 Transesophageal echocardiography (TEE). Standard planes through the heart. The probe is positioned for the transgastric view. By moving it we obtain the other two views.

This is probably the shortest description of a subject that has spawned uncounted papers, chapters, and books with exhaustive explanations. Studying them will introduce the reader to the complexities of the topic, but fairly intensive practice will be required to become facile with this increasingly popular monitoring modality.

The electroencephalogram and evoked responses

In anesthesia, we expend much more effort in monitoring the cardiovascular and respiratory systems than the nervous system; even though anesthesia is all about putting nervous function out of commission long enough to abolish awareness or at least the perception of pain. The reason for our bias against monitoring nervous activities is that we can afford to overdose the nervous functions and put them completely to rest as long as we continue to satisfy the basal needs for glucose and oxygen to brain and nerves. Hence, we worry more about the circulation than about the brain. However, when the systemic circulation is doing well but blood supply to all or parts of the central nervous system (brain and spinal cord) is threatened, we need to monitor

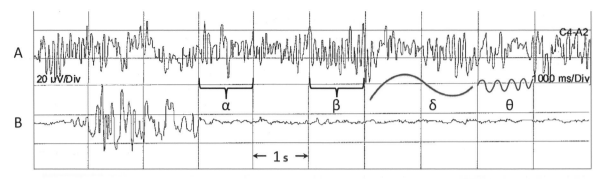

Fig. 7.7 (A) Electroencephalogram patterns comprise superimposed waves of delta (0–4 Hz), theta (4–7 Hz), alpha (8–13 Hz), beta (14–30 Hz), and gamma (above 30 Hz) frequencies.

(B) Burst suppression patterns exhibit spindles of activity among runs of isoelectric quiescence. When we induce burst suppression to decrease cerebral metabolism, we typically administer high doses of barbiturates and try to limit bursts to about 10% of total time (i.e., 90% burst suppression suffices and avoids dangerous cardiovascular side effects of even higher doses). Burst suppression resulting from hypoxic or ischemic hypoxia is never intentional.

their function. Two methods are available: the electroencephalogram and evoked responses.

The EEG as recorded by experts requires a montage with many electrodes. In anesthesia, that is not practical and in the operating room, you will rarely see more than a couple of leads plus a ground. The typical EEG of an awake individual shows rapid fire wiggles of low amplitude. With increasing depression of the central nervous system, the frequency of the wiggles decreases, and the amplitude increases. Before the EEG becomes flat, showing no electrical activity, it goes through a stage of burst suppression in which brief electrical activity alternates with longer periods of electrical silence. Figure 7.7 shows these typical patterns, which can be described by the frequency of their waves and the amplitude of their excursions.

The EEG can be processed to make interpretation more convenient. Several methods have been published. A commercial success has been the BIS® (bispectral index) monitor, which translates an automatic analysis of the EEG waveforms (obtained from forehead leads) into a unit-less number between 0 and 100 – the higher the number, the more awake the patient. In general, a BIS of 60 or less is associated – most of the time – with general anesthesia. However, even in physiologic (not pharmacologic) sleep, the BIS can dip well below 60. Thus, we still need to consider the context (drugs, surgical stimulation) in which we observe BIS values. It will have served us well if it helps us to avoid excessively deep anesthesia – which might be harmful – and all too light anesthesia – which carries the risk of intra-operative awareness. Anesthesia

that is neither too deep nor too light can speed postoperative recovery (wake-up and PACU time).

When we need to monitor the integrity of specific neuronal pathways, we use the evoked potential. Here, we apply a volley of either somatic, auditory, or transcranial stimuli. The system then automatically overlaps the EEGs (for afferent sensory stimulation) that immediately follow the stimuli. For example, with a sensory evoked potential there may be a tiny 1 microvolt response occurring about 10 ms after the stimulus. This response, however, is buried inside a 50 microvolt EEG squiggle. The summation technique allows the minuscule signal to grow to 1000 microvolts (1 mV) over 1000 summated stimulus–response cycles while all the random EEG produced by brain activity unrelated to the stimuli, like doing math, dreaming of vacation, or simply sleeping, adds progressively to zero. What results is an evoked potential response with characteristic hills and valleys that are described by their latencies and amplitudes of positive and negative deflections. Categorically, we can say that a central response to a peripheral stimulus signifies that the sensory pathways (mostly posterior spinal cord) between periphery and brain are conducting impulses and that the brain is capable of responding. Furthermore, peripheral muscle twitch responses to several hundred volt transcranial stimuli to the motor strip of the brain reassures us that the involved motor pathways (mostly anterior spinal cord) are also conducting and the brain is working. The responses are delayed or muted when the pathways have been affected or the brain depressed, for example by anesthetics, low blood pressure, or anemia. You can imagine that the monitoring of evoked responses can also be helpful when the integrity of the pathways is jeopardized by trauma or surgical manipulation, e.g., retraction, excision, or distraction.

Invasive monitors

Arterial catheter

The ease with which a small catheter can be inserted into an artery, usually the radial, has caused many patients to be monitored with arterial catheters (often called "lines" which is not an ideal term, as a line has no lumen, something arterial and venous catheters distinctly possess). Before inserting a catheter into a radial artery, some clinicians like to check the patency of the volar arterial arch that connects radial and ulnar arteries. In the so-called Allen's test, the hand is blanched, both arteries occluded by external pressure, then one occluded artery is freed. If now the entire hand, rather than the vascular bed of just one artery, turns pink, we accept the idea that the volar arch is patent and should one artery become obstructed by a clot or through damage to the intima, the other artery will prevent necrosis of fingers. Both the reliability and the necessity of pre-arterial catheter Allen's test have come into question.

For this and all other invasive pressure measurements, we use saline ± heparin-filled non-compressible (pressure) tubing connected to a transducer, which converts the pressure waveform into an electrical signal. We need to make sure that the instrument is properly calibrated and that the zero level (open to air) is at the level of the patient's heart. Two problems can cause the system to report faulty systolic and diastolic – but usually correct mean – pressures. When the signal is damped, for example owing to an air bubble somewhere in the tubing, the systolic pressure will read falsely low, and the diastolic pressure falsely high. When the system is not damped enough, it might ring (like a bouncing spring on a doorstop), now reporting falsely high systolic (and low diastolic) pressures (see Fig. 7.8).

Arterial catheters give ready access to arterial blood and thus to an analysis of blood gases and other chemistries. When drawing arterial blood for analysis, be sure you are not diluting the blood with the fluid in the system, that you remove any air bubbles from the syringe, and that you have the analysis performed without delay so that normal cellular metabolism does not affect the results.

Central venous catheter

Placement of a central venous catheter offers not only the ability to determine the central venous pressure but also a central avenue for infusion of potent medications and fluid (see Chapter 3). Because no valve separates the vena cava from the atrium, central venous pressure (CVP) reflects right atrial pressure. Similarly, when the tricuspid valve is open, and pressure has equalized between the atrium and ventricle (end-diastole), the CVP will also reflect right ventricular end-diastolic pressure (RVEDP). If we assume a normal ventricular compliance (pressure–volume relationship), we now have an indication of the end-diastolic volume or pre-load. However, because of its intrathoracic location, the central venous catheter also records pressures in the thorax as a whole, and thus, CVP fluctuates with ventilation. In a spontaneously breathing patient, normal pressures might range from –2 to +12 mmHg. If we then mechanically ventilate that patient's lungs, pressures of +6 to +15 mmHg (or more with high peak inspiratory pressures) can be expected – this without changing his intravascular volume and, in fact, likely *lowering* his preload as venous return is hampered by high intrathoracic pressure. The shape of the CVP waveform reflects the cardiac cycle (Fig. 7.9) and may suggest conditions that limit the extrapolation of pre-load from CVP, such as tricuspid valve disease or a poorly compliant ventricle. As with all monitors, when interpreting CVP data we must consider the clinical scenario and look more at trends in a given patient than the actual values.

Pulmonary artery (PA) catheter

Once the catheter is properly positioned, best in an area where the balance between blood flow and ventilation favors flow (below the level of the left atrium or zone III according to West),[5] the cuff can be gently inflated, blocking the vessel so that the tip of the catheter no longer senses PA pressure. Instead, it now looks downstream and registers pressures submitted retrograde from the left atrium. This PA occlusion or wedge pressure helps to identify situations affecting left ventricular preload. However, as with the CVP, many factors can influence the readings, e.g., mitral valve disease, pulmonary hypertension. Normal data appear in Table 7.2.

A number of refinements add utility to the PA catheter. For one, a thermistor at the tip of the catheter can record the temperature of the blood flowing past. After the injection of cold saline through a port situated in

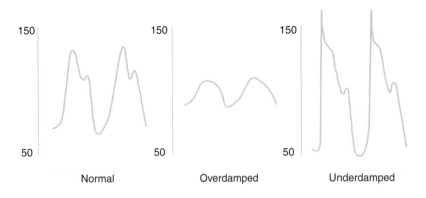

Fig. 7.8 Arterial pressure waveform patterns. Note the flattened peak of an overdamped waveform, often corrected by removing small bubbles in the pressure tubing and/or flushing the arterial catheter. In an underdamped waveform, an extreme peak introduces error in the systolic and diastolic data.

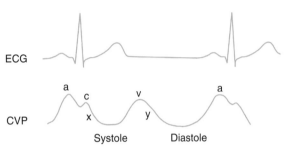

Fig. 7.9 Central venous pressure waveform. The *a* wave is from atrial contraction, *c* from closure of the tricuspid valve and ventricular contraction; *v* from venous filling of the atrium. The *x* descent represents relaxation of the atrium with downward movement of the tricuspid valve and the *y* descent is the emptying of the atrium when the tricuspid valve opens.

Table 7.2. Normal pulmonary artery catheter pressure data

Location	mmHg
Right atrium	5–12
Right ventricle	25/5
Pulmonary artery	25/10
Pulmonary artery occlusion or wedge pressure	8–12

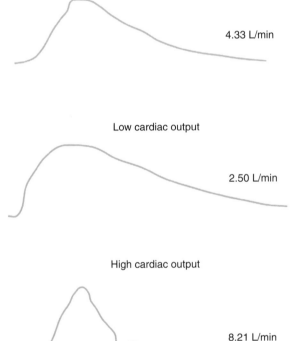

Fig. 7.10 Thermodilution cardiac output curves.

the vena cava, the observed temperature changes at the tip of the catheter make it possible to estimate the cardiac output. When the output is low, blood will flow slowly past the thermistor, and a large temperature change (thermodilution) curve will result. Conversely, with a large cardiac output, the thermodilution curve will be small (Fig. 7.10).

We can also monitor the oxygen saturation of mixed venous blood either intermittently by drawing samples for the laboratory, or continuously by incorporating an oximeter in the catheter. When oxygen content of arterial blood and oxygen consumption are constant, a drop in venous oxygen saturation indicates a decrease in tissue blood flow (cardiac output) or O_2 delivery (e.g., anemia).

PA catheters have come under much criticism because they may not reveal as much as originally hoped for, and they are highly invasive and saddled with a measurable rate of sometimes life-threatening complications including but not limited to dysrhythmias, thrombosis, infection, and devastating pulmonary artery rupture. Much less invasively, transesophageal

Table 7.3. Monitoring in anesthesia

	Qualities measured	Pros	Cons
Cardiac			
Palpation	Pulse rate, rhythm and quality; thrill; point of maximal impulse	Inexpensive, non-invasive	
Auscultation	Rate, rhythm, S3, S4, murmur, air embolism	Inexpensive, non-invasive	
Non-invasive blood pressure	Blood pressure	Non-invasive	May have a problem with arrhythmias
ECG	Rate, rhythm, ischemia	Non-invasive	Non-specific
TEE	Structure, function, volume, ischemia	Few confounding factors	Expensive, requires expertise, uncomfortable for the awake patient, no alarm capability
Arterial catheter	Blood pressure, arterial blood gases	Beat-to-beat blood pressure, easy access to arterial blood, low risk	Invasive
Central venous catheter	Preload	High volume catheter useful for resuscitation	Invasive
Pulmonary artery catheter	Preload, cardiac output, right heart pressures, mixed venous oxygen saturation	Gold standard for cardiac output, availability of mixed venous O_2	Invasive, significant rate of potentially severe complications, expensive
Pulmonary			
Auscultation	Breath sounds	Inexpensive, non-invasive	
Pulse oximetry	Hemoglobin saturation, heart rate	Continuous, inexpensive, non-invasive	Inaccurate with carbon monoxide, severe anemia
Capnography	Inhaled and exhaled carbon dioxide	Gold standard to document tracheal position of ETT, continuous	Not quantitative unless intubated
Arterial blood gas	Oxygenation, ventilation, acid–base status	Accurate measure, multiple parameters	Invasive, highly intermittent
Neurologic			
Twitch monitor	Neuromuscular blockade	Inexpensive	Insensitive unless at least 70% of receptors blocked
Processed EEG (BIS)	"Depth of anesthesia"	Non-invasive	Not always a leading indicator of light anesthesia
Evoked potentials	Specific neuronal pathways	Relatively specific for the pathway investigated	Expensive, requires technical expertise for interpretation, affected by many anesthetic agents

echocardiography offers a great advantage over the PA catheter. PA catheters generate pressure and flow data; TEE shows volumes and function of all four chambers and valves.

Thus we have many monitors at our disposal (Table 7.3), with new ones arriving regularly. Each has strengths, weaknesses, risks, and potential benefits. No monitor is therapeutic in itself but requires the skill and vigilance of a trained observer to interpret the information in the context of the ever-changing clinical picture.

Notes

1   www.anest.ufl.edu/EA.

2   The conversion from cmH$_2$O (or blood) to mmHg is 1.0 cmH$_2$O = 0.7 mmHg. So for each rise of 10 cm of the heart over the monitored location, the pressure will increase by 7 mmHg.

3   Radiation: loss of heat to the atmosphere; evaporation: loss of heat as fluids absorbed from surface (airway, exposed viscus); convection: loss of heat to a cold air mass moving across the body; conduction: transfer of heat to a colder object in direct contact (OR table).

4   Eponymous for the Austrian mathematician and physicist Christian Doppler who proposed the phenomenon in 1842, not from observations of train whistles barreling past, but in an effort to explain the colors of binary stars. We take advantage of his discovery in analyzing the speed of blood in the heart, submarines in the ocean, weather patterns overhead, and galaxies much further overhead.

5   John B. West (1928–) described ventilation and perfusion inequality in the lung, and wrote a very nice and readable textbook reviewing the concepts. *Respiratory Physiology: The Essentials*, 8th edn, 2008.

Clinical management

The anesthesia machine

As anesthetic agents and techniques have evolved, so have the delivery systems. Modern anesthesia requires the ability to administer gases and vapors in the desired combinations, often while mechanically ventilating the patient's lungs. Here we present step-by-step the concepts on which anesthesia machines are based. We start with systems that sport neither valves nor means to store gases, advance to systems that can store gases – which requires a couple of valves – and then advance still further to systems in which the patient rebreathes his exhaled gas, but without the previously exhaled carbon dioxide. Thus, we will have set the stage for the modern anesthesia machine. A nice interactive computerized diagram can be found at www.anest.ufl.edu/EA.

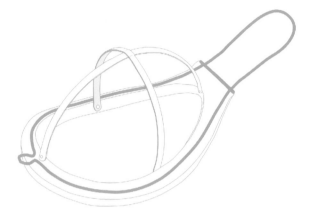

Fig. 8.1 A Schimmelbusch mask; used to keep gauze off the patient's face while administering open drop ether anesthesia. (Named for Curt Schimmelbusch [1860–1895], a German surgeon.)

Systems without gas storage

If we have to give anesthesia at the North Pole (in a comfortable, if barren, igloo), and we have nothing but a can of diethyl ether, we can give a fine anesthetic by dripping the ether on a cloth held over the patient's mouth. That will work also with halothane and sevoflurane. Early anesthetists used masks (Fig. 8.1) on which to drape the cloth.

Back from the North Pole, assume we have a patient who weighs 70 kg, has a tidal volume of 500 mL, a respiratory rate of 10 breaths/min, and an I:E (inspiratory to expiratory) ratio of 1:2; that is, he spends twice as much time exhaling (and pausing between breaths) as inhaling. Assume his trachea to be intubated. All his respired gases flow through the tubing connecting his endotracheal tube to the source of oxygen (Fig. 8.2). We wish to provide his lungs with 100% oxygen. To achieve this, his exhaled gas needs to be vented through a T near the mouth. This T will also allow him to pull in room air during inspiration, diluting his FiO_2. What oxygen flow rate will prevent such entrainment of room air? The easy answer: the oxygen flow rate must match his inspiratory flow rate (which, by the way, is not constant). The total amount of oxygen the system must

deliver then will equal his minute ventilation of 5000 mL, but this volume must be given over only one-third of a minute (with an I:E of 1:2). The technology for such an arrangement, i.e., to flow oxygen only during inspiration, exists in ICU ventilators. In anesthesia machines, we instead have continuous gas flow throughout the respiratory cycle. In the example above, during exhalation the continuing oxygen flow has nowhere to go but to escape, together with the patient's exhaled gas, to the atmosphere. We still must meet his inspiratory flow demand, delivering his minute volume during inspiration (in one-third of a minute), and we would lose all of the oxygen (two-thirds of the total) flowing during expiration. Thus, using this simple system in a patient with a typical I:E ratio of 1:2, we would need a fresh gas flow at least three times as large as his minute volume.

Single-valve system with gas storage

In order to save gas, we can provide for storage of the gas. Well known is the Mapleson system,[1] often used during resuscitation and during transport of a patient who requires mechanical ventilation. The system shown in Figure 8.3 is properly called a Mapleson

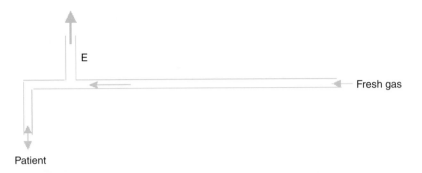

Fig. 8.2 The simplest arrangement of delivering gas to the patient. Fresh gas flows throughout the respiratory cycle. If its flow matches the patient's inspiratory gas flow, the patient will not inhale room air through the T of the expiratory limb (E); however, the fresh gas flowing throughout exhalation will be lost to the atmosphere.

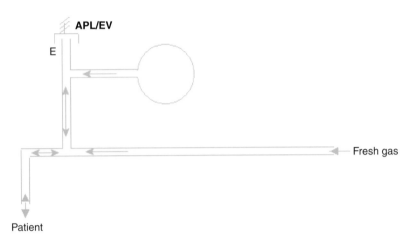

Fig. 8.3 The arrangement of Fig. 8.2 has been expanded to include an adjustable one-way valve (APL: adjustable pressure-limiting; EV: expiratory valve) that, when open, lets the patient exhale to the outside and, when partially closed, enables the anesthesiologist to generate pressure by squeezing the bag and thus inflating the patient's lungs while spilling some gas to the outside. Depending on the fresh gas flow, more or less of the patient's carbon dioxide will be vented to the outside. In other words, with inadequate fresh gas flow, the patient will re-inhale some or much of his exhaled carbon dioxide. E: expiratory limb.

D (as there are different arrangements lettered A through F).

Figure 8.4 shows the real thing. It is light and deceptively simple. To prevent rebreathing of exhaled carbon dioxide requires a relatively high fresh gas flow, both to meet inspiratory demand and to wash exhaled CO_2 out of the tubing. Here, the excess gas escapes through an adjustable one-way (pop-off) valve that prevents entrainment of room air. The pressure required to open the spring-loaded valve can be varied, enabling us to generate enough pressure (by squeezing the bag) to inflate the patient's lungs. Slow respiratory rates help because, during a long pause between inspirations, the fresh gas will push the exhaled gas toward the pop-off valve. During spontaneous ventilation, the fresh gas flow should be as high as 200–300 mL/kg/min; for our patient, that would be 14–21 L/min. With manually controlled ventilation, 100–200 mL/kg/min will do. We will occasionally observe lower flow rates in clinical usage, causing unintended rebreathing of carbon dioxide. To be sure, err on the high side – which wastes a little gas (but oxygen is cheap) and has no disadvantage to the patient – rather than on the low side, which

causes rebreathing of carbon dioxide, the very problem patients in respiratory distress should be spared. Keep in mind, however, that running out of oxygen during transport, especially when using a Mapleson system, which depends on a pressurized gas source, may be disastrous. When transporting a patient we note carefully the volume of gas in the tank: an E-cylinder (normal transport size) contains nearly 700 L of oxygen when full (pressure = ~2000 psi). This decreases linearly with oxygen usage.

Multi-valve system with gas storage

A self-inflating bag provides an alternative that enables the resuscitator to ventilate the patient's lungs with room air or, if oxygen is available, with air enriched with oxygen. For the latter to succeed, the self-inflating bag must have a reservoir in which oxygen can accumulate during inspiration (see Fig. 8.5). An interactive version of this is available at www.anest.ufl.edu/EA. In Figure 8.6 we add this inspiratory valve to our circuit from Figure 8.3, fresh gas accumulates in the bag during exhalation when the inspiratory valve closes and the expiratory valve opens (venting CO_2-laden gas to

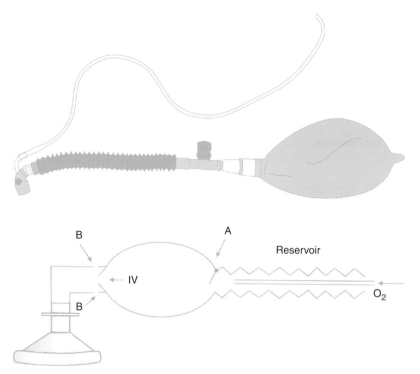

Fig. 8.4 Line drawing of a Mapleson system. The Mapleson (D) system finds extensive use in anesthesia. While simple, the system requires a source of compressed oxygen. See text.

Fig. 8.5 The self-inflating bag. Conceptual diagram of a self-inflating resuscitation bag that prevents rebreathing of exhaled gas but enables the clinician to ventilate the patient's lungs either with room air or with oxygen delivered into a reservoir. B denotes the exhalation ports, which become occluded during inspiration when the inspiratory valve (IV) opens. The one-way valve, A, closes when the bag is squeezed, forcing gas toward the face mask during inspiration. The valve opens as the bag re-expands, allowing oxygen-rich reservoir gas to fill the breathing bag (if using the system without an oxygen source, the reservoir gas will consist of room air).

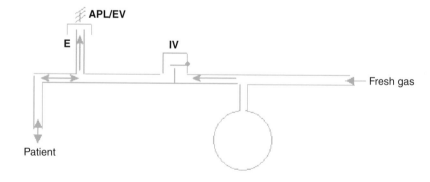

Fig. 8.6 After adding another one-way valve to Fig. 8.3, and moving the bag, we arrive at a system that reduces the required fresh gas flow to that of the patient's minute ventilation. During exhalation, the inspiratory valve (IV) closes, enabling the continuously flowing fresh gas to accumulate in the breathing bag. E: expiratory limb; APL: adjustable pressure-limiting valve; EV: expiratory valve.

the atmosphere). During inspiration the valves swap roles: the inspiratory valve opens and the expiratory one closes. Such valves have little resistance, perhaps 1 or 2 cmH$_2$O, and thus will easily open during the respiratory cycle. This also works for a patient breathing spontaneously as long as the mask is snugly enough applied so that the patient can generate the negative pressure required to open the inspiratory valve.

Systems with carbon dioxide absorption

In anesthesia, because of the cost (and ozone-depleting qualities) of volatile anesthetic agents, we prefer to conserve even more gas. Furthermore, the patient does not consume all inhaled oxygen (at rest, a patient consumes only a small portion of the inhaled oxygen,

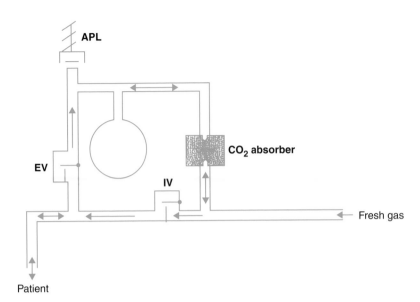

Fig. 8.7 A circle system has been formed by tapping into the expiratory limb to attach the reservoir bag so that it can collect exhaled gas. During inspiration, the gas will now be drawn out of the reservoir bag, pass through the carbon dioxide absorber, and then join the fresh gas. For abbreviations see Fig. 8.6.

reducing the FiO_2 of 0.21 to an FeO_2 of 0.17). Thus, we save a lot if we do nothing more than replace the oxygen the patient consumes (for the average adult at rest – 3.5 mL/kg/min or about 250–300 mL/min). We need to remove the carbon dioxide, of which our resting patient generates almost as much (depending on his respiratory quotient) as he consumes oxygen. Figure 8.7 shows the arrangement. We simply formed a circle (conceptually, if not diagrammatically) by connecting the expiratory and inspiratory limbs. The two valves in the circle assure a one-way flow of gases in the circuit. We still have the adjustable pressure-limiting (APL) valve and the breathing bag, but we have incorporated a carbon dioxide absorber. Now we can reduce the inflow of oxygen (and anesthetic gases) into the circle quite drastically. In point of fact we could literally reduce the oxygen inflow to match the amount of oxygen consumed, i.e., 250–300 mL/min (plus whatever leaks out or is pulled into a gas analyzer).

With this circle system, we have the basic anesthesia machine. Now, all we need to add are flow meters for other gases (nitrous oxide, air) and vaporizers that let us introduce anesthetic vapor to the fresh gas flowing into the breathing system. We also have the option of switching on a mechanical ventilator.

Using a handy diagram of a modern anesthesia machine (Fig. 8.8), we point out several features. The system receives compressed gases from the hospital's gas supply; it has a back-up gas supply stored in cylinders; it reduces the high pressure in the cylinders and pipeline to manageable levels in the machine; it

has adjustable vaporizers for halogenated anesthetics (isoflurane, desflurane, and sevoflurane – but permits only one agent to be administered at a time); and it funnels the anesthetic-laden fresh gas into the breathing circuit, which has a carbon dioxide absorber. The system makes it possible for the patient to breathe spontaneously with a breathing bag reservoir, which can be compressed by hand if necessary, to manually ventilate the patient's lungs. While all systems have mechanical ventilators, the design of these differs markedly among manufacturers of anesthesia machines.

The hospital system also provides suction that is put to work removing waste gases. Such scavenging keeps the air in the operating room virtually free of anesthetic agents presumed to present a hazard to personnel, particularly pregnant women. Collectively, only minuscule amounts of gas leak out around the face mask or from the breathing system during induction/intubation, from gas vented into the room if high fresh gas flows exceed scavenging vacuum capacity, and from the patient's breath after extubation. Modern ORs successfully limit waste gas concentrations to below the 25 parts per million (ppm) for N_2O and the 2 ppm for halogenated agents considered safe for OR personnel by the National Institute for Occupational Health and Safety.

Modern anesthesia machines have a bevy of safety features:

- All gas hoses have connectors specific to the gas, preventing plugging the machine's oxygen supply hose into the hospital supply of another

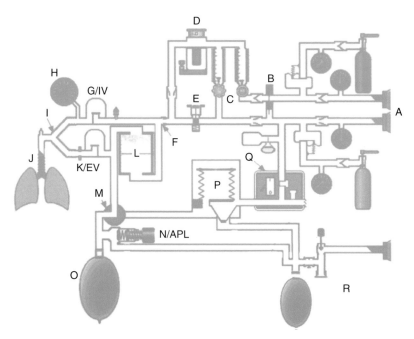

Fig. 8.8 Diagram of a traditional anesthesia machine. To view this diagram as a helpful computer animation, and for explanation and operating instruction, please check: www.anest.ufl.edu/EA. A: The gases enter the anesthesia machine either from hospital piping or from cylinders attached to the anesthesia machine (nitrous oxide on top, oxygen below); B: the so-called fail-safe system that stops the flow of nitrous oxide should the pressure in the oxygen pipe drop; C: the flow meters with which to set the flow rates for gases – here only oxygen and nitrous oxide. On many machines, there will be a flow meter for air and sometimes even one for heliox; D: the vaporizer. Many machines carry more than one vaporizer but they are always arranged so that we can use only one at a time; E: the oxygen flush button, which admits a high flow of oxygen under pressure to the system. If pressed during the ventilator's inspiratory phase, excessive pressure can build up in the breathing system with the potential for causing barotrauma to the patient's lungs; F: fresh gas inlet to the breathing circuit; G/IV: the inspiratory one-way valve; H: manometer registering the pressure in the breathing circuit; I: the "Y" piece, named after its shape. It connects the breathing circle to the patient; J: trachea and lungs of the patient; K/EV: the expiratory one-way valve. As long as this and the inspiratory valve function properly, the breathing circle imposes no significant apparatus deadspace, extending only into the "Y" piece; L: the carbon dioxide absorber; M: the selector valve, which funnels the gas either into the breathing bag – as shown here – or to the ventilator; N/APL: the "pop-off" or APL (adjustable pressure-limiting) valve enables gas to escape when the pressure in the breathing circuit exceeds a selected value; O: breathing bag; P: ventilator bellows; Q: ventilator controls; R: scavenging system.

gas. It does not guarantee, however, that oxygen comes out of the oxygen pipeline should the pipes have been switched during hospital construction or repairs, an occurrence unfortunately not all that rare and why all anesthesia machines have an oxygen analyzer with an audible low oxygen alarm.

- One-way valves prevent gas from flowing from the accessory gas cylinders into the anesthesia machine as long as the system is connected to the pipeline. The pipeline pressure exceeds the reduced cylinder pressure. This arrangement prevents drainage of the cylinders while the machine is connected to the wall supply. This also means that one has to disconnect the machine from the wall should it become necessary to use gas from the cylinders.

- A safety valve closes the flow of nitrous oxide should the pressure in the oxygen conduit drop below a critical level. This so-called *fail-safe valve* makes it impossible to give nitrous oxide without oxygen, hopefully preventing a hypoxic mixture.
- A back-up to the fail-safe valve is the linkage between nitrous oxide and oxygen, which prevents the delivery of less than 25% oxygen.
- The gases in the breathing system are monitored and their concentration displayed.

Anesthesia breathing circuits have come a long way since the open-drop ether days; however, with increased sophistication also comes a need for heightened awareness. These systems, if improperly used, e.g., inadequate fresh gas flow, inappropriately tightened APL valve, faulty expiratory valve, incorrect setting of the ventilator, undiscovered disconnection, can and do cause significant injury. Because of these many potential dangers, we monitor gas flows and pressures in the breathing circle, tidal and minute volumes, inspired oxygen, inhaled and exhaled carbon dioxide, and anesthetic agent concentrations. These variables come with alarms that sound at adjustable thresholds.

Note

1   His department head at the University of Wales assigned William Wellesley Mapleson (1926–) to study gas flows through five existing breathing systems in 1954. Mapleson was surprised to later hear his name attached to the alphabetic labels he had conjured up.

Section 2

Applied physiology and pharmacology

Chapter

9

Anesthesia and the cardiovascular system

Surgical procedures and anesthesia confront the cardiovascular system with a triple threat: trauma, blood loss, and depressant drugs. Trauma triggers a cascade of hormones; if that were not enough, the surgeon might constrict the vena cava, compress the heart or a lung, trigger reflexes, and handle the gut, causing sequestration of fluid in traumatized tissue. Exposed pleural and peritoneal lining lets water evaporate, not to mention blood loss and the potential for small clots. To this onslaught, anesthesia adds depressant drugs, induces ventilation/perfusion mismatches with mechanical ventilation (which turns respiratory mechanics upside-down by imposing positive pressure during inhalation), and then infuses cold solutions that are never quite the same as the real thing. Aware of all of these factors, the anesthesiologist appreciates the stresses imposed on the patient and does his or her best to keep the system as close as possible to "how Mother Nature intended it." To that end, we must have a firm grasp of physiology. Let's start with the most visible outward sign of the cardiovascular system: blood pressure.

Blood pressure and its determinants

To understand how surgery and anesthesia affect blood pressure, we must consider its basic components (Fig. 9.1). First, *afterload*, the combination of all resistances against which the heart must eject. Its aliases include systemic vascular resistance (SVR) and total peripheral resistance (TPR). This parameter cannot be measured, but rather is calculated based on the relationship of pressure to flow:[1]

$$ SVR = \frac{(MAP - CVP)}{CO} \times 80 $$

where MAP = mean arterial pressure, CVP = central venous pressure, and CO = cardiac output.

The vasomotor center influences the diameter of peripheral vessels through sympathetic α_1 innervation. SVR, then, changes with anything that affects the vasomotor center (the baroreflex [see below], anesthetics),

the sympathetic chain (neuraxial[epidural or spinal] anesthesia), α_1 receptors (catecholamines, vasopressors), or smooth muscle of the vessel wall directly (histamine, anesthetic agents, nitric oxide).

Cardiac output, the other determinant of blood pressure, depends on heart rate and stroke volume. *Heart rate* is somewhat more complex than it may first seem, with both sympathetic (β_1) and parasympathetic innervation "battling it out" for supremacy. Here the baroreflex exerts its influence, as well as the majority of pharmacologic agents we use to manipulate the heart rate.

For *stroke volume*, there are multiple factors in play, beginning with *Starling's law of the heart*[2] (Fig. 9.2). Basically, it states that the heart tends to pump out all the blood it receives, in essence maintaining the same end-systolic volume. Note the normally sloped Starling curve: stroke volume increases directly with the filling volume (measured as left ventricular end-diastolic pressure [LVEDP], central venous pressure [CVP], or pulmonary artery occlusion pressure [PAOP]). Think of the actin and myosin filaments having an optimal overlap. With little ventricular volume, they are completely overlapped and can generate little pressure. Similarly, at some point they become over-stretched, beyond their optimal overlap, causing a reduction in force, represented by the flat or downward sloping portion at the right-most end of the curve. Notice the flatness of the heart failure curve; increasing preload does not really help these patients. From the Starling curve we see that, if a patient becomes hypotensive but has an abnormally *high* CVP, something must be wrong with the ejection of the blood – either systolic dysfunction, perhaps from ischemia, or diastolic dysfunction from ischemia, left ventricular hypertrophy, or some other cause like tricuspid insufficiency.

Starling's law is in evidence when anesthetics cause venodilation, either directly or through inhibition of the sympathetic nervous system (there are α_1 receptors on the venous side). This increased *venous capacity*

95

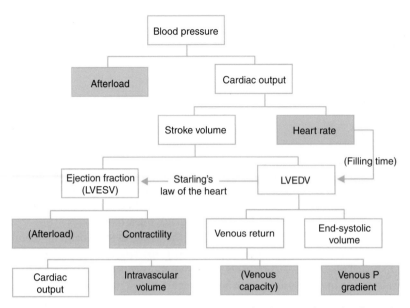

Fig. 9.1 Determinants of blood pressure. Each successive level gives its dependent factors (e.g., blood pressure depends on cardiac output and afterload). For all but the parameters in parentheses, the relationship is direct; for example, increasing afterload *increases* blood pressure but *decreases* ejection fraction. Some interrelationships are identified (e.g., as heart rate increases, it adversely affects filling time [shortened diastole], lowering the LVEDV). The flowchart can be helpful in recognizing the effects of pathologic changes. For example, hemorrhage (decreased intravascular volume on the bottom row, and following the chart toward the top) decreases venous return, LVEDV, stroke volume, cardiac output, and blood pressure. We can improve the blood pressure through any of the independent parameters (shaded): increase after-load (α_1 or vasopressin), heart rate (β_1), contractility (β_1 or phosphodiesterase inhibitor), intravascular volume, venous pressure gradient (e.g., Trendelenburg's position), and/or *reduce* venous capacity (α_1 or vasopressin). In fact, the baroreflex and Starling's forces start working on all this even before we intervene. LVEDV: left ventricular end-diastolic volume; LVESV: left ventricular end-systolic volume; venous P gradient: venous pressure gradient from distal to proximal – a larger gradient encourages more blood return to the heart.

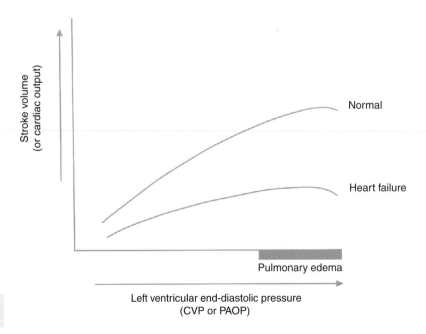

Fig. 9.2 The Starling curve. Demonstrating the Frank–Starling law of the heart: the heart ejects what it receives. Thus stroke volume increases with filling pressure. In heart failure the relationship shifts downward – increased ventricular filling fails to increase stroke volume and the high filling pressure eventually causes pulmonary edema. CVP: central venous pressure; PAOP: pulmonary artery occlusion pressure.

causes peripheral pooling of blood away from the heart and reduces the venous pressure that ordinarily pushes blood back toward the right atrium. Functionally, this results in a reduced preload, limiting the stroke volume via Starling's law of the heart. Thus, managing anesthesia-induced hypotension with intravenous fluids or an alpha agonist like phenylephrine makes a lot of sense. The specific approach weighs the subsequent need to mobilize excess fluids once the anesthetic effects are removed against the potential for renal perfusion problems and kidney injury from pressors.

Remember that Starling's law is "length-dependent shortening" of heart muscle fibers and should not be confused with the energy-consuming *contractility* (although it is often difficult to distinguish these). For a given filling pressure, increasing contractility will shift the Starling curve upward, resulting in increased stroke volume (decreased end-systolic volume). Such a shift can be achieved via β_1 receptors, either endogenously through the sympathetic nervous system and/or the baroreflex, or pharmacologically with many agents. Some anesthetics (particularly the volatile agents) are direct myocardial depressants and will cause a dose-dependent downward shift and flattening of the Starling curve. Thus, not only is there less central blood volume due to venodilation, more is required to achieve the same stroke volume.

The other factor beneath ejection fraction in the blood pressure determinant diagram (Fig. 9.1.) is "*Afterload*" surrounded by the parentheses. Its effect here is actually the inverse. While increasing afterload directly raises blood pressure, increasing afterload reduces stroke volume by closing the aortic valve earlier in the ejection process. This partially explains why afterload reduction, e.g., via angiotensin-converting enzyme (ACE) inhibitors, benefits the patient in cardiac failure. A failing heart can eject blood more readily into a low-resistance circuit.

Other basic physical concepts to understand when thinking about the cardiovascular system include the following:

- *Compliance.* The change in pressure resulting from a change in volume ($\Delta V/\Delta P$). As blood flows into a vessel, the highly compliant veins will gladly dilate to accommodate the volume, while the less compliant arteries dilate less, resulting in a great increase in pressure. In many ways, compliance and resistance are simply the inverse of each other.

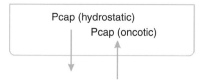

Fig. 9.3 Starling's forces. Hydrostatic pressure is exerted by fluid, while proteins that cannot cross the vessel wall generate oncotic pressure. These forces exist on both sides of the vessel wall, but under physiologic conditions the intracapillary oncotic forces dominate over those exerted by the interstitium.

- *Starling's forces.* Not to be confused with his law of the heart (Dr. Starling, 1866–1927, was a busy man!). No vessel wall is entirely impermeable. Two main forces push and pull fluids across membranes (see Fig. 9.3). On the arterial end of a vascular bed, the hydrostatic pressure on the luminal side of a capillary pushes fluid through the wall, while on the venous side, oncotic pressure (one could almost better call it the oncotic vacuum) of the intravascular proteins pulls fluids back into the vessel. You can readily imagine how increased capillary pressure and decreased oncotic pressure (low albumin) lead to the accumulation of fluids outside the capillary, i.e., edema.

So, putting it all together, the right atrium/ventricle receives oxygen-poor blood from the periphery and pumps it through the low-resistance vascular bed of the lungs for a swap of carbon dioxide for oxygen. Meanwhile, the left atrium and ventricle stand by to receive the oxygenated blood and pump it on its way to the periphery. Upon taking leave of the heart, the blood travels through the aorta and peripheral arteries. The speed with which it is propelled forward depends not only on the cardiac output but also on the character of the arterial vessels. If hard and inelastic (an old aorta can have poor compliance; atheromatous vessels in the periphery offer high resistance), the stroke volume from a cardiac contraction will cause a substantial increase in pressure.

The venous side represents a quintessential low-resistance bed. It accommodates large volumes of fluid with little rise in pressure, at least up to a point. A number of factors can increase the pressure and decrease flow in the vena cava: the surgeon with a hand in the abdomen, the uterus with a baby inside, the ventilator running up a high peak inspiratory and, consequently, intrathoracic pressure, the patient performing a Valsalva maneuver, the abdomen insufflated with gas

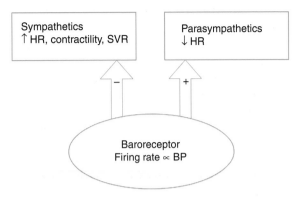

Fig. 9.4 Baroreflex. The baroreceptor in the carotid sinus fires in proportion to the blood pressure (more rapid with hypertension, slower with hypotension). Knowing the expected response (tachycardia with hypotension and vice versa), we recognize the baroreceptor must inhibit the sympathetics (less inhibition during hypotension) and stimulate the parasympathetics (less bradycardia with hypotension).

for a laparoscopy, or the heart if it is stiff from diastolic dysfunction, or if it cannot expand because of fluid in the pericardial sac (tamponade).

Finally, we must briefly discuss the control mechanisms that keep everything running smoothly.

Blood pressure control

So blood pressure can take a major hit with decreases in preload (blood/fluid loss, venodilation), contractility, and afterload. The body, however, has reflexes to try to fix this. For short-term blood pressure control, the baroreflex bears the brunt of the responsibility.

Baroreceptor

Located in the carotid sinus, the baroreceptor provides the most important immediate feedback mechanism for short-term control of blood pressure. These pressure receptors have a basal firing rate, stimulating the vagal center and inhibiting the vasomotor center (Fig. 9.4).

Hypertension increases the firing rate, amplifying the vagal effects. Conversely, hypotension results in *decreased* baroreceptor firing (a little counterintuitive), resulting in reduced stimulation of the vagal centers and less inhibition (as opposed to stimulation) of the vasomotor center. The end result is increased sympathetic outflow, resulting in increased heart rate, contractility, and SVR with decreased venous capacity. This reflex requires an intact sympathetic nervous system, that is, one that has not been destroyed by the ravages of diabetes, blocked with neuraxial anesthesia,

inhibited by a drug like propofol, or depleted with illicit drugs, e.g., cocaine.

Atrial stretch receptors

Stretch on the atria, particularly the sinoatrial node, results in reflex vasodilation and decreased blood pressure, as well as increased heart rate. Simultaneously, atrial stretch receptors elicit the *Bainbridge reflex*[3] with a vagal afferent to the medulla and efferents through the vagus and sympathetics to increase heart rate and contractility.

Chemoreceptors

Located in the carotid and aortic bodies, the chemoreceptors are stimulated by decreasing oxygen and increasing carbon dioxide and hydrogen ions. They affect the vasomotor center to increase blood pressure, as well as stimulate breathing. Causing occasional consternation, receptors in the ventricles also can elicit a vasodepressor (vasodilation and bradycardia) response to decreased ventricular volume (vasovagal reflex) or certain chemical or mechanical stimuli (Bezold–Jarisch reflex).[4]

Long-term control

Long-term blood pressure control occurs through the kidney and aldosterone, renin, and angiotensin, which alter the volume of fluid in the system and modulate vascular resistances as well.

Anesthesia in the patient with cardiovascular disease

Hypertension

When we do not know the etiology, we hide behind the technical term "essential." Thus, we call "essential" the hypertension afflicting some 95% of patients. The pathophysiology of essential hypertension is probably multi-factorial including renal, vascular, cardiac, and neurohumoral factors – with reflex control problems thrown in for good measure.

Chronic hypertension leads to left ventricular hypertrophy with consequent stiffening of the ventricle. A "stiffer," less compliant ventricle will exhibit a large rise in intraventricular pressure during diastole. This increased diastolic pressure (wall tension) both increases myocardial oxygen demand and limits coronary perfusion. All organ perfusion depends on the upstream and downstream pressures. Thus, for the coronary perfusion pressure (CorPP):

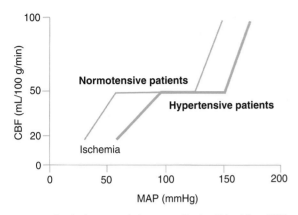

Fig. 9.5 Cerebral autoregulation curve. Cerebral blood flow (CBF) is maintained over a range of mean arterial pressures (MAP). The curve shifts with chronic hypertension, increasing the potential for inadequate cerebral blood flow with marginal MAP. Ischemia results when the CBF falls below 20 mL/100 g/min.

$$CorPP = DBP - RAP \text{ or } LVEDP$$

where DBP = diastolic blood pressure (because the majority of coronary perfusion occurs during diastole), RAP = right atrial pressure (where the coronaries empty, measured as central venous pressure, CVP), and LVEDP = left ventricular end-diastolic pressure. With a stiff left ventricle, LVEDP may exceed RAP and limit coronary perfusion, particularly in the subendocardium. This combination leads to an increased risk of myocardial ischemia (oxygen supply < demand). In addition to its deleterious effects on the heart, chronic hypertension leads to aortic, cerebral, and peripheral vascular disease, as well as strokes and renal dysfunction.

In all patients, particularly those we are going to anesthetize, we worry about cerebral perfusion. The cerebral vasculature autoregulates to maintain a stable blood flow over a range of mean arterial pressures. Chronic hypertension causes a rightward shift of this cerebral autoregulation curve (see Fig. 9.5). An unfortunate side effect of this shift is intolerance of low blood pressure. That is, a normotensive patient can maintain cerebral blood flow down to a MAP of 60 mmHg; with chronic hypertension, such a MAP might result in decreased cerebral perfusion and possibly ischemia (decreased CNS function or even a stroke). While a conscious patient might complain of dizziness and perhaps become confused, under general anesthesia we find it difficult to assess the adequacy of cerebral perfusion. Thus, we apply a general, albeit conservative, rule of thumb: maintain a patient's blood pressure within 30% of their baseline pressure (see Chapter 1).

The anesthetic management of hypertension includes the following:

(i) Pre-operative control of blood pressure. We have data showing that grossly hypertensive patients do poorly peri-operatively; we have no data that would enable us to pinpoint the optimum of controlled hypertension.

(ii) Continuation of antihypertensive medication in the peri-operative period, with the possible exception of ACE inhibitors and angiotensin receptor blockers, which have been linked to refractory post-induction hypotension during anesthesia.

(iii) Intra-operative control of blood pressure swings. Hypertensive patients are often volume-depleted from chronic vasoconstriction or diuretic use. Most anesthetics are vasodilators, and blood pressure can fall precipitously. Furthermore, the presence of antihypertensive drugs and some anesthetics may interfere with the normal reflex response to hypotension. As already mentioned, hypotension presents a particular risk to chronically hypertensive patients because they require increased diastolic pressure to maintain coronary perfusion and may have impaired cerebral autoregulation with rightward shift of that curve (Fig. 9.5).

Ischemic heart disease

Patients with ischemic heart disease face significant risks when undergoing anesthesia and surgical procedures. In our pre-operative assessment, we must weigh measures to protect them from peri-operative ischemia (see Chapter 1). Diagnosing ischemia by electrocardiography (ST segment depression) can be difficult if a bundle branch block pattern obscures ST segment changes. Transesophageal echocardiography (TEE), which is minimally invasive (but unpleasant if awake), can be quite helpful as it reveals wall motion abnormalities, an early sign of ventricular dysfunction from coronary insufficiency. TEE requires expensive equipment, a skilled examiner, and an experienced interpreter (see Chapter 7).

If we suspect ischemia, remember physiology: ischemia means oxygen supply does not meet demand. By looking at the factors affecting supply and demand, we can try to improve conditions (Table 9.1).

First, consider *supply*. Because the coronary arteries are perfused during diastole, we want to maximize

Table 9.1. Factors affecting myocardial oxygen supply and demand

Factors increasing supply
↓ Heart rate
↑ Diastolic blood pressure
↓ Intraventricular pressure
↑ Oxygen saturation
↑ [Hemoglobin]
Factors decreasing demand
↓ Heart rate
↓ Wall tension
↓ Contractility

diastolic time (lower heart rate) and coronary perfusion pressure (see above). For each amount of blood that gets through, we want it to contain as much oxygen as possible (see oxygen content equation in Chapter 10). Surprisingly, the optimal hematocrit is actually only 30 mg/dL; at higher concentrations, fluidity of blood decreases.

Now for *demand*. Cardiac contraction is "expensive" in an oxygen consumption sense, and the more contractions, the more "expense." Thus, tachycardia has a dramatic impact on the supply:demand ratio, increasing oxygen consumption while at the same time reducing its supply (remember a high rate steals the time previously available between heartbeats, i.e., diastole). For this reason, heart rate reduction is a primary target during ischemic episodes. In addition, myocardial oxygen demand increases with increasing wall tension and, more importantly, contractility.

As of this writing (and the previous edition for that matter), peri-operative beta-receptor blockade receives much attention. It may have the potential to reduce cardiac deaths and complications (see Chapter 12), though random application is not warranted due to an increased risk of stroke.

Pacemaker/AICD

More and more patients are presenting with these life-saving devices (AICD, automatic internal cardioverter defibrillator) in place for heart rhythm disturbances (see Pacemaker/AICD section in Chapter 1, for advance evaluation). Intra-operatively, there are general rules for surgery in these patients:

(i) Enlist the help of cardiology colleagues to check on the pacer function following the operation, if there is any question.

(ii) Have a magnet on hand. This nifty low-tech device reverts pacemakers into a back-up paced-only mode at a rate dependent on the manufacturer, program, and remaining battery life. If the device is also an AICD then the magnet does not affect the pacer function at all but, more importantly, it turns off the AICD detection and shocking function. Because electrocautery makes a signal that looks very much like ventricular fibrillation to the ECG monitoring program of the AICD, it is vitally important to disengage this feature if cautery is to be used. An erroneous intra-operative cardiac shock from the AICD during an operation could stop a perfectly functioning heart.

(iii) Avoid electromagnetic interference. We do not want the pacemaker to become part of the electrocautery circuit, so we consider the route between the surgical site and the electrocautery return electrode (often incorrectly called "grounding pad") and make sure it does not cross the pacemaker or its leads.

(iv) With rate-responsive pacemakers, we might avoid agents that fool the device into thinking its owner is running a marathon (succinylcholine-induced fasciculations, shivering).

(v) Keep electrolytes normal, particularly K^+ and Mg^{2+}.

Following conclusion of the operation, the pacer may require reprogramming, and the AICD should be reactivated by either removing the magnet or turning it back on if it was turned off by a cardiologist prior to the operation.

Congestive heart failure

Congestive heart failure (CHF) describes a heart that is not pumping well. Ordinarily, the heart dilates to accept blood at a low filling pressure, then propels it forward forcefully with each contraction. CHF can result from pathology at several points in the pump's function:

(i) Poor *ventricular compliance*. A non-compliant ventricle, as may occur with ischemia or hypertrophy, will exhibit substantial increases in pressure even at "normal" filling volumes. This will impede ventricular filling and increase the pressure in the venous system. In approximately one-third of CHF patients, this *diastolic dysfunction* predominates as the mechanism for their disease.

(ii) The descending limb of *Starling's curve*. Though a bit controversial, there may be a point at which further increasing diastolic filling actually results in a *decreasing* stroke volume. Here, substantial increases in ventricular pressure can result in pulmonary congestion and edema. A reduction in preload can move the heart back to the more functional side of the curve (see Fig. 9.2) and reduce the filling pressure sufficiently to alleviate pulmonary congestion.

(iii) *Contractility*. In Fig. 9.2 the Starling curve of the CHF patient resides lower and runs flatter than normal, reflecting the high filling pressures required to generate even a marginal stroke volume.

(iv) *Afterload*. Increased afterload is the most common cause of hypertension. The increased force of contraction required to eject against this afterload is deleterious to a failing heart.

The importance of these influences suggests the current treatment regimen for the most common cause of CHF (left ventricular systolic dysfunction), namely inotropic support with digoxin, diuretics to decrease preload, and especially afterload reduction as with an ACE inhibitor.

Cardiovascular problems during anesthesia

Hypotension

Picture the acutely hypotensive, tachycardic patient (BP 80/50, HR 120 beats/min), a fairly common observation. How should you go about treating this patient? After the ABCs,[5] we recommend a physiologic approach, rather than a mnemonic laundry list of possible causes. First, there are three main ways a patient can become hypotensive: low preload (not enough blood to push forward through the system), low contractility (inadequate force pushing the blood), and low resistance (dilated vascular bed). Other categories are less common and include lack of atrial kick as with atrial fibrillation, and valvular anomalies. To distinguish between these, we start with situational awareness. Did the cross-clamp just come off the aorta? Are the suction

canisters filling rapidly with blood? Did we just induce a sympathectomy with a high spinal anesthetic? Add to that a quick physical examination to rule out abnormal rhythm or valvular or cardiac dysfunction, and review of the patient's medical history (chronic CHF or recent myocardial infarction [MI]?). If these do not lead to a high-probability diagnosis, invasive or TEE monitoring (if you are really modern and fortunate enough to have access to it) may be indicated.

The invasive monitors we have available, in addition to the arterial catheter for blood pressure monitoring, include:

- filling pressure as an inference of ventricular volume/preload: central venous pressure (CVP), pulmonary artery occlusion pressure (PAOP);
- cardiac output: thermodilution via a pulmonary artery catheter (PAC) or, less invasively, peripheral arterial waveform analysis.

For example, consider the hypotensive, tachycardic patient above. Assume a CVP of 1 mmHg (normal 5–12 mmHg) and cardiac output of 7.5 L/min. A low filling pressure (low preload) translates into low ventricular volume – but contractility appears to be good (a cardiac output of 7.5 L/min is not consistent with a poorly contracting or very empty heart). With a look at the systemic vascular resistance (SVR) equation above, we see that a low MAP (small numerator) and high cardiac output (denominator) implies a very low SVR. The baroreflex, though, should be railing against the low BP and *raising* the SVR – we cannot measure the baroreflex activity but assume that it is straining to raise resistance, without success. Thus, our attention is drawn to vasodilation (via endotoxin as in septic shock, or deep anesthesia, or blockade of sympathetic outflow as in spinal shock or neuraxial anesthesia).

Such a physiologic approach allows tailoring of intervention to the specific problem. While intravenous fluid administration is routinely our first choice in a hypotensive patient – particularly in the post-operative setting – and proves the correct choice 99 times out of 100, it does no favor for the patient hypotensive from CHF. Thus, with an unclear etiology or a troubling response to initial treatment, invasive or TEE monitoring may be helpful (Table 9.2).

We see from the table that the typical general inhalation anesthetic can affect blood pressure from top to bottom, decreasing preload by venous pooling, decreasing contractility by a direct negative inotropic

Table 9.2. Differentiating causes of hypotension

	CVP	CO	SVR	TEE	Treatment
Low preload: hemorrhage, increased intra-abdominal pressure, sympathetic block, anesthetics	↓	↓↔	↑	Empty ventricle	Fluids; Trendelenburg's position
Low contractility: ischemia, CHF, anesthetics	↑	↓	↑↔	Poor systolic motion (WMA for ischemia)	Inotrope; ? vasodilator/diuretic; If ischemia: oxygen; beta-blocker, NTG, ASA
Low SVR: anaphylaxis, sepsis, spinal shock, anesthetics	↓	↑	↓	Hyperdynamic ventricle	Vasoconstriction, e.g., α_1 agonist, vasopressin

Until the preload is very low, there is usually sufficient cardiac reserve (increased heart rate and contractility) to maintain cardiac output. With low contractility, initial baroreflex-mediated stimulation will cause vasoconstriction – not such a good idea in a heart already having difficulty ejecting! Over time, this response dissipates, and SVR returns toward normal.
CVP: central venous pressure; CO: cardiac output; SVR: systemic vascular resistance; TEE: transesophageal echocardiography; WMA: wall motion abnormalities; NTG: nitroglycerin; ASA: aspirin.

Table 9.3. Causes of intra-operative hypertension

Underlying hypertension (exacerbated by missing antihypertensive doses while awaiting surgery):

- rebound hypertension (especially from missing beta-blockers or clonidine)
- pre-eclampsia

Elevated catecholamines:

- anxiety
- inadequate anesthetic depth for level of stimulation (surgery, laryngoscopy, emergence)
- iatrogenic (drug error, inadvertent intravascular injection or absorption)
- drugs (cocaine, monoamine oxidase inhibitors [MAOIs], ephedra)
- bladder distension
- pheochromocytoma

Reflexes:

- hypoxia
- hypercarbia
- Cushing's reflex (from elevated intracranial pressure)
- autonomic hyperreflexia (from spinal reflexes after cord transection)

Elevated preload (volume overload)

Elevated afterload:

- drugs (decongestants)
- aortic cross-clamp

Rare events:

- malignant hyperthermia
- thyroid storm
- delirium tremens

effect on the heart, decreasing SVR by depressing sympathetic outflow and, with some agents, even decreasing the baroreceptor reflex. The treatment of hypotension under anesthesia – when not attributed to primary heart disease, hypovolemia from hemorrhage, or sepsis – still consists of "filling up the tank" by giving fluids, lightening anesthesia to improve cardiac function, and giving sympathomimetic drugs, such as phenylephrine, or even vasopressin, to raise SVR. If we want also to augment contractility then we instead use ephedrine.

Arrhythmias

Rhythm disturbances occur in up to 70% of patients subjected to general anesthesia. Fortunately, the majority of these, in the otherwise healthy patient, are benign and transient. A number of factors can be blamed: the effects of anesthetic agents on the SA and AV nodes, peri-operative ischemia, and increased sympathetic activity during light anesthesia, e.g., laryngoscopy, hypoxemia, and hypercarbia (not uncommon during induction of general anesthesia). In addition to adhering to ACLS protocols, potential triggers must be sought and eliminated: correct ventilation, check for electrolyte abnormality (especially potassium), alter anesthetic agent selection, increase oxygenation, deepen anesthetic, etc.

Hypertension

The differential diagnosis of intra-operative hypertension is lengthy, but should be approached by considering the patient and procedure first (Table 9.3).

Management of intra-operative hypertension should focus on three things:

(i) Fix the underlying problem: correct anesthetic depth, treat hypercarbia, drain the bladder, etc.

(ii) Where correction is not possible, treat according to the physiologic derangement. For example, volume overload should not be treated with beta-blockade nor anxiety with diuretics.

(iii) Consider the time course of the treatment: if a patient's hypertension results from a transient surgical stimulus, a long-acting antihypertensive

may cause refractory hypotension when the stimulus ends.

See Chapter 12 to review a selection of the myriad antihypertensive agents at our disposal.

Notes

1 You might (at least the engineers in the crowd) recognize this equation as a corollary to Ohm's law ($V = IR$) with blood pressure drop over the body circuit replacing the voltage drop, cardiac output replacing current (I), and SVR in the role of resistance (R). The "$\times 80$" part corrects the units into the dubious "dynes s cm^{-5}."

2 Actually more correctly the (Otto) Frank – (Hermann) Straub – (Ernest) Starling law of the heart – to give credit where credit is due.

3 Francis Arthur Bainbridge (1874–1921), an English physiologist particularly interested in the physiology of exercise.

4 Albert von Bezold (1836–1868) described the slowing of the heart in response to veratrine (an irritant). Upon his untimely death at age 32 from rheumatic heart disease, his work was greatly furthered by Austrian Adolph Jarisch, Jr. (1891–1965).

5 Airway, Breathing, Circulation.

And the Lord God formed man from the dust of the ground and breathed into his nostrils the breath of life; and man became a living soul

(Genesis 2:7)

The concept of breath and soul reverberates through many languages in which spirit and breath share overlapping meanings. For example, in English, to *inspire* can have a physiological or psychological connotation, while to *expire* can mean nothing more than to exhale, or it can describe the moment when your spirit leaves you with your last breath. In anesthesia, we deal with both; on the one hand, the breath that needs to be provided for patients who cannot breathe by themselves and, on the other hand, the spirit – in a larger sense – which we subdue with drugs. Small wonder, then, that the linkage of breath and life gives us awesome responsibilities. In our practice no function is more important than ventilation, and no organ more integral to our practice than the lungs. Failure of ventilation has always been, and continues to be, the single most important cause of anesthesia-related mortality. An understanding of basic pulmonary physiology and pathophysiology, therefore, is vital to the safe practice of anesthesia.

Basic pulmonary physiology

Purpose of breathing

Breathing brings in oxygen necessary for cellular respiration and eliminates the resulting carbon dioxide. If oxygen supply does not meet demand, desperate cells revert to anaerobic metabolism, resulting in lactic acidosis.[1] Our oxygen requirement depends on the metabolic rate, but for a resting individual 3–4 mL O_2/kg/min should suffice. Meanwhile, we generate CO_2 at a rate dependent on the respiratory quotient "R":

$$R = \frac{\dot{V}_{CO_2}}{\dot{V}_{O_2}}$$

where $\dot{V}_{CO_2}$ and $\dot{V}_{O_2}$ are the minute production of carbon dioxide and consumption of oxygen, respectively. R depends on the energy source (carbohydrates, proteins, fat). It approaches 1 in several conditions including pregnancy and patients on total peripheral nutrition (TPN), but we usually peg it at 0.8.

Control of breathing

Can you commit suicide by simply not breathing or by willing your heart to stop? Even though we have voluntary muscular control over ventilation, we cannot stop breathing. We are hard-wired so that, in response to rising carbon dioxide tensions in the medulla, carbon dioxide-sensitive neurons stimulate ventilation to keep the arterial partial pressure of CO_2 ($PaCO_2$) near 40 mmHg. In physiological sleep, they let the $PaCO_2$ drift up to 45 mmHg, while in pregnancy they are reset by the controller to maintain 30 mmHg. Within physiological limits, ventilation and $PaCO_2$ (Fig. 10.1) keep a linear relationship.

We can restrain the center pharmacologically with opioids or deep inhalation anesthesia. In some diseases resulting in high $PaCO_2$, the respiratory center fatigues permanently and these "CO_2 retainers" must then rely on hypoxemia to drive their ventilation.

Perhaps surprisingly, oxygenation is not detected in the brain at all, but rather is sensed by peripheral chemoreceptors in the carotid and aortic bodies. These receptors do not really kick in until the PaO_2 falls below about 60 mmHg. Thus, our "CO_2-retaining" patients with chronic obstructive pulmonary disease (COPD) are not only chronically hypercarbic, they are also (at least borderline) hypoxemic. We often hear it said that such a patient will become apneic if given supplemental oxygen. Please do not take this to mean that, in an emergency, oxygen should be withheld from a hypoxemic patient for fear of apnea! Instead, give oxygen and ventilate the patient's lungs. Once

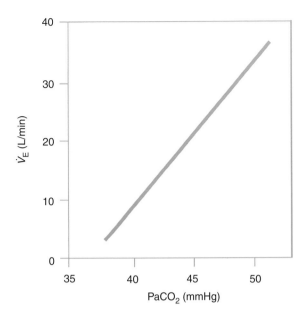

Fig. 10.1 Ventilatory response to changing $PaCO_2$. $\dot{V}_E$ = exhaled minute ventilation.

on top of the emergency, turn down the FiO_2 (fraction of inspired oxygen) step by step and remind the patient to breathe (no small task) until the oxygen saturation falls to a point where hypoxic drive takes effect (around 90%, which corresponds not surprisingly with a PaO_2 of about 60 mmHg). Similarly, when weaning these patients from mechanical ventilation, they might not start to breathe until returned to the hypoxic and hypercarbic state to which they are accustomed (another curse of smoking).

Mechanics of ventilation

Spontaneous ventilation at rest involves generating negative intrathoracic pressure (by lowering the diaphragm and expanding the chest wall), causing air to be drawn into the lungs. This requires that the upper airway remains patent. In the presence of an obstruction, e.g., tongue, mass, soft tissue, or mechanical, we observe retractions, particularly around the clavicles and the jugular notch and, in children, the intercostal spaces. An early sign is a *tracheal tug*, a little downward movement of the larynx with each inspiration. A reliable sign of airway obstruction, the tracheal tug signals the recruitment of accessory muscles to maintain gas exchange. Similarly, pulmonary cripples (advanced emphysema) and patients still partially paralyzed after

anesthesia will show a tracheal tug. Hypoxemic patients weakened by drugs or muscle disease require immediate assisted ventilation with bag and mask and, if necessary, establishment of a patent airway via intubation.

At rest, exhalation should be passive and, if it is not, consider asthma or airway obstruction.

The work of breathing

The medullary centers control the $PaCO_2$ by altering the minute ventilation ($\dot{V}_E$):

$$\dot{V}_E = V_T \times f$$

where V_T = tidal volume and f = frequency of breaths or respiratory rate. How these parameters change to maintain minute ventilation depends on the work of breathing. Because inhaling requires the work of muscles, it is "costly," in an energy expenditure sense, to breathe. In general, a few large breaths are more efficient than many small ones because all breaths must move the same amount of deadspace volume (about 150 mL for the average adult, see below).

Endotracheal tubes offer much resistance and can greatly increase the work of breathing. We borrow from J. L. M. Poiseuille (1799–1869), a French physician and physiologist, who described the factors affecting blood flow in tubes to understand exactly how. A simplified and restructured version of his equation shows that the resistance (R) to flow is proportional to the tube length (L), fluid (or gas) viscosity (η), and inversely proportional to the radius (r) to the fourth power:

$$R \propto \frac{\eta . L}{r^4}$$

Simply put, a change in ETT size of only 1 mm, from 8.0 mm to 7.0 mm ID (internal diameter), nearly doubles the resistance to flow of the same gas down the same length tube, and if it were from 4.0 mm to 3.0 mm ID, resistance would more than triple. Patients, and especially babies, may struggle to breathe if left unassisted on a too small, kinked, or partially obstructed (with inspissated secretions) ETT. Fortunately, a ventilator will ease this burden by doing the inspiratory work for the patient. Just as with all other muscles, disuse leads to reduced strength and stamina. Several investigators continue to study the optimal amount of respiratory muscle loading to prevent muscle atrophy and weaning difficulties.

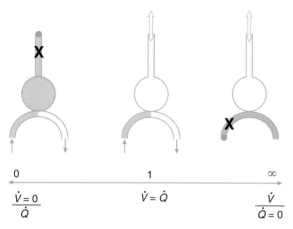

Fig. 10.2 Ventilation–perfusion mismatch. The ideal is perfect matching of ventilation and perfusion ($\dot{V}/\dot{Q} = 1$). To the far left, the numerator falls to zero ($\dot{V} = 0$), representing no ventilation but plenty of perfusion; this is termed shunt. Deadspace ventilation is the opposite. Thus deadspace ventilation and shunt represent the extremes on the continuum of $\dot{V}/\dot{Q}$ matching. See text.

Patients with low pulmonary *compliance*, e.g., pulmonary fibrosis, tend to breathe rapidly with low tidal volumes because of the great work required to expand a stiff lung. Compliance (C) describes the relationship between changes in volume (ΔV) and the associated changes in pressure (ΔP) in any enclosed space (lung, cardiac ventricle):

$$C = \frac{\Delta V}{\Delta P}$$

Conversely, a patient with high *airway resistance* cannot move air rapidly through the bronchial tree and tends to breathe slowly, which decreases turbulence. The resulting shift toward laminar movement of air increases flow and reduces the work of breathing.

Since resistance increases as the fourth power of the shrinking radius, we can easily see why even a small amount of bronchospasm so drastically affects air movement, and why babies with subglottic edema present us with such great difficulties.

Matching of ventilation and perfusion

All the tubes leading to the alveoli – ETT, trachea, large and small bronchi – serve only as a conduit. These make up the deadspace volume: areas with bidirectional airflow but no gas exchange. There are three types of deadspace:

- physiologic – areas of the normal lung with ventilation but no perfusion – as found in the apices in the upright subject;
- anatomic – trachea and bronchi, which lack alveoli altogether;
- apparatus – the endotracheal tube and other pieces of tubing with bidirectional gas flow.

An endotracheal tube will replace the anatomic deadspace generated by the pharynx, nose, and mouth. Applying a face mask will increase deadspace, but an anesthesia breathing circuit will add relatively little to the deadspace as long as the valves in the circuit function normally. The deadspace to tidal volume ratio is measured as:

$$V_D/V_T = (P_A CO_2 - P_{\bar{E}} CO_2)/P_A CO_2$$

where V_D = deadspace volume, $P_A CO_2$ = alveolar CO_2, and $P_{\bar{E}} CO_2$ = mixed expired CO_2. A normal V_D/V_T ratio should not exceed 0.3.

When pulmonary arterial blood manages to pass through the lungs without picking up oxygen or delivering carbon dioxide, we are faced with a shunt. A shunt wastes perfusion. Typically, the difference between arterial and end-expired gases increases when ventilation and perfusion are mismatched, owing either to deadspace ventilation (inspired gas is exhaled without having picked up carbon dioxide or delivered oxygen) or to shunting (pulmonary arterial blood bypasses alveoli and then dumps blood high in CO_2 and low in O_2 into the pulmonary venous blood, see Fig. 10.2). Even normal lungs have some deadspace ventilation and shunting. When either becomes excessive, we refer to a $\dot{V}/\dot{Q}$ mismatch evident in blood gas values.

Tissue oxygenation

Once we get both air and blood into the lungs, oxygen must traverse the alveolar membrane. Oxygen diffusion across this membrane depends on the Fick[2] equation:

$$Diffusion = \frac{SA}{T} \times D \times (P_{alv} - P_{bld})$$

where SA = surface area of the alveoli (decreased in emphysema), T = membrane thickness (increased with pulmonary edema), D = diffusion constant for a given gas,[3] and $P_{alv} - P_{bld}$ = the gas pressure difference across the membrane dividing alveolus from blood.

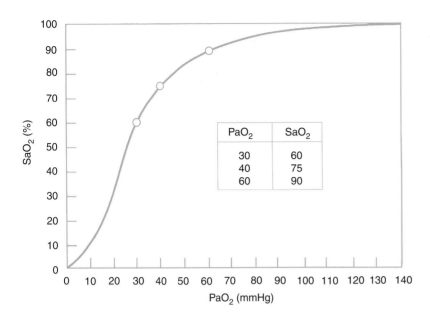

PaO$_2$	SaO$_2$
30	60
40	75
60	90

Fig. 10.3 The oxyhemoglobin dissociation curve for normal adult hemoglobin. SaO$_2$ is saturation of hemoglobin with oxygen; PaO$_2$ is partial pressure of oxygen in arterial blood.

After traversing the alveolar and capillary wall membrane, oxygen dissolves in plasma (not much; $0.003 \times$ PaO$_2$) and binds with hemoglobin (a bunch), and the arterial oxygen content (CaO$_2$) becomes:

$$CaO_2 = (1.34 \times [Hgb] \times SaO_2) + (0.003 \times PaO_2)$$

where CaO$_2$ = volume of oxygen in 100 mL blood, [Hgb] = hemoglobin concentration, and SaO$_2$ = arterial hemoglobin saturation with oxygen.

Oxyhemoglobin dissociation curve

The amount of oxygen bound to hemoglobin depends on the qualities of the hemoglobin molecule. The familiar oxyhemoglobin dissociation curve appears in Fig. 10.3. Observe the steep portion of the curve where small changes in PaO$_2$ result in large shifts in saturation. The point of 50% saturation (P$_{50}$) provides a helpful reference. In adults, it hovers around 26 mmHg (hemoglobin will be 50% saturated with oxygen at a PaO$_2$ of 26 mmHg). For a fetus to pull needed oxygen from its mother's blood, his hemoglobin must have a higher affinity for oxygen. In fact, the left shift of fetal hemoglobin (Hgb F) brings its P$_{50}$ to 19–21 mmHg.

A simple mnemonic helps to define several points on the oxyhemoglobin dissociation curve: 30–60; 60–90; 40–75 (Fig. 10.3). It does not sound much like a mnemonic, but put it to a beat and it works quite well. The first number of each pair cites the PaO$_2$, followed by the SaO$_2$. We use this to estimate (roughly) the PaO$_2$ from

the SpO$_2$ (obtained from the pulse oximeter). A PaO$_2$ of 60 mmHg or less defines hypoxemia (SpO$_2$ ~90%), and 40 mmHg is the normal mixed venous PO$_2$.

Four factors influence the position of the oxyhemoglobin dissociation curve. For ease of memorization, we cite those factors that shift the curve to the right: *increasing* temperature, CO$_2$, H$^+$, and 2,3-diphosphoglycerate (DPG). Remember pH decreases with increasing [H$^+$]. For the curious, the mechanism by which fetal hemoglobin maintains its leftward shift is a distaste for 2,3-DPG.

Alveolar air equation

The PO$_2$ we expect to find in arterial blood depends, in large part, on the inspired concentration. Oxygen makes up approximately 21% of the volume of dry air. If we assume the ambient (sea level) pressure to be 760 mmHg, the partial pressure of oxygen in dry air would be 160 mmHg (760×0.21). The warm and moist airways add water (water vapor pressure is temperature-dependent, and at 37°C it is 47 mmHg). Thus, breathing room air, our inspired oxygen concentration (PiO$_2$) on its way through the nose and upper airway will be diluted by water vapor:

$$PiO_2 = (760 - 47) \times 0.21 = 150 \text{ mmHg}$$

Once it arrives in the alveolus, this inspired oxygen will be diluted by carbon dioxide and taken up into the bloodstream. Summarized mathematically, the

107

resulting equation is too cumbersome for clinical application.[4] Instead, we use the approximation commonly referred to as the alveolar air equation:

$$P_A O_2 = P_i O_2 - \frac{P_A CO_2}{R}$$

where the "A" subscript denotes alveolar gas and R is the respiratory quotient described above.

If we take the trouble of calculating for a person breathing room air ($PiO_2 = 150$ mmHg), assuming $R = 0.8$ and $P_A CO_2 = 40$ mmHg, we arrive at a $P_A O_2$ of about 100 mmHg. You can easily see that many factors affect the results: altitude, retention or rebreathing of CO_2, changing the concentration of oxygen in the inspired gas, changing the respiratory quotient, or changing the patient's temperature. To get an even better handle on this concept we encourage you to play with the interactive equation in both simplified and fancy form at the link provided at www.anest.ufl.edu/EA.

Clinical relevance of the oxyhemoglobin dissociation curve

Notice on the curve (Fig. 10.3), if a patient has an oxyhemoglobin saturation of 100%, we know that the PaO_2 must be at least 100 mmHg, but it could be anywhere from about 100 to 600 mmHg or more! We see the importance when administering supplemental oxygen in two different scenarios that follow.

The hypoxemic patient

When a patient becomes hypoxemic, we first apply supplemental oxygen. Wonderfully, the patient's saturation usually responds. Should it fall again, we can simply increase the inspired oxygen concentration once again – but we are not solving the problem. The adequate saturation may lull us into an inappropriate sense of security regarding the well-being of the patient.

Assume this patient requires 50% inspired oxygen to maintain an SpO_2 of 90%, much less than we would expect with that FiO_2. We estimate the degree of the oxygenation problem by looking at the difference between the alveolar and arterial oxygen concentrations. With an SpO_2 of 90%, we can assume the PaO_2 to be around 60 mmHg (from Fig. 10.3).

Next, we need to know what the alveolar concentration of oxygen would be in a healthy patient breathing 50% oxygen. The alveolar air equation comes to our aid. We estimate $P_A CO_2$ and R to be 40 mmHg and 0.8, respectively.

$$P_A O_2 = FiO_2 \times (P_B - P_{H_2O}) - \frac{P_A CO_2}{R}$$
$$P_A O_2 = 0.50 \times (760 - 47) - \frac{40}{0.8} = 306 \text{ mmHg}$$

Therefore, we would expect the PaO_2 to be close to 300 mmHg instead of the observed 60 mmHg. This "A–a difference" (often mislabeled an A–a gradient) may be due to a problem with oxygen diffusion and/or matching of ventilation and perfusion ($\dot{V}/\dot{Q}$). In healthy patients some 4% of the venous blood will manage to make it through a right (venous blood in the pulmonary artery) to left (arterial blood in the pulmonary vein) shunt. Thus, normally we expect to see a slightly lower partial pressure of oxygen in arterial blood than in alveolar gas. However, a patient requiring 50% inspired oxygen to barely maintain an SpO_2 of 90% should worry us greatly.

If a patient is hypoxemic on room air, giving supplemental oxygen is a great first step, but the *source* of the hypoxemia should be sought and appropriately treated.

Conscious sedation

The patient receiving intravenous sedation presents another situation in which the alveolar air equation can help. Some physicians routinely place these patients on supplemental oxygen by nasal cannula, resulting in a PaO_2 of 150 mmHg or more in the normal, awake patient. This puts them well into the flat part of the oxyhemoglobin dissociation curve: Fig. 10.3. If the patient now hypoventilates, his $PaCO_2$ will rise (please try this for yourself at www.anest.ufl.edu/EA) and PaO_2 will fall, but his SpO_2 can stay deceptively normal. Thus, *not* giving supplemental oxygen (to a patient with normal oxygenation) will make the SpO_2 a sensitive indicator of respiratory depression. Once a drop in saturation occurs, we need to treat the patient's hypoventilation.

A final concept regarding oxygenation deserves mention: just as oxyhemoglobin saturation does not instruct us on ventilation (the value of the $PaCO_2$), an SpO_2 of 100% does not guarantee delivery of oxygen to brain and other organs. SpO_2 is, after all, simply the fraction of oxygenated hemoglobin present in the blood passing the sensor, but tells us little about how many "box cars," or hemoglobin molecules, are doing the work. Both the arterial oxygen content mentioned above, which includes the hemoglobin concentration, and cardiac output determine oxygen delivery. A global problem with oxygen delivery might be detected as a lactic acidosis on an arterial blood sample. Even more specifically, perfusion of individual organs, the kidney for example, determines availability of oxygen for metabolic activity in that tissue. If the surgeon has cross-clamped the aorta above the level of the renal artery, a comforting high-pitched beep noting 100% SpO_2 at the right middle finger tells us nothing about the oxygenation of the nephron. In addition to monitoring the oxyhemoglobin saturation, we seek reassurance of adequate oxygen delivery to observable end-organs with the ECG, BIS, cerebral oximetry, urine output, evoked potentials, and others.

Studies of pulmonary function

Spirometry

Pulmonary function tests (PFTs) are rarely indicated in preparation for anesthesia, though they can tell us whether a patient with severe lung disease has been optimally prepared. Pulmonary restrictive and obstructive diseases worry us. Short of treating infection, we cannot do much about restrictive disease; however, it can coexist with obstructive bronchospasm, which is common and can be treated with bronchodilators. Of the many pulmonary function studies, we pay particular attention to forced vital capacity (FVC). FVC values below 15 mL/kg are problematic. How much the patient can exhale in 1 second (FEV_1 for forced expiratory volume), and whether this can be improved by bronchodilators determine obstructive disease. Typically, PFT results are reported as "% of predicted," based on population studies that consider the patient's height, age, and gender. We accept values of at least 80% predicted as normal. With obstructive disease, the patient experiences airway closure during exhalation, measured as a low FEV_1 (Table 10.1). With advanced disease and air trapping, the FVC might also decline, though not as much as the FEV_1; thus the hallmark of obstructive disease is a reduced ratio of FEV_1 to FVC. With age, this ratio declines as well (to perhaps 0.7), so again we look at the percent predicted. Flow volume loops (Fig. 10.4) can also be helpful. It is only a small exaggeration to say that a PFT demonstrating a reduced FEV_1/FVC is worthless without also assessing the patient for response to bronchodilators.

Table 10.1. Pulmonary function test interpretation

	FEV_1	FVC	FEV_1/FVC
Normal	>80%	>80%	>0.8
Obstruction	↓	↔↓	↓
Restriction	↓	↓	↔↑

% of predicted; FEV_1: forced expiratory volume in 1 s; FVC: forced vital capacity. In obstructive disease, FVC may decline due to air trapping.

Arterial blood gas analysis

When we call for an analysis of arterial blood gases (ABG), we are really asking about the function of two organs: lungs and kidneys. An ABG reports the partial pressures of oxygen and carbon dioxide in arterial blood, both clearly related to lung function, but also provides the pH and bicarbonate concentration, which tells us something about how the kidneys are handling non-volatile acids and bases.

In the laboratory, the ABG values are corrected to 37°C. This facilitates interpretation of data because of the complexities introduced by temperature changes: in addition to a direct effect on pH, both the dissociation constants and solubility of gases are temperature-dependent. For example, a $PaCO_2$ of 40 mmHg at 37°C, will drop to 25 mmHg when temperature falls 10°C. The total carbon dioxide content stays the same, but the distribution of the components of the CO_2–carbonic acid–bicarbonate complex changes (see below). Thus, if not corrected in the laboratory, a drop in temperature from 37°C to 27°C would raise the reported pH of the blood sample from 7.4 to about 7.54.

Oxygen

The lab reports the partial pressure of oxygen in arterial blood as PaO_2 in mmHg, and the saturation of arterial hemoglobin with oxygen as % SaO_2. Most ABG analyzers *calculate* the SaO_2 based on a standard, adult oxyhemoglobin dissociation curve. When we have reason to suspect an erroneous result by this method, e.g., elevated levels of carboxyhemoglobin (fire survivor, suicide attempt, or an extremely heavy smoker), we must order co-oximetry (see Chapter 7). This method analyzes the transmission of several wavelengths of light, the better to distinguish reduced from oxygenated hemoglobin, as well as met- and carboxyhemoglobins. Please observe the convention of writing SaO_2 for the laboratory calculation of arterial hemoglobin

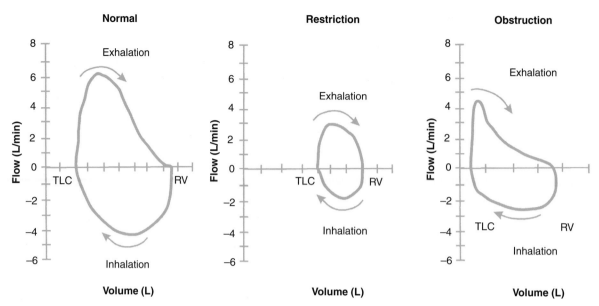

Fig. 10.4 Flow volume loop obtained in a normal patient, compared with those with restrictive and obstructive pulmonary diseases. With restriction, the flow volume loop has a slightly more convex shape and small volume. Note the rapid decline in flow rate in the patient with moderate obstruction. TLC: total lung capacity; RV: residual volume. To read these loops, we must keep in mind that the x-axis is conventionally written backwards, with the 0 for volume to the *right*, and that inhalation is the area below the x-axis, and exhalation above.

saturation, SpO$_2$ for the estimation of this value by pulse oximetry, and specify SaO$_2$ by co-oximetry if available. These values are rarely, if ever, identical but usually agree within a percent or so.

Carbon dioxide

Carbon dioxide in blood affects the pH because CO$_2$ in an aqueous medium (i.e., blood) will form carbonic acid, which dissociates into bicarbonate and hydrogen ions:

$$CO_2 + H_2O \leftrightarrow H_2CO_3 \leftrightarrow H^+ + HCO_3^-$$

We often describe this relationship with the *Henderson–Hasselbalch*[5] equation:

$$pH = pKa + \log\left(\frac{HCO_3^-}{PCO_2 \times 0.03}\right)$$

where *pKa* = the dissociation constant for carbonic acid (~6.1), that is, the pH at which 50% of the weak carbonic acid is ionized into equal amounts of HCO$_3^-$ and H$_2$CO$_3$ (for which PCO$_2$ × 0.03 is substituted). Thus the *ratio* of bicarbonate to PCO$_2$ determines pH, not their individual concentrations.

From this equation, we see that if we add carbon dioxide, the pH drops (respiratory acidosis). The interaction of CO$_2$ with water will lead to the generation of carbonic acid, which will lower the pH while increasing bicarbonate, without which the pH would be even lower. Slowly (over 1–2 days), the kidneys retain extra bicarbonate to further offset the acidosis, although never completely correcting it. When faced with an ABG demonstrating respiratory acidosis (decreased pH and increased PCO$_2$), we can use the 1–2–4–6 Rule of Ten (see Table 10.2), which simply states that the indicated acute or chronic respiratory disturbance will cause the bicarbonate to change. If that change did not take place or is exaggerated, we need to look for metabolic explanations.

Bicarbonate

The addition of acids, e.g., keto acids in diabetes, will also lower the pH. From the Henderson–Hasselbalch equation, we predict that the addition of hydrogen ions (lower pH) will cause the bicarbonate to gobble up some of the H$^+$ (lowering the concentration of HCO$_3^-$), leading to the generation of more carbonic acid, which can then dissociate into CO$_2$ and water. The CO$_2$ gas can be exhaled, thus reducing the effect of having added hydrogen ions.

Table 10.2. Bicarbonate response to acute or chronic respiratory disturbances

	The $^1_2{^4_6}$ Rule of Ten	
	Change in bicarbonate during hypercapnia above 40 mmHg	**Change in bicarbonate during hypocapnia below 40 mmHg**
Acute respiratory disturbance	**Up 1** mmol/L for every **10** mmHg $PaCO_2\uparrow$	**Down 2** mmol/L for every **10** mmHg $PaCO_2\downarrow$
Chronic respiratory disturbance	**Up 4** mmol/L for every **10** mmHg $PaCO_2\uparrow$	**Down 6** mmol/L for every **10** mmHg $PaCO_2\downarrow$

Anion gap

The addition of many acids will increase the anion gap. Recognizing that there must always be electroneutrality, if we add up all the cations (Na^+, K^+, Ca^{2+}, Mg^{2+}), they must equal all the anions (HCO_3^-, Cl^-, PO_4^{3-}, SO_4^{2-}, proteins, organic acids). Since we do not routinely measure the proteins and organic acids, these become the "anion gap," the difference between cations and anions.[6] We simplify all this math by only counting sodium, chloride, and bicarbonate and accepting as normal an anion gap of 12 ± 4 mEq/L, thus:

$$\text{Anion gap} = Na^+ - \left(Cl^- + HCO_3^-\right).$$

Buffers

Were it not for buffers in blood and tissue, any change in hydrogen ion concentration would cause large swings in pH. The buffers in blood (primarily hemoglobin) avidly sop up hydrogen ions, mitigating shifts in pH; therefore, a severely anemic patient will experience greater shifts in pH than a patient with normal hemoglobin values. When buffering proves insufficient, and correcting a low cardiac output fails to help, we must treat serious metabolic acidosis with the titration of bicarbonate. We calculate the initial dose[7] as

$$\frac{0.3 \times \text{wt (kg)} \times \left(24 \text{ mEq/L} - \text{actual } HCO_3^-\right)}{2}$$

which should not fully correct the acidemia. We then look at repeated blood gas values presenting pH, bicarbonate, and PCO_2, realizing that the addition of bicarbonate will increase the pH while also liberating CO_2, which must (if possible) be exhaled.

ABG interpretation

A normal room air[8] arterial blood gas in a non-pregnant[9] patient should look something like:

pH $7.35 - 7.45$, PCO_2 $35 - 45$ mmHg,

PO_2 $75 - 100$ mmHg, HCO_3^- $22 - 26$ mmol/L.

Other values include methemoglobin (metHb) <2%, carboxyhemoglobin (COHb) <3%, and base excess –2 to 2 mEq/L.

When the laboratory reports abnormal results, we ask several questions:

(i) Is the PO_2 OK? As discussed above, we look not at the value in isolation, but in the context of the inspired oxygen concentration; thus we apply the alveolar air equation.

(ii) Is the pH OK? If not, is there a metabolic or respiratory disturbance with or without compensation or is it a mixed disturbance? (See Table 10.3.)

Two clinical examples

Case 1: A PACU nurse calls because a post-operative patient has a low SpO_2, which did not normalize by giving the patient oxygen by face mask.

The findings:

(i) SpO_2 of 90% on FiO_2 of 0.5.

The alveolar air equation estimates (presuming – probably falsely – a normal arterial CO_2 of 40 mmHg) an alveolar oxygen tension of 306 mmHg ($0.50 \times [760 - 47] - [40/0.8]$). An SpO_2 of 90% corresponds to a PaO_2 of approximately 60 mmHg. Thus there is a *large* A–a difference.

(ii) ABG: pH 7.28, $PaCO_2$ 55 mmHg, PO_2 60 mmHg, HCO_3^- 26 mmol/L.

The measured PaO_2 corresponds (miraculously exactly) with the estimated PaO_2 using the SpO_2 data. The elevated $PaCO_2$ of 55 mmHg indicates hypoventilation, which would partially explain the low PaO_2. In addition, there must also be a substantial ventilation/perfusion inequality as

Table 10.3. Interpretation of acid–base disorders from an arterial blood gas analysis

1. Is the pH low (acidemia <7.35) or high (alkalemia >7.45)?

2. Compare the pH with the $PaCO_2$ and HCO_3^-:

   Acidemia: $PaCO_2$ >45 mmHg = respiratory

       $[HCO_3^-]$ <20 mmol/L = metabolic

   Alkalemia: $PaCO_2$ <35 mmHg = respiratory

       $[HCO_3^-]$ > 28 mmol/L = metabolic

3. If the primary disturbance is respiratory, is it acute or chronic?

   Acute: pH changes 0.08 units per 10 mmHg change in $PaCO_2$

   Chronic: pH changes 0.03 units per 10 mmHg change in $PaCO_2$

   Confirm with the bicarbonate; it will not have had time to change much in an acute disturbance (Table 10.2)

4. If the primary disturbance is metabolic, is the respiratory response appropriate?

   Acidemia: $PaCO_2 = (1.5 \times HCO_3^-) + 8 \ (\pm 2)$ mmHg

   Alkalemia: $PaCO_2 = (0.7 \times HCO_3^-) + 21 \ (\pm 1.5)$ mmHg

   If the $PaCO_2$ is higher than expected, there is a coexisting primary respiratory acidosis; if lower, there is a respiratory alkalosis

5. If there is a metabolic acidosis, is the anion gap >12?

   $AG = [Na^+] - ([Cl^-] + [HCO_3^-])$

6. Consider the differential diagnosis for the resulting disorder(s) (see Table 10.4 for a representative [non-exhaustive] list)

can come from shallow breathing and atelectasis where the blood flowing through the atelectatic alveoli acts as shunt.

Step 1: The pH of 7.28 indicates acidemia.

Step 2: The elevated arterial carbon dioxide tension implies a respiratory contribution.

Step 3: The CO_2 is increased (55 – 40 = 15 mmHg). The pH fall of 0.12 (7.40 – 7.28) is consistent with an acute respiratory acidosis (0.08 per 10 mmHg rise in the CO_2). In confirmation, according to Table 10.2, an acute elevation of $PaCO_2$ by 15 mmHg should be associated with a rise in bicarbonate of 1.5 mEq/L. The patient's bicarbonate confirms our suspicion that we are dealing with an acute, i.e., so far uncompensated, respiratory acidemia.

We must now determine whether obstruction (is the airway patent? Do bandages impede ventilation?), weakness (is there a muscle relaxant hangover?), or central depression and shallow or slow breathing (effects of narcotics?) can explain the hypoventilation and shunt. Therapy will depend on what we find.

Case 2: The ambulance brings a trauma patient to the Emergency Department. The patient has a fractured pelvis. As a routine, a nurse applies a face mask delivering 50% oxygen. SpO_2 is 100%. An ABG reveals: pH 7.23, $PaCO_2$ 25 mmHg, PaO_2 250 mmHg, HCO_3^- 12 mmol/L.

(i) We welcome the SpO_2 of 100% but realize that the patient can still have a ventilation/perfusion abnormality. However, the PaO_2 of 250 mmHg confirms a small A–a difference ($P_AO_2 = 0.5 \times [760 – 47] – 25/0.8 = 325$ mmHg).

(ii) *Step 1*: The pH of 7.23 shows acidemia.

    Step 2: The low $PaCO_2$ and HCO_3^- describe a metabolic source (with significant hyperventilation).

    Step 3: The respiratory response is appropriate ($PaCO_2 \approx 25 \approx [1.5 \times 12] + 8$ mmHg).

We follow up with additional studies, such as determining the patient's volume status, hemoglobin, lactate and electrolyte levels (the latter to calculate the anion gap), to identify the cause of the patient's trouble and establish a plan for therapy (Table 10.4).

Providing supplemental oxygen

If breathing room air, a patient's FiO_2 will be 0.21. FiO_2 is the *fraction* of inspired oxygen (0.21 at sea level as well as on Mount Everest) – frequently confused with the percentage of oxygen (21%) – frequently muddled with the partial pressure of oxygen (about 150 mmHg at sea level and much less on Mount Everest). We have several devices to increase the spontaneously breathing patient's FiO_2 (Fig. 10.5):

- Nasal cannula increases FiO_2 about 3–4% per liter (thus 2 L delivers about 28% oxygen). Flow rates above 5 L/min irritate the nose without further increasing the FiO_2.

- A loosely fitting oxygen mask with an oxygen flow rate of 6–8 L/min may bring the inspired oxygen percentage to 60–80%.

- A non-rebreathing face mask with a reservoir can deliver ~95% oxygen (the bag should be inflated … unlike what the flight attendants tell us).

Table 10.4. Differential diagnosis of metabolic disorders (non-exhaustive list)

Anion gap metabolic acidosis: MUDPILERS:

M   Methanol[a]

U   Uremia

D   Diabetic or alcoholic ketoacidosis[a]

P   Paraldehyde (a rarely used hypnotic and anticonvulsant)

I   Iron, isoniazid, isopropyl alcohol[a]

L   Lactic acidosis

E   Ethylene glycol,[a] ethanol[a]

R   Rhabdomyolysis

S   Salicylates, strychnine

Non-anion gap metabolic acidosis:

Hyperchloremia (as with large-volume infusions of normal saline)

Diarrhea

Renal disease

Carbonic anhydrase inhibitors

Hyperalimentation

Many others …

Metabolic alkalosis:

Emesis

Administration of bicarbonate

[a] Often with an increased osmolar gap.

For each device we need an oxygen cylinder,[10] a reducing valve to bring the high pressure of a full cylinder to a manageable 40 psi (12 atm), and a flow meter that lets us select a flow rate anywhere from about 100 mL/min to 10 000 mL/min. The actual inspired concentration of oxygen will depend on the flow rate of oxygen, as well as the patient's peak inspiratory flow rate.

Pre-oxygenation/denitrogenation

Generally, tracheal intubation in adults is made easier with muscle relaxation, which causes apnea. An apneic healthy adult (previously breathing room air) will begin to desaturate (decreasing oxyhemoglobin percentage, SpO_2) within 2 minutes. Young and healthy patients usually maintain close to 100% oxygen saturation while breathing room air. Increasing the inspired oxygen concentration will raise the arterial oxygen tension, but add relatively little to the overall oxygen content of blood, as explained above.

However, to provide a reservoir of oxygen in the lungs, we apply a tight-fitting mask and have the patient breathe 100% oxygen before inducing apnea. This reservoir occupies the functional residual capacity (FRC) of the lung (the volume remaining after normal exhalation, see Fig. 10.6). Notice that little of the total lung volume is actually exchanged with normal tidal ventilation; therefore, several minutes of pre-oxygenation, or four to five full vital capacity breaths, are required to maximize the oxygen depot in the FRC. Two requirements for effective denitrogenation: (i) we need to let the patient inhale pure oxygen, which means the anesthesia machine must deliver a fresh gas flow rate of at least a minute volume of oxygen to the patient in order to prevent the rebreathing of exhaled nitrogen (the carbon dioxide absorber takes care of the CO_2). (ii) The patient must breathe 100% oxygen long enough to wash out the nitrogen in the lungs. We usually think of this process in terms of time constants (volume/flow), that is to say that it will take about four time constants to approach near complete denitrogenation of the lungs (there will still be nitrogen in solution in the body). One time constant is the time required to deliver a volume of gas equal to the volume of the lungs. After one time constant, we will have replaced 63% of the gas in the lungs (with additional time constants we get to 86.5%, 95.0%, 98.2%, and 99%, respectively). In a healthy, non-obese adult, with adequate pre-oxygenation (end-tidal oxygen concentration of >85%), this reservoir will provide 5–8 minutes of oxygen before the apneic patient's blood begins to desaturate.

Some factors can increase the rate of desaturation:

- A smaller reservoir: decreased FRC as in obesity, pregnancy, infancy.
- Increased oxygen consumption: hyperthermia, obesity, pregnancy, infancy.

Mechanical ventilation

Many patients require mechanical ventilation in the operating room or intensive care unit. While an intubated patient can breathe spontaneously through an endotracheal tube (which imposes significant resistance), many operative procedures require muscle relaxation, making mechanical ventilation mandatory. Most anesthesia machines are equipped with ventilators capable of providing volume- or pressure-controlled ventilation. For volume-controlled ventilation, the operator sets a tidal volume, respiratory rate, and inspiratory to expiratory time ratio (*I:E* ratio),

113

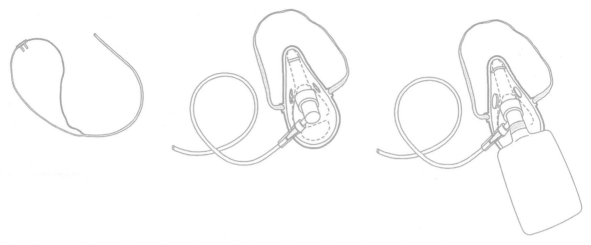

Fig. 10.5 Devices that provide supplemental oxygen. Nasal cannula (prongs), face mask, non-rebreather face mask.

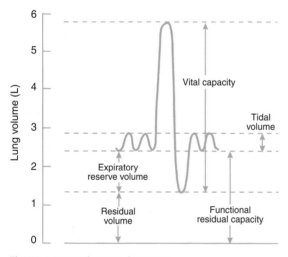

Fig. 10.6 Lung volumes and capacities.

and the ventilator does its best to comply. If compliance deteriorates, the machine will generate additional pressure (up to a set limit) in an attempt to deliver the desired tidal volume. In pressure-controlled mode, as the name suggests, the selected pressure will be maintained for a set time, which might mean variable tidal volumes, depending on the patient's pulmonary compliance and resistance.

In general, ventilators used in the ICU offer more options than anesthesia machine ventilators. For example, they might offer SIMV (synchronized intermittent mandatory ventilation), in which the mechanical breath is synchronized with the patient's inspiratory effort, and the patient can breathe spontaneously between mechanical breaths. SIMV is often combined with pressure support ventilation (PSV), in which spontaneous respiratory efforts are reinforced with a set level of positive pressure, assisting with inhalation and designed to overcome the resistance imposed by the endotracheal tube and ventilator.

Another ventilator mode that requires explanation is continuous positive airway pressure (CPAP) and its fraternal twin (with which it is often confused) positive end-expiratory pressure (PEEP). Ordinarily, when we exhale, some gas remains in the lungs (the FRC – see Fig. 10.6). Supine positioning and anesthesia reduce the FRC, potentially resulting in hypoxemia. Normal FRC can be restored with the addition of end-expiratory pressure, PEEP. It becomes particularly useful if increased intra-abdominal pressure or extravascular fluid (pulmonary edema, atelectasis, aspiration of gastric contents or adult respiratory distress syndrome [ARDS]) decreases FRC or causes collapse of alveoli. Two major factors limit the amount of PEEP that we can apply: (i) the increase in intrathoracic pressure, to the extent it is transmitted to the mediastinum, will impede venous return; and (ii) the inspired tidal volume is administered on top of this baseline positive pressure, causing increased peak inflation pressure and possibly baro/volutrauma (lung damage from high pressures and/or volumes). CPAP, as the name implies, continues throughout the respiratory cycle, rather than only at exhalation, and is often applied through a mask to a spontaneously breathing patient with, for example, obstructive sleep apnea.

Anesthesia in the patient with pulmonary disease

Patients with lung disease arrive at respiratory patterns optimal for their condition. This can include the recruitment of auxiliary muscles and changes in inspiratory and expiratory flow rates, respiratory rate, and arterial carbon dioxide tension. Because anesthesia can disturb these delicate adjustments, many anesthesiologists prefer to resort to regional anesthesia, where practical. Two major issues must be considered, however:

(i) The potential respiratory effects of the intended regional anesthetic. For example, a thoracic-level epidural anesthetic block begins to compromise intercostal muscle activity, reduces FRC, limits the patient's ability to cough, and theoretically can stimulate bronchospasm by blocking dilatory sympathetic innervation to the bronchi. Some approaches to the brachial plexus (especially interscalene blocks) have a high incidence of unilateral phrenic nerve paralysis and an occasional pneumothorax. While the average patient can tolerate the loss of intercostal muscles, a "pulmonary cripple," who at rest uses accessory muscles to breathe, might be left with inadequate respiratory muscle strength.

(ii) The respiratory depressant effects of sedative medications might be accentuated in these patients. While it is preferable to attempt an anesthetic that avoids airway instrumentation, this preference turns into a liability if the need for emergent tracheal intubation arises should the patient slip into respiratory failure.

Asthma

The patient with well-controlled asthma should sail through general anesthesia without much difficulty. All asthma medications, and particularly steroids, should be continued pre-operatively. Nebulized albuterol (or another β_2 agonist) administered in the pre-operative holding area provides bronchodilation just before anesthesia. Because instrumentation of the airway can stimulate bronchospasm, patients with refractory asthma might benefit from anesthetic techniques that avoid airway manipulation, such as regional or local anesthesia with gentle intravenous

sedation. Should general anesthesia be required, several options for induction and airway management are available. A small dose of propofol (much better than thiopental in this population) can ease the patient to sleep, at which point one of the halogenated inhalation anesthetics can be slowly introduced. These agents are bronchodilators. Ketamine is a bronchodilator as well and may be used, provided its potential side effects can be accepted. A laryngeal mask airway (LMA) is a lesser stimulus to bronchospasm than an endotracheal tube. When tracheal intubation becomes necessary, the goal at induction will be to completely block the airway reflexes that stimulate bronchospasm. Intravenous lidocaine (0.5–1.0 mg/kg) can also prove helpful. Intravenous opioids (but perhaps not morphine, which tends to release histamine) can be used. But remember that some patients develop respiratory difficulties (earlier reported as a "stiff chest" but recently discovered to be from laryngospasm) in response to large doses of opioids, the treatment of which requires muscle relaxation.

Intra-operatively, warm and humidified gases can reduce bronchospasm. Mechanical ventilation requires consideration of the pulmonary pathology. Bronchospasm limits airflow rates and causes a prolonged expiratory phase. If we do not give enough time for exhalation, air will be trapped ("dynamic hyperinflation"), resulting in increased intrathoracic pressures. This "auto-PEEP" reduces venous return and cardiac output. A prolonged expiratory time allows for full exhalation. Simply lengthening the exhalation time steals time from inhalation, however, which in turn might require high inspiratory pressures (the same tidal volume must be given over a shorter time). Reducing the tidal volume and/or respiratory rate would help, but will necessarily reduce minute ventilation and introduce the potential for hypercarbia. "Permissive hypercapnia" can become necessary when minute ventilation cannot be maintained without risk of barotrauma (e.g., pneumothorax).

Because stimulation of the trachea can trigger bronchospasm, making sure the tube is not in contact with the carina is important and in some cases removal of the endotracheal tube may be best accomplished during deep anesthesia. This is only appropriate in patients at low risk for aspiration and obstruction of the upper airway. Prophylactic supplemental oxygen in the post-operative period can prevent hypoxia-induced airway reactivity.

Obstructive sleep apnea

Obstructive sleep apnea (OSA) occurs when the soft tissues of the pharynx collapse during sleep, obstructing the airway and resulting in hypoxemia. Sleep apnea plagues obese patients who snore heavily with intermittent bouts of obstruction to the point of apnea (reported by partner), desaturation (not reported by partner but determined in a sleep study), and repeated awakening. During the day, they are often somnolent. The apneic periods cause hypoxemia and hypercarbia, resulting in (i) cardiac irritability with bradycardia and premature ventricular contractions (PVCs), (ii) vasoconstriction, both peripherally (leading to increased systemic vascular resistance and chronic hypertension) and in the pulmonary circulation (with pulmonary hypertension and potentially right heart failure), and (iii) erythropoiesis (resulting in polycythemia in an effort to increase oxygen-carrying capacity). Because of the potential for thrombosis and unfavorable rheology, a polycythemic patient should be phlebotomized if the hematocrit is too high (>55%).

Should you obtain a history of OSA during the anesthesia pre-operative evaluation, you may have to order further studies including ECG and possibly echocardiogram to look for evidence of pulmonary hypertension and right heart compromise. In a subset of patients ("Pickwickians[11]"), ABG analysis might demonstrate daytime CO_2 retention with potentially impaired hypercarbic respiratory drive (this is the sort of patient who might experience decreased respiratory drive if you give supplemental oxygen to the point of normalizing the SpO_2). Therapeutic interventions include nasal CPAP during sleep, weight loss, and surgical correction. OSA patients are particularly sensitive to opioids and sedatives and we worry about airway obstruction with even low doses of respiratory depressants. We thus understandably like to keep them continuously monitored with a pulse oximeter postoperatively while administering parenteral narcotics. In fact, obstructive episodes cause us to delay by several hours their discharge to a ward setting. Finally, patients with excess pharyngeal tissue and obesity present difficulties with airway management. Not only can intubation be tough, we may be unable to mask–ventilate or even use an LMA. Thus ventilation may be very difficult to provide once we render the patient unconscious and paralyzed.

Pulmonary problems during anesthesia

Once the airway is secured, many things can still go wrong with the pulmonary system. Often – but not invariably – pulse oximetry gives the first signal of trouble:

(i) We have to provide oxygen into the airway. Problems arise when (inadvertently) another gas is substituted for oxygen, or when a mechanical problem affects the delivery mechanism (like failure to turn on the ventilator or disconnection of the ventilator from the breathing circuit).

(ii) We need to have adequate alveolar ventilation, i.e., tidal volumes in excess of deadspace. Problems include a kinked or plugged ETT, a leak somewhere (allowing the gas to vent to the atmosphere), bronchospasm, pneumothorax, a plug (mucus, blood, tissue, foreign body) in a bronchus, decreased lung compliance, increased intrathoracic pressure (as with insufflation of carbon dioxide into the abdomen for laparoscopy), mainstem intubation, or increased apparatus deadspace as from machine valve failure.

(iii) When the oxygen arrives at the alveolus, it has to be able to get into the bloodstream. Problems here include a diffusion block in the alveolus (pulmonary edema fluid), lack of blood flow to the alveolus (pulmonary embolism), or inability of the blood to pick up oxygen, e.g., carbon monoxide poisoning – though this would fool the SpO_2 into reporting normal saturation; see Chapter 7.

(iv) Finally, the oxygenated blood has to make it to the location of the pulse oximeter for analysis. Problems here would include dilution of the oxygenated blood with venous blood (shunt), flow blockade to the location of the pulse oximeter (distal to an inflated blood pressure cuff or tourniquet), presence of dyes that can alter the color of the blood (methylene blue), inaccurate probe placement (only partially on the finger), or failure of the oximeter probe itself.

So, in addition to calling for help:

(i)   Check FiO_2 (if unexpectedly low, disconnect from wall oxygen source and use oxygen from a cylinder or room air).

(ii) Increase FiO_2, e.g., turn off air or nitrous oxide, increase fresh gas flow with oxygen.

(iii) Check capnogram shape of $ETCO_2$ waveform – beyond confirming adequate gas exchange, the shape of the waveform provides information, e.g., lack of a plateau suggests uneven alveolar emptying as in bronchospasm, inspired CO_2 suggests absorbent depletion or valve failure.

(iv) Check pulse oximeter waveform and probe. Pulse oximeters are remarkably simple and robust devices. When they sound an alarm, we should reflexively believe them and seek a cause for the distress signal. But the devices can be fooled (e.g., some i.v. dyes, high-intensity infrared light from a frameless navigation system flooding the detector, or probe malposition). Reposition the probe only for an erroneous waveform or after eliminating the critical conditions as a cause.

(v)   Listen to breath sounds bilaterally – mainstem intubation? Pneumothorax? Inadvertent extubation?

(vi) Check peak inspiratory pressure – if low, there may be a leak, perhaps even at the level of the ETT cuff; if high, an obstruction somewhere between the ventilator and the alveoli such as a crimp or plug in the ETT, increased airway resistance, or decreased lung compliance.

  (a) Give several manual breaths – while it turns out that even "educated hands" cannot gauge compliance and resistance well, a few slow, deep manual breaths allow control over the pattern of inspiration, which may improve the situation. In fact, briefly sustained airway pressure at the peak of inspiration can facilitate recruitment of alveoli that may have become atelectatic. However, we must not tie our hands squeezing the bag, to the exclusion of handling other needs. Anesthesia machines and ventilators inflate lungs with aplomb.

  (b) Suction ETT – confirms patency and removes secretions.

  (c) Observe the capnogram – as noted above, a severely sloped waveform suggests uneven alveolar emptying (e.g., from bronchospasm).

  (d) Listen to breath sounds – if unilateral we suspect endobronchial tube placement or pneumothorax.

  (e) Look at the surgical field – compression of the thoracic cavity from abdominal retractors, high abdominal insufflation pressures, or sleepy medical students leaning on the patient's chest during a long case cause increased inspiratory pressures.

(vii) Check exhaled tidal volume (to ensure there is no leak and the majority of inhaled gas makes it back out the expiratory limb).

(viii) Consider obtaining an arterial blood gas and chest radiograph.

(ix)   PEEP – administering PEEP may improve the saturation, since often the cause is decreased FRC. Inspiratory pressures and/or venous return can constrain the level of PEEP tolerated.

Notes

1 In the presence of oxygen, cells metabolize glucose through the Krebs cycle and electron transport chain, netting 36 ATP. Without oxygen, glycolysis proceeds, but nets only 2 ATP and a bunch of lactic acid.

2 Adolph Eugen Fick (1829–1901), a German physician, physiologist, and physicist. He came up with this diffusion equation when just 26 years old! He is even more famous for describing the calculation of cardiac output still in use today (cardiac output = oxygen consumption/arterial-venous oxygen content difference).

3 $D = \dfrac{S}{\sqrt{MW}}$; S = solubility, MW = molecular weight.

4 $P_AO_2 = P_IO_2 - P_ACO_2 \times [FiO_2 + (1 - FiO_2)/R]$, which corrects for the fact that an $R < 1$ results in a lower volume of exhaled gas.

5 Lawrence Joseph Henderson (1878–1942) linked $[H^+]$ and buffers as $[H^+] = Ka([acid]/[salt])$; later Karl Albert Hasselbalch (1874–1962) coupled this with Søren Sørensen's pH scale to produce the now famous equation: $pH = pKa + \log([A^-]/[HA])$.

6 Albumin contributes the most to the gap. A fall in albumin concentration by 1 gram lowers the anion gap by 2.5–3 mmol/L. Thus hypoalbuminemia must be considered when calculating the anion gap.

7 This equation determines the missing bicarbonate (normal – actual), and its normal distribution in the extracellular fluid ($0.3 \times$ body weight in kg), then replaces only half that amount.

8 It is common to specify "room" air which, when dry, contains 20.947% oxygen, 78.084% nitrogen, 0.934% argon, and 0.033%

carbon dioxide. The rest is made up of – in decreasing concentrations – neon, helium, krypton, sulfur dioxide, methane (oops), hydrogen, nitrous oxide, xenon, ozone, nitrogen dioxide, iodine, carbon monoxide and ammonia. Medical compressed air often contains a little more carbon dioxide (up to 0.05%) than room air and trace amounts of oil (up to 0.5 g per cubic meter). Clinically these differences can be ignored.

9   Pregnant women lower their $PaCO_2$ to minimize any respiratory acidosis in their little angel (parasite, really). Thus a normal arterial blood gas in pregnancy includes pH 7.44, $PaCO_2$ 30 mmHg, HCO_3^- 20 mEq/L. This must be taken into account when interpreting a maternal ABG.

10   Oxygen cylinders contain gaseous oxygen under pressure to 2000 psi (pounds per square inch) or ~140 atm. They are painted green in the USA and white in much of Europe.

11   The term Pickwickian refers to a character in Charles Dickens' 1837 novel *The Posthumous Papers of the Pickwick Club*. The obese Joe suffers uncontrollable daytime sleepiness.

Anesthesia and other systems

If you are reading this, you are not a neurologist, gastro-enterologist, hepatologist, nephrologist, or hematologist. Yet, anesthesiologists need to worry about some features and functions of the stomach, liver, kidneys, blood, and particularly the brain. Here is a short perspective on the why and how.

The brain

General anesthesia is, ultimately, about putting the central nervous system (CNS) to sleep. We choose this or that agent in an effort to optimize the patient's intra-operative course, but in reality the nuances of the different agents make little difference a few days after minor surgery in a healthy patient. However, in the patient with intracranial pathology, a thorough understanding of neurophysiology and the implications of anesthesia take center stage. Because we do not know which patients have undiagnosed cerebral aneurysms or tumors, we like to apply our understanding to all patients.

The brain is an amazing organ. Despite weighing only about 1.3 kg, just 2% of total body weight, it receives 15% of the cardiac output, consumes 20% of the oxygen used by the body, and watches over it all! Formulating some mental models of this metabolic workhorse will help to explain its dynamic workings. Conveniently, the spinal cord behaves physiologically similarly to the brain.

Compared to other organs, cerebral hemodynamics have both similarities and unique features. Numerous factors affect the cerebral vascular system (Table 11.1). The brain autoregulates cerebral blood flow (CBF) to maintain it stable at cerebral perfusion pressures (CPP) between 65 mmHg and 150 mmHg. But similar to virtually all other organs, it also couples flow to metabolism to assure active areas of the brain receive enough oxygen and glucose to sustain their activities. The cerebral vascular network, curiously, has few alpha-1 receptors. This makes phenylephrine a preferred choice for correcting hypotension without constricting cerebral

Table 11.1. Effect of systemic and local factors on cerebrovascular resistance

Cerebral vasoconstriction is observed with:

Increased blood pressure (autoregulation)

Hyperoxia (PaO_2 >300 mmHg produces 12% decrease in CBF)

Decreased $PaCO_2$ (every 1 mmHg reduction in $PaCO_2$ decreases CBF 4%)

Decreased blood viscosity

Decreased cerebral metabolic demands:

    Barbiturates (decrease CBF up to 60% by producing isoelectric EEG)

    Lowered temperature

Cerebral vasodilatation is observed with:

Decreased blood pressure (autoregulation)

Increased $PaCO_2$

Increased blood viscosity

Hypoxia (PaO_2 <60 mmHg)

Vasodilators (nitroglycerin, nitroprusside)

Ketamine

Increased cerebral metabolic demands:

    Stress state

    Fever

Vessels surrounding brain tumors lose CO_2 responsiveness and remain maximally dilated

vessels. Opposite to the pulmonary artery's response, brain vascular responsiveness to hypercarbia causes vasodilatation while hypocarbia produces vasoconstriction and, in extreme cases, can produce cerebral ischemia.

The skull rigidly constrains the volume of the intracranial space and its three constituents: brain tissue (1100 g or mL), blood (75 mL), and cerebrospinal fluid (CSF, 150 mL). The falx cerebri divides the brain into a left and right hemisphere, while the tentorium

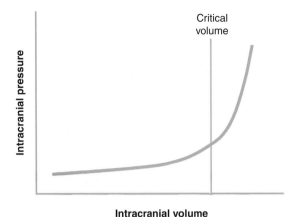

Fig. 11.1 Intracranial pressure with increasing intracranial volume. Initially, an increase in one constituent volume causes a decrease in another (increased tissue, e.g., tumor, causes decreased CSF). At the critical volume the compensatory mechanisms have been exhausted.

cerebelli separates the cerebellum from the rest. If any of the brain components increases in volume, either the others must shrink by a similar amount, or the intracranial pressure (ICP) increases (Fig. 11.1). This increased pressure may manifest as papilledema on fundoscopic examination of the eye, and as narrowed ventricles or midline shift on an imaging study. Clinical signs include nausea, vomiting, ataxia, altered mental status or the seldom seen Cushing's triad[1] of bradycardia, hypertension, and bradypnea.

Intracranial hypertension poses a significant threat. Because the brain has no stored oxygen, it withstands limited ischemic exposures only by increasing its blood flow or increasing oxygen extraction from hemoglobin. As the ICP increases beyond a critical point, blood flow to the brain decreases. A metabolic engine that uses only glucose (or ketones) and oxygen for energy, the brain spends 60% of its energy performing electrophysiologic functions and 40% preserving cellular integrity. Thus, defending cerebral perfusion and oxygen delivery are intrinsic to the anesthetic management of patients with intracranial masses and elevated ICP. As with all organs, perfusion depends on the pressure difference across the organ:

$$CPP = MAP - (CVP \text{ or } ICP)$$

where CPP is cerebral perfusion pressure; MAP, mean arterial pressure; CVP, central venous pressure; ICP, intracranial pressure (normal mean <15 mmHg). Thus CPP depends on both arterial blood pressure, and the higher of CVP or ICP.

When ICP continues to rise, the increasing pressure on the brain must eventually "pop off" into another area. This spontaneous decompression, termed "herniation," can occur via several routes: transtentorial, uncal, subfalcine, across the foramen magnum (tonsillar) or out of the skull, when a fracture offers an opening. Tonsillar herniation pushes the brainstem through the foramen magnum, a life-threatening emergency. Herniation is a critical event; beyond the implications of local ischemia (from which a recovery may be possible), the sheer forces of herniation produce irreparable mechanical disruption.

With general anesthesia, we aim to produce a sleeping, well perfused and oxygenated brain. Unfortunately we possess little information about actual brain function, and use surrogate data based on sound physiologic understanding. For example, we know that the EEG begins to demonstrate an ischemic pattern when the CBF decreases below about 20 mL/100 g brain/min, a reduction of over 50% from its normal 50 mL/100 g brain/min perfusion. Hence, hypotension in this setting must be treated even in the absence of cardiac ischemia.

In the presence of intracranial pathology, we intentionally address each of the intracerebral volumes to optimize the operative course: (1) We lower the brain blood volume by placing the patient in a slightly head-up position to facilitate venous drainage. Barbiturates given for induction cause an isoelectric EEG (always, but only briefly at standard doses) and a subsequent autoregulated decrease in CBF. We avoid ketamine and halothane because they increase CBF and dramatically increase ICP. We may induce mild hyperventilation to produce arterial vasoconstriction. (2) Under specific circumstances, we might have to remove CSF perioperatively via a ventriculostomy or spinal drain. (3) In the presence of edema or a large mass, we might use steroids and diuretics (mannitol and/or furosemide) to reduce the interstitial volume and, through oxygen free radical scavenging, protect the brain from ischemic insult. When confronted with a high ICP we must maintain CPP, for example by increasing the mean arterial pressure with phenylephrine, which can find no alpha receptors in the brain's blood vessels to interact with.

An aneurysm or arteriovenous malformation challenges us to maintain stable pressures across the vascular wall by balancing the ICP against the MAP. We might lower temperature when we anticipate regional ischemic events, as can occur when temporary clips

Table 11.2. Methods to reduce intracranial pressure

- Hyperventilation – in the short term, hyperventilation to a $PaCO_2$ of 25 mmHg can reduce cerebral blood flow, reducing ICP. This must be balanced, however, against the increased intrathoracic pressure required to hyperventilate the patient's lungs, which can reduce venous return causing hypotension. Meanwhile vasoconstriction in the areas under carbon dioxide control might decrease compensatory blood flow.

- Mannitol – bolus administration of this 6-carbon sugar has three effects: (i) it expands the blood volume and decreases viscosity, improving cerebral blood flow; (ii) it generates an osmotic gradient in the brain, drawing water out of brain tissue; and (iii) it scavenges oxygen free radicals. The net effect – an acute reduction in ICP. However, the subsequent diuresis can exacerbate hypovolemia, and in the presence of poor renal perfusion the high osmolality can trigger acute tubular necrosis.

- Elevating the head of the bed and keeping the neck in a neutral position – these simple maneuvers can reduce ICP. Head elevation can also impair venous return from the lower extremities. Trauma patients are often placed in Trendelenburg position (with the head below the level of the legs) to increase venous return, a maneuver best avoided in patients with high ICP.

- Fluid management – hypotonic solutions and those containing glucose clearly worsen neurologic outcome by encouraging brain swelling. With an intact blood–brain barrier, hypertonic solutions might provide an advantage by *reducing* brain swelling.

- Glucocorticoids – these drugs reduce edema associated with brain tumors and are also used by many for the treatment of acute spinal cord injury; but steroids do not reduce edema from traumatic brain injuries.

- Hypothermia – oxygen consumption depends on temperature (in the absence of shivering, basal metabolic rate falls by 7% per 1°C of temperature reduction). But hypothermia raises other problems: the patient might shiver, which dramatically raises oxygen consumption; coagulation is profoundly disturbed, which can worsen intracerebral hemorrhage; arrhythmias can be triggered with temperatures below 30°C; and wound infections become slightly more likely.

- Barbiturate coma – reserved for the most severely injured who have failed to respond to more conservative therapy; high barbiturate plasma levels reduce cerebral metabolic rate and cerebral blood flow thus lowering ICP until the injury can heal. Unfortunately, barbiturates depress the cardiovascular system.

- CSF drainage – after a ventriculostomy has been placed, we can readily reduce the CSF volume. Care must be taken in the presence of brain swelling and elevated ICP, however, as draining CSF from a lumbar tap can result in brain herniation into the foramen magnum. Hence the admonition to look for clinical signs and symptoms of elevated ICP before performing a lumbar puncture or neuraxial anesthetic.

are placed to facilitate definitive aneurysm clipping. Otherwise, we strive to keep patients warm. The potent inhalational anesthetics all uncouple metabolism-flow autoregulation, causing a decreased metabolic rate but increasing the CBF. Hence, we use the halogenated vapors in modest concentrations during intracranial vascular surgery.

Consider how one might approach a trauma patient with both arterial hypotension and increased ICP from a subdural hematoma (SDH). We will work feverishly to increase his MAP but must also reduce ICP (Table 11.2). We treat low blood pressure in a trauma patient with the infusion of fluids and, as mentioned above, intravenous phenylephrine. In addition to CPP, arterial oxygen and carbon dioxide tensions affect CBF and therefore ICP (Fig. 11.2). We might acutely manipulate $PaCO_2$ in an effort to reduce ICP in the short term; however, aggressive hyperventilation to decrease ICP can worsen outcome, probably by decreasing CBF.

Until the last decade of the twentieth century, the brain remained an organ that could not be easily monitored. We had to be guided by changes in heart rate, blood pressure, urine output, and the patient's motor responses. Today, we monitor raw and processed EEG, e.g., BIS®, to aid us in titrating our drugs, avoiding and treating cerebral ischemia, and reducing intra-operative awareness.

The stomach

The stomach should ideally be empty before we give general anesthesia because regurgitating or vomiting and then, because of obtunded reflexes, inhaling the stuff found in the stomach can lead to serious trouble. The aspirated particulate matter can lodge

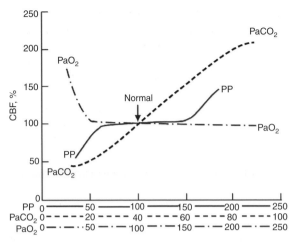

Fig. 11.2 Cerebral blood flow in a changing environment. Cerebral blood flow (CBF) responds to changes in perfusion pressure (PP = MAP – [ICP or CVP]), as well as arterial oxygen (PaO₂) and carbon dioxide (PaCO₂) tensions. MAP: mean arterial pressure; ICP: intracranial pressure; CVP: central venous pressure.

in a distal bronchus causing harm both immediately (shunt) and long term (post-obstruction pneumonia or lung abscess). A large particle can block a main-stem bronchus or the trachea with obvious dire consequences. Even in the OR, a patient can be treated with the Heimlich maneuver. Given an unconscious patient and the worry about more regurgitation and aspiration, tools such as a bronchoscope and suction available in the OR might be better suited for retrieval of foreign matter in the trachea or upper bronchial tree.

More common than particulate aspiration is the aspiration of gastric juice. If it has a pH under 2.5 and a volume of more than 0.4–1.0 mL/kg, the aspirate can cause the infamous Mendelson[2] syndrome, a nasty chemical burn of the lungs that can be fatal. Treatment consists of support of oxygenation and ventilation, often with positive end-expiratory pressure (PEEP) to expand the bronchioles and alveoli, reduce edema, and improve gas exchange.

The fearsome potential of gastric acid aspiration leads us to take precautions. The idea of emptying the stomach with help of a gastric tube comes to mind. While it might decompress a full stomach by removing gas and liquid, it cannot *empty* the stomach and is rather poorly tolerated in the awake patient. For elective surgery, we ask patients to take nothing by mouth for several hours before anesthesia. We also have drugs available to increase gastric pH and reduce volume as indicated. Even with such preparations, for patients with a full stomach or frank gastroesophageal reflux, we resort to a rapid-sequence induction (see Chapter 5).

The liver

We expect this large organ to do its biotransformation magic on many of the drugs we give. For example, the liver avidly removes propofol, which is said to have a hepatic extraction ratio (HER) of close to 1. Reduced liver blood flow will, therefore, reduce the rate of propofol biotransformation. The rate of biotransformation of drugs with a low HER, such as thiopental, will be less affected by changes in liver blood flow. Remember that the liver normally receives about 25% of cardiac output, roughly two-thirds of that via the low-pressure portal system, the rest by way of the hepatic artery delivering oxygenated blood. General anesthesia tends to reduce cardiac output and, proportionally, hepatic arterial blood flow more than portal blood flow. The hepatic circulation is also richly supplied with alpha receptors; hence the administration of alpha active vasopressors will reduce hepatic blood flow. Because of the enormous reserves of the liver, we rarely see the consequences of reduced liver blood supply. Even in the face of mild to moderate hepatic failure, the liver attends to its biotransformation job. There are limits, however, to what even the most faithful of livers can accomplish.

Liver enzymes

The liver attacks many drugs with mixed function oxidases of which the cytochrome P450 system represents a well-known member. In this first phase of hepatic biotransformation, drugs may be degraded to ineffective compounds (e.g., the benzodiazepines and barbiturates) or to active substances (e.g., meperidine becomes normeperidine). In the second phase, drugs undergo conjugation, often leading to more water-soluble compounds prepared for renal elimination.

When drugs such as ethanol, anti-seizure medications or barbiturates stimulate the production of enzymes, we speak of enzyme induction, which often affects one or more of the isoforms of the P450 system. With more enzyme available, the biotransformation of some drugs will be accelerated, leading to greater tolerance and reduced drug effect. Some drugs, such as cimetidine, can inhibit the P450 system and thus enhance the effect of drugs dependent on the system's detoxifying activity.

Liver function studies

We assess liver function by searching for liver enzymes spilled into the blood. We often ask the simple question: is the patient's hepatic disease brought about by biliary obstruction (elevated bilirubin and alkaline phosphatase) or hepatocellular dysfunction (prolonged prothrombin time, low plasma albumin, and elevated SGOT and SGPT)?[3]

Halothane hepatitis

Soon after halothane was introduced in the late 1950s, concerns arose about a new entity called halothane hepatitis. Several case reports described sometimes fatal acute hepatitis in patients exposed to the drug. In the meantime, other halogenated anesthetics have also been implicated. Suspicion was directed at the potentially toxic effects of the products of biotransformation of the halogenated vapors, particularly if they arose during hypoxic conditions. Because patients repeatedly exposed to the drug appeared to have a higher incidence of "halothane hepatitis," a sensitivity reaction was suspected. However, uncounted patients had many repeated halothane anesthetics without ill effect. Many investigators believe that most cases of so-called halothane hepatitis have nothing to do with the anesthetic agent and are instead evidence of a post-operative recrudescence of viral hepatitis. Others think that the products of anaerobic biotransformation, particularly those involving fluoride (trifluoroacetic acid), can cause trouble in sensitive patients. As of this writing halothane has disappeared from the USA but remains popular elsewhere due to its bargain price.

The kidneys

The kidneys concern us when drugs or their products of biotransformation need to be eliminated in urine. For this route out of the body, the substances must be non-protein-bound so they can slip through the glomeruli, then they must become ionized so as to escape tubular reabsorption.

Impaired renal function becomes relevant with advancing years (creatinine clearance declines with age), with low cardiac output and decreased glomerular filtration, and with renal disease. The elimination of some drugs can be affected by decreased renal function. Of greatest interest to the anesthesiologist are a number of muscle relaxants such as pancuronium and doxacurium and their antagonist, neostigmine. Thus for patients in renal failure, we might elect atracurium or cisatracurium, muscle relaxants that undergo hydrolysis in plasma, making them independent of renal excretion.

Patients in renal failure present special challenges not only because they cannot eliminate drugs in urine, but also because their water and electrolyte balance goes through roller-coaster swings with intermittent dialysis. Ideally, the patient should have undergone dialysis the day before the anesthetic. Intra-operatively we manage intravenous fluids carefully, as the patient has no mechanism to eliminate excess water or electrolytes. These patients tend to be somewhat anemic with a reduced oxygen-carrying capacity, which puts an extra burden on the heart should it be called on to increase cardiac output to compensate for reduced delivery of oxygen to the tissues. Vascular access is often a problem in patients with arteriovenous fistulas.

In patients at risk of major changes of renal perfusion (operations with anticipated great blood loss, cardiac insufficiency, vascular procedures affecting renal blood flow or ureteral function), we often monitor urine with the help of an indwelling urinary catheter (Foley). We consider normal a urine flow of at least 0.5 mL/kg/h, though renal failure may occur at even higher rates of urine output, and often enough, patients make less urine intra-operatively without sliding into acute renal failure or tubular necrosis. After all, complex physiologic mechanisms enable the kidney to reduce urine production and to conserve blood volume. ADH (antidiuretic hormone, also known as vasopressin), whose job it is to retain fluid in the face of hypovolemia, is secreted during anesthesia even without the normal triggers. Regardless, if fluid deficits cannot account for reduced urine production, and there is no reason to assume reduced kidney blood flow, for example secondary to hypotension or low cardiac output or because of mechanical interference with renal blood flow, and we confirm the Foley catheter is intact (not kinked or compressed), we begin to worry about acute tubular damage, for which a number of direct- or indirect-acting toxins (including antibiotics, chemotherapeutic agents, and contrast dyes) can be responsible. Acute tubular damage, if not too severe, can undergo spontaneous repair over days to weeks.

The blood

Three functions of the blood demand attention: its volume, its oxygen-carrying capacity, and its ability or propensity to clot. More information is available in the chapter on vascular access and fluid management (Chapter 3).

Volume

Blood volume varies with age, weight, and sex (see Chapter 3). As we know from donating blood, the average adult can easily lose 500 mL without conspicuous consequences. Indeed, healthy patients can readily tolerate a blood loss of 20% of their total blood volume. The body compensates for such loss by mobilizing interstitial and eventually even intracellular water to replenish the decreased intravascular volume. In the process, the hematocrit will fall gradually over a couple of days.

Oxygen-carrying capacity

With a loss of blood volume, the patient also loses oxygen-carrying capacity. Compensatory increases in cardiac output can insure uninterrupted delivery of oxygen, even in the anemic patient. As hematocrit decreases to about 30%, fluidity of blood increases, which improves flow and thus aids in the delivery of a higher cardiac output. There are limits to how much anemia can be tolerated. If the anemia develops over weeks or months, astonishingly low hematocrit values can be compatible with an active life, though the patient will have to deal with easy fatigability. Thus, we cannot with confidence identify a certain hematocrit value that compels us to administer red cells. The idea that a hematocrit below 30% would lead us to administer packed cells has long been abandoned; even 18% is now often accepted. Instead of picking a threshold at which we would call for a transfusion, we take many factors into account. We might merely watch an anemic patient with a good cardiovascular system and normal CNS and renal function, while the same hematocrit in a patient with congestive failure and arrhythmias or confusion signals an urgent need to increase oxygen-carrying capacity. Generally, we expect a single transfusion (450 mL packed cells) to increase the hematocrit by 3 volume % in the average adult.

Clotting

Like everything in life, too much of a good thing can be as bad as not enough. Thus, we find ourselves time and again in the position of interfering with the clotting mechanism to prevent thrombosis, or stimulating the system when the patient is at risk of bleeding into vital organs. To approach this problem in a rational manner, we need to recapitulate the normal clotting cascade. We will not delve into the details that fascinate hematologists and instead focus on specific points of common interest to anesthesiologists.

The normal clotting mechanism prevents uncounted (and unnoticed) bleeding opportunities in everyday life. This normal clotting mechanism is extraordinarily complex with a dizzying array of factors and steps, the most important to anesthesia being the following:

Platelets

Normally we have 150 000 to 450 000 platelets/microL. Surgical bleeding becomes a problem with counts below 50 000/microL, and spontaneous bleeding occurs below 20 000/microL. In patients with thrombocytopenia, we can increase the platelet count by 5000 to 10 000/microL with every platelet "unit" transfused, necessitating multiple units in most patients (order 1 unit/10 kg body weight). Platelets have a limited survival of up to 5 days if properly stored. Note that, unless specifically requested, platelets are "random donor pooled", meaning the patient is exposed to MANY donors at once with platelet transfusions. In contrast, one single donor pheresis unit is equivalent to about 6 units of pooled platelets.

Calcium

Calcium plays a crucial role in the clotting cascade (where it is honored as factor IV). In stored blood, the calcium is bound up and deactivated by citrate. With massive (equivalent to an entire blood volume or more) and rapid blood transfusion, the liver may not be able to keep up the metabolism of calcium citrate. Plasma citrate can rise and interfere with calcium's function as a coagulation factor. Citrate intoxication will also cause hypotension, cardiac depression, and prolonged QT intervals.

Congenital hemorrhagic diseases

- von Willebrand's disease is the most common inherited bleeding disorder. It comes in various degrees of severity and is associated with a decreased or qualitatively abnormal von Willebrand's factor (VIII: vWF).

- Classic hemophilia (A), a genetic disease affecting males, is a factor VIII deficiency. Patients often suffer hemarthroses and have hematuria.
- Hemophilia B or Christmas disease clinically resembles hemophilia A but is caused by a deficiency of factor IX.

Before anesthesia, these patients are treated with specific drugs, e.g., desmopressin (DDAVP[4®]) for von Willebrand's disease, or factor transfusion.

Heparin

The drug exhibits a medley of effects resulting in the inhibition of thrombin. Heparin is frequently given in the OR when coagulation must be stopped – as in vascular and cardiovascular procedures. In small subcutaneous doses, it is given to patients at risk for perioperative thrombosis. We measure the effect of heparin with the activated partial thromboplastin time (aPTT) and reverse it with the administration of protamine, a highly positively charged molecule that binds the negatively charged heparin. Of note, the effect of low-molecular-weight heparins (LMWH, e.g., enoxaparin) cannot be assayed by aPTT, and is not completely reversed by protamine.

Warfarin-type agents

These oral anticoagulants inhibit vitamin K-dependent factors (II, VII, IX, and X). Their activity is assayed by the prothrombin time (PT-INR [see below]), with a therapeutic range of 1.5–4 times normal. These agents can be reversed by the administration of vitamin K, or acutely by transfusing fresh frozen plasma (FFP).

Coagulation studies

The coagulation status of a patient can be assessed clinically: is there evidence of bleeding (bloody urine, black stools (blood in upper GI tract), bleeding gums and/or easy bruising)? There are several laboratory tests to evaluate the clotting cascade.

Prothrombin time (PT)

This tests the extrinsic coagulation cascade and is prolonged when tissue factors are involved. Because there are differences between labs, an international normalized ratio (INR) has been adopted, with a normal value of 1.0.

Activated partial thromboplastin time (aPTT, normally 25–40 s)

This tests the intrinsic pathway of coagulation and almost all the factors except VII and XIII. We use this test to monitor unfractionated heparin activity.

Activated clotting time (ACT, normally <120 s)

This is commonly used in the OR to test therapeutic heparin anticoagulation, e.g., during cardiopulmonary bypass or vascular surgery. We mix 2 mL of the patient's blood in a test tube containing an activator of coagulation, such as celite (diatomaceous earth), kaolin, or glass particles. We then stir the blood and monitor the time to clot formation. An ACT >200 s indicates adequate anticoagulation for vascular procedures and ACT >450 s enables cardiopulmonary bypass. Note ACT is not a good monitor for lesser levels of heparin anticoagulation, e.g., deep venous thrombosis (DVT) prophylaxis.

The thromboelastogram (TEG)

This is used much less frequently. A clever machine scrutinizes the whole clotting process by analyzing the patient's blood in an oscillating cup as it clots around a piston. Developing fibrin between cup and piston transmits the oscillations, which are then recorded. As the clot forms, the device records the transmitted oscillations, assuming the shape of a bomb (no fins!) in a normally clotting patient. Abnormal clotting because of the presence of anticoagulants or thrombocytopenia or fibrinolysis causes the bomb to look spindly or skinny, or leaf-shaped. Cognoscenti can read these shapes like a book. If you are not in that league you can find interactive details and pictures in: www.anest.ufl.edu/EA.

We detail replacement of clotting factors in Chapter 3.

Notes

1 Harvey Williams Cushing (1869–1939), an American pioneer in neurosurgery, also lends his name to several syndromes with CNS pathology, a surgical clip, and even an ulcer.

2 Curtis Mendelson, MD, an obstetrician/gynecologist and, later, cardiologist, described and studied gastric acid aspiration, pioneering translational research, improved preparation of patients for cesarean delivery (NPO), preferential

use of regional anesthesia in obstetrics, and the employ of anesthesiologists to handle airways. He accomplished all this before the age of 46, at which time he retired to a tiny Caribbean island where he served as the sole physician and veterinarian.

3   SGOT is serum glutamic-oxaloacetic transaminase, also known as AST = serum aspartate aminotransaminase. SGPT is serum glutamic-pyruvic transaminase, also known as ALT = serum alanine aminotransaminase.

4   DDAVP = 1-deamino-8-D-arginine vasopressin, also known as desmopressin.

Chapter

12

A brief pharmacology related to anesthesia

Approaching the anesthesia task with drugs

The basic approach

Many different approaches to general anesthesia are possible. Often, pre-operative preparation includes the administration of drugs to (i) minimize the chance of aspiration of gastric juice, (ii) minimize anxiety, and (iii) provide analgesia, immediate and/or planning ahead for subsequent need. Once the patient is in the operating room, we aim to denitrogenate the patient's lungs, followed by induction of anesthesia. One technique is to induce sleep with propofol, give a paralyzing dose of succinylcholine to facilitate intubation of the trachea, and then maintain anesthesia with a halogenated anesthetic vapor administered together with nitrous oxide and, of course, oxygen. Muscle relaxation during the operation might be accomplished with one of the non-depolarizing neuromuscular junction blockers, frequently called "muscle relaxants." Another technique might start with etomidate instead of propofol and it might rely on large doses of an opiate, such as fentanyl and, to assure amnesia, a low concentration of a halogenated inhalation anesthetic. Many different combinations of these approaches are in use.

At the end of anesthesia and if the patient is still weakened from the muscle relaxant, the neuromuscular blockade has to be reversed with, for example, neostigmine given together with an anticholinergic drug. When the patient responds to commands and meets extubation criteria, we remove the endotracheal tube and return the patient to the post-anesthesia care unit (PACU).

Drug interaction

The practice of anesthesia involves the administration of several drugs, some of them with overlapping effects. For example, premedication with midazolam (Versed®,

a benzodiazepine) will make the patient more sensitive to the side effects of narcotic analgesics; neuromuscular blockade can be more readily achieved if the patient is in surgical anesthesia from a halogenated vapor than if anesthesia relies on nitrous oxide and narcotics. The degree of surgical stimulation will influence the patient's response to anesthetic drugs. During a small-bowel anastomosis, which does not represent major noxious stimulation, less anesthesia will be required than when stimulating the carina with a suction catheter, for example. An elderly or debilitated or abstentious patient will require less depressant drug for the same effect than a young and vigorous person accustomed to regular alcohol intake, or a redhead – really. Drugs that undergo biotransformation with the help of enzymes that had been induced may have a shorter duration of action (some barbiturates) or more side effects, e.g., halothane biotransformation liberating hepatotoxins, than in the absence of induced enzymes. Repeated exposure to a drug can induce marked tolerance to the medication, as is well known for narcotics. In other words, our brief discussion of pharmacology cannot cover all factors that might influence the patient's response to a cited dose.

In this chapter, we will look at the drugs typically used in anesthesia. First, however, a word about the theories of anesthesia.

Theories of anesthesia

Please note that we are speaking of theories (in the plural!). This simply reflects the fact that a single theory could not possibly explain the phenomenon of induced coma: there are simply too many different substances (and events) that can render a person reversibly unconscious. In some instances, we can imagine a mechanism; for example, lack of oxygen will stop the functioning of cells dependent on oxygen. But then think of a knock on the head, very high or low blood sugar, alcohol, sleeping pills, noble gases (xenon), inorganic gases (nitrous oxide), acetone, organic solvents such as chloroform, carbon tetrachloride, trichlorethylene, ethylene, diethyl ether, and a slew of halogenated compounds, not to mention narcotics, benzodiazepines, barbiturates, steroids, phenols, etc. To complicate matters, one fluorinated hydrocarbon, hexafluorodiethyl ether, is a convulsant (in the past used instead of electroconvulsant therapy in the treatment of depression) while several of its close relatives (isoflurane, desflurane, sevoflurane) are in common use as anesthetics. Isoflurane and enflurane are isomers, both being di-fluoromethyl-trifluorochloroethyl-ether (see formulae below) but, despite their close relationship, only enflurane can sometimes elicit minor convulsive motions. The same yin–yang kinship exists among barbiturates, which can be turned into convulsants with a chemist's sleight of hand.

Investigators of the mechanism by which drugs produce reversible coma have focused on the cell membrane where lipids and proteins can be affected by substances that alter the wonderful order of these complex structures. Some theorists stress the lipid solubility (think grease stain removers) of anesthetics, others their ability to insinuate themselves in the intricate ways proteins coil up and trap water. Some anesthetics may work by changing the membrane, expanding it, altering its fluidity, and by one or the other or a combination of effects changing cell membrane function and responses to transmitter substances. Many of the organic intravenous drugs, such as propofol, barbiturates, and the benzodiazepines, appear to increase the inhibitory action of GABA receptors, while opiates have their Greek alphabet of receptors (see below). From all of this, it must be apparent that we really do not understand all that much about reversibly induced coma or indeed about consciousness itself.

Pharmacologic preparation for anesthesia[1]

Reduce the risk of aspiration (Table 12.1)

The aspiration of acidic gastric juice can lead to a nasty chemical burn of the trachea and bronchi and to bronchospasm and pneumonitis and, potentially, to death. We aim to reduce gastric volume and limit acidity. Gastric juice with a pH of 2.5 or less causes dangerous chemical burns when aspirated. We have several methods to reduce the hazards of aspiration of acidic juice:

(i) Buffer the gastric acid with an antacid. Many different agents are available. We prefer a non-particulate liquid, which not only mixes more readily in the stomach but also causes less harm when aspirated than would be true for a particulate antacid. Sodium citrate (trisodium citrate) or Bicitra® (sodium citrate and citric acid) – which are liquid – find common use in anesthesia. We give 15–30 mL by mouth within 30 minutes before induction of anesthesia.

(ii) Enhance gastric emptying. Metoclopramide (Reglan®) works both locally – acetylcholine-like and thus enhancing lower esophageal sphincter tone, gastric motility, and emptying – and centrally as a dopaminergic blocker. We do not know how much the CNS action contributes to the desired GI effect, but we do know that the drug can cause undesirable CNS effects, including extrapyramidal symptoms; it might contribute to early post-operative delirium.

(iii) Inhibit gastric secretion. We have several drugs that antagonize H_2 receptors and thus inhibit secretion of gastric acid. While they start working rapidly, they do not affect the acid already in the stomach. We prefer to administer these agents an hour before anesthesia. Proton pump inhibitors (among them omeprazole [Prilosec®], esomeprazole [Nexium®] and pantoprazole [Protonix®]) can also reduce gastric acidity. Because of their slow onset of action (hours), proton pump inhibitors are not routinely prescribed as antacids in anesthesia.

Reduce anxiety (Table 12.2)

Benzodiazepines

To allay fear and induce antegrade amnesia, many patients receive a benzodiazepine before induction of anesthesia. Several different benzodiazepines are on the market. Prominent among them are diazepam (Valium®) and midazolam (Versed®); the latter is about three times as potent as diazepam.

In most adults, small (1–2 mg) intravenous doses of midazolam produce not only a calming effect, but also antegrade amnesia. The effect sets in over 2–3 minutes. Benzodiazepines work through GABA receptors, much like alcohol, and therefore, those who are not alcohol-naïve might require additional doses. However, we separate the doses by at least 5 minutes

Table 12.1. Gastrointestinal drugs

Class and agent	Trade name	Dose	Comments
Antacid			
Sodium citrate		p.o.: 15–30 mL	Immediately neutralizes stomach acid
H₂ blockers i.v. at least 1 h before induction			
Cimetidine	Tagamet®	p.o.: 400 mg i.v.: 300 mg	More side effects than alternatives
Famotidine	Pepcid®	p.o./i.v.: 20 mg	
Ranitidine	Zantac®	p.o.: 150 mg i.v.: 50 mg	
Pro-kinetic			
Metoclopramide	Reglan®	p.o./i.v.: 10 mg	Dopamine antagonist to enhance gastric emptying and increase LES pressure

LES: lower esophageal sphincter.

Table 12.2. Anxiolytics

Agent	Trade name	i.v. dose	Duration	Comments
Diazepam	Valium®	2–10 mg	2–6 hours	Slow i.v.; anticonvulsant, sedative
Lorazepam	Ativan®	1–2 mg	6–8 hours	Sedative
Midazolam	Versed®	0.5–5 mg	2–6 hours	Amnestic
Benzodiazepine antagonist				
Flumazenil	Romazicon®	0.2–1 mg	60–90 min	Risk of seizures; benzodiazepine withdrawal
Non-benzodiazepine sedative				
Dexmedetomidine	Precedex®	0.2–0.7 mcg/kg/h	Infusion	Some analgesia; maintain ventilation; expensive

to avoid drug-induced respiratory depression and even apnea. The elimination half-life is about 3 hours. Midazolam can reduce the incidence of recall of intra-operative events.

Midazolam has also been used to induce anesthesia. We slowly administer 0.2–0.3 mg/kg intravenously, and anticipate respiratory depression. Even in small doses, e.g., 1 mg for the average adult, the drug serves as a good anticonvulsant.

As with all CNS active drugs, we use great care for fear of drug interaction, as may occur at the extremes of age or in the debilitated patient.

Flumazenil (Romazicon®) antagonizes the effects of benzodiazepines (see Table 12.2). When we wish to reverse a slight excess sedation before or during anesthesia (e.g., during a simple sedation anesthetic) or perhaps to reverse a residual effect produced by synergism with opioids post-operatively, we titrate flumazenil, starting with 0.2 mg given slowly i.v. and not more than a total of 1 mg for the average adult. In case of midazolam-induced respiratory depression, we manually ventilate the patient's lungs rather than start with an antagonist. Flumazenil can trigger convulsions in patients poisoned with tricyclic antidepressant overdose or chronically on high doses of benzodiazepines.

Dexmedetomidine (Precedex®)

Dexmedetomidine stimulates α_2-adrenoreceptors in areas of the brainstem (locus coeruleus) and spinal cord producing a remarkable (and unique) constellation of sedation, analgesia, anxiolysis, and sympatholysis all without much respiratory depression. Its short

129

Table 12.3. Anti-emetics

Agent	Trade name	i.v. dose	Comments
Droperidol	Inapsine®	0.625 mg	Butyrophenone; dopamine antagonist, anxiolytic
Promethazine	Phenergan®	25 mg	Phenothiazine
Ondansetron	Zofran®	4 mg	Serotonin blocker
Granisetron	Kytril®	1 mg	Serotonin blocker
Dolasetron	Anzemet®	12.5 mg	Serotonin blocker

6-minute context-sensitive half-life[2] makes dexmedetomidine infusions a popular choice for many applications such as awake craniotomy, awake intubation, radiological exams, and intensive care unit sedation – but not exceeding 24 hours.

Dexmedetomidine is a more potent sedative than analgesic and when used in surgery, it is usually necessary to supplement with small doses of narcotic. Despite its wide therapeutic index, cases of profound hypotension, bradycardia, asystole, intra-operative recall, and increased anxiety with bolus and infusions have been described. Airway obstruction can also occur as sedation deepens, even as ventilatory drive remains nearly unaffected. Acquisition costs remain prohibitive for many economy-minded facilities.

Prevent nausea and vomiting (Table 12.3)

Even though modern anesthesia techniques have decreased the frequency of early post-operative nausea and vomiting, these two disagreeable complications still trouble patients greatly. A number of drugs help to suppress or minimize the occurrence.

Droperidol (Inapsine®)

This butyrophenone is a dopamine antagonist. It has been around for nearly 50 years and has been used extensively during anesthesia and for the prevention or treatment of nausea and vomiting. We start with 0.625 mg i.v. to the average adult. The question has been raised whether it would be justifiable to give droperidol prophylactically, which would mean giving it to many patients who would not have developed nausea and vomiting. Such across-the-board prophylaxis can only be defended when the drug adds little cost and poses no risk but offers considerable benefits. Droperidol is inexpensive and offers the benefits, but not without risks. In 2001 the FDA published a warning implicating droperidol in the prolongation of the QT interval (normal between 0.38 s and 0.42 s, with fast or slow heart rates, respectively). It quoted studies describing patients who developed widening QT intervals exceeding 0.45 s and ending in torsade de pointes, a malignant arrhythmia. Many drugs have been shown to prolong the QT interval, more frequently in women than men. The list includes (but is not limited to) amiodarone, cisapride, erythromycin, ondansetron, sevoflurane, quinidine, and sotalol. We must be particularly concerned in patients with existing prolongation of the QT interval. We mention the worry about QT prolongation even though in anesthesia a dangerous prolongation of QT intervals had not been linked to droperidol. However, the issue raised by the FDA has caused considerable discussion in anesthesia circles.

Droperidol has other side effects that may be quite troublesome, if not lethal. Very few patients develop extrapyramidal symptoms, others a feeling of terror which they cannot express. Due to the concerns about droperidol's side effects and our inability to reliably identify patients in whom the drug may pose an additional risk, it is no longer the recommended drug of first choice for treatment of nausea.

Serotonin receptor blockers

Among these are ondansetron (Zofran®), granisetron (Kytril®), and dolasetron (Anzemet®). These serotonin receptor blockers have found use in patients undergoing chemotherapy and in the prevention of nausea and vomiting post-operatively. Fortunately, these agents are not burdened with a list of disagreeable side effects (unless you count their cost!) – other than constipation in 11% of patients, something of concern to patients undergoing chemotherapy, and even less frequent headaches and elevated liver enzymes. A 40–60% efficacy rate along with a tolerable side-effect profile have made this class of anti-emetics the new recommended first-choice therapy.

Table 12.4. Intravenous anesthetics

Agent	i.v. induction dose	$T_{1/2}$ elim.	Pros	Cons
Etomidate	0.2–0.5 mg/kg	2–5 h	Minimal CV depression	Lowers seizure threshold; pain on injection; myoclonus; inhibits steroid synthesis
Ketamine	1–2 mg/kg i.m.: 5–10 mg/kg	1–2 h	Maintain ventilation and airway reflexes; excellent analgesia; does not blunt sympathetic nervous system	Dissociative anesthesia → hallucinations; increased salivation; hypertension/tachycardia
Methohexital	1–2 mg/kg	4 h	Short half-life oxybarbiturate	Lowers seizure threshold; myoclonus
Propofol	1–2.5 mg/kg	0.5–1.5 h	Anti-emetic; short half-life, great for conscious sedation (25–75 mcg/kg/min) and TIVA (50–200 mcg/kg/min)	Pain on injection; no analgesia; culture medium for bacteria; rare propofol infusion syndrome[3]
Thiopental	2–5 mg/kg	12 h	Reliable, inexpensive	Long elimination half-life; histamine release

Intravenous anesthetics (Table 12.4)

Barbiturates

The drugs with the longest history of intravenous use in anesthesia are the barbiturates. While many different barbiturates have been synthesized and used, the drugs most commonly found in current anesthesia practice are thiopental (Pentothal®) and methohexital (Brevital®). These drugs share the basic barbituric acid foundation (Fig. 12.1), which by itself has no CNS depressant effect. Substitutions on position 5 give us pentobarbital, a slow- and long-acting hypnotic. Simply substituting sulfur for the oxygen on position 2 turns the drug into the highly lipid soluble, fast-acting thiopental.

After an intravenous thiopental bolus, e.g., 4 mg/kg, the patient falls asleep in less than a minute and comes around again within a few more minutes. The drug owes its rapid onset of effect to the S= substitution on position 2 and to the fact that the "vessel rich group" (tissues with a high blood flow; especially the brain) gets the first lion's share of the drug. Then the other body compartments pick up more and more drug during the distribution phase, and brain levels fall off rapidly (see Fig. 12.2). For an animated mental model of this type of drug distribution, see a simulation for a muscle relaxant; the depicted principle applies to other drugs (www.anest.ufl.edu/EA).

You will appreciate that much drug not contributing to the primary and desired drug effect lingers in other body compartments. The drug in these "silent" compartments will trickle back into the circulation and the brain for a hangover effect. Eventually, all of the drug will undergo biotransformation and excretion, but the elimination half-life of thiopental is about 12 hours. Some of the biotransformation will convert the drug back into an oxybarbiturate (O= instead of S= in position 2), reducing lipid solubility and extending the depressant effect.

Drugs other than thiobarbiturates can have a rapid onset, as exemplified by methohexital, which is a little more potent and more rapidly metabolized than thiopental.

All barbiturates used in anesthesia reduce sympathetic control of the peripheral vasculature, thereby increasing the capacitance of the venous system, which in turn leads to reduced preload. Coupled with a negative inotropic effect on the myocardium, blood pressure falls. In compensation, the baroreceptors will accelerate heart rate and mitigate the reduction in cardiac output. Respiration is also depressed. These negative effects do not play a major role in anesthesia of healthy patients where hydration with intravenous fluids can

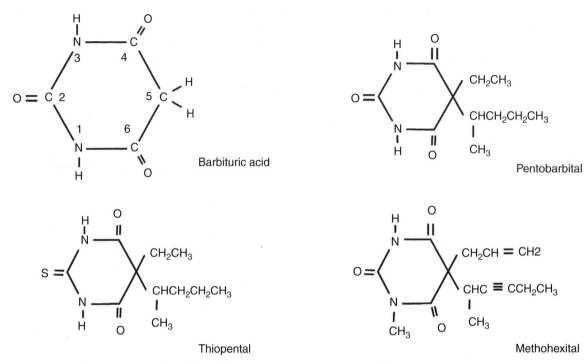

Fig. 12.1 Barbiturate structural relationships. All based on barbituric acid; see the text for a description of the seemingly minor structural variations.

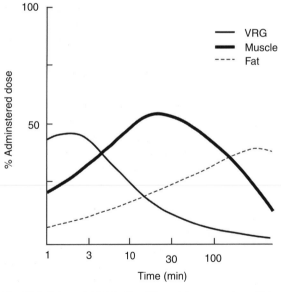

Fig. 12.2 Thiopental distribution. After an intravenous dose of thiopental at Time 0, the patient's blood levels rise rapidly (not shown here). The blood then distributes the drug according to the hierarchy of blood flow: first to the best perfused vessel rich group (VRG), which includes the brain (also heart, liver, kidneys) where thiopental will exert an early (sleep and cardiovascular effects) and fleeting effect. The other compartments (muscle and fat) then pick up the drug, depending on blood flow and solubility of the drug in the respective tissues. The last compartment, the fat, finally accumulates the drug after the other compartments are already seeing a decline in drug concentration. The fat compartment thus becomes the depot from which the drug trickles back into the blood to be disposed of by biotransformation and excretion.

compensate for the reduced preload from venous pooling, and where we routinely overcome depressed ventilation by manual or mechanical ventilation. In addition, the barbiturates constrict blood vessels in the brain (as a result of decreased metabolic rate and an active metabolism-flow coupling mechanism), a welcome side effect when increased intracranial pressure concerns us in patients with tumors or head trauma.

The following non-barbiturate induction agents also possess anticonvulsant effects, even in relatively small dosages.

Propofol (Diprivan®)

Propofol is another frequently used intravenous anesthetic. As a phenol, it belongs to an entirely different category of drugs. Not being water soluble, it is presented in a milky-white emulsion of oil, glycerol, and lecithin ("Milk of Amnesia"), an ideal culture medium for bacteria. Sterile technique, of course, is mandatory for all intravenous injections; however, with propofol, we dare not keep an open vial for later use. Even a drawn syringe can be kept for only 6–12 h depending on the preservative. Because an injection of slightly acidic propofol into a small vein smarts, we often elevate the arm during injection and give it together with a local anesthetic, systemic narcotics, a tiny dose of thiopental or ketamine, or just buffer it with a little sodium bicarbonate. A typical induction dose might be 1 to 2.5 mg/kg. Propofol, 20 to 200 mcg/kg/min, as a continuous infusion provides sedation or sleep, for example when a child must hold still for radiation treatment. Together with nitrous oxide (nitrous oxide provides the analgesia, propofol the sleep), it also serves well for short surgical procedures because patients awaken rapidly from this technique and rarely suffer nausea or vomiting.

Propofol also lowers the blood pressure by a negative inotropic myocardial effect, vasodilatation, venous pooling, and reduced preload. It depresses ventilation and airway reflexes (preferred agent in asthmatic patients), and reduces cerebral perfusion. Occasionally, patients show mild myoclonic movements during propofol infusion. The drug is cleared from the plasma much more rapidly than thiopental, and the lack of a hangover and freedom from nausea after recovery have secured propofol a place in outpatient anesthesia.

Etomidate (Amidate®)

Chemically unrelated to barbiturates and propofol, this drug enjoys the (perhaps overrated) reputation of causing little cardiovascular depression. It finds use primarily in patients with heart disease where 0.2 to 0.5 mg/kg is given for induction of anesthesia – preferably into a large vein with a rapidly running infusion in order to minimize pain from venous irritation. Etomidate lowers the seizure threshold. In up to half of all patients it triggers a myoclonus, which appears to be harmless. The drug inhibits cortisol and aldosterone synthesis (via dose-dependent inhibition of 11β-hydroxylase), a feature that makes it unsuitable for long-term intravenous sedation in the ICU.

Ketamine (Ketalar®)

This drug occupies a peculiar position between the induction agents on the one hand and the narcotic analgesics on the other. It provides both sleep and analgesia – but at a cost. The drug is the grandchild of phencyclidine, a nasty compound that made a brief appearance as an intravenous anesthetic, soon abandoned, and now mainly encountered as a psychedelic drug on the street and known under a medley of colorful names (PCP, Angel Dust, Dust, Sherm, Super Weed, Killer Weed, Elephant, Embalming Fluid, Hog, PCE, Rocket Fuel, TCP). Ketamine has shed almost all of the psychedelic effects of phencyclidine. It provides excellent analgesia (via stimulation of both NMDA[4] and opioid receptors), particularly of the integument and less so of the intestinal tract. It is classified as a dissociative anesthetic because, in low doses, the patient may appear to be awake (perhaps with open eyes and nystagmus) but unresponsive to sensory input. Only in deep anesthesia does the drug obtund airway reflexes, while in light anesthesia with spontaneous ventilation, bronchodilation is a welcome side effect, although increased secretions are bothersome. Unlike the other common anesthetic agents, ketamine *stimulates* the sympathetic nervous system, tending to increase heart rate and blood pressure. As such, it is often the drug of choice in the hypovolemic trauma patient. However, in cardiac patients in congestive failure whose sympathetic system may be exhausted, the drug can reveal its direct myocardial depressant effect. Ketamine is relatively contraindicated for patients at risk of high intracranial pressure, as its sympathetic stimulation increases cerebral blood flow. On awakening from the effect of the drug, many adults, but usually no pediatric patients, experience visual hallucinations and delirium.

In increasing dosages, we use ketamine for analgesia (0.1–0.3 mg/kg i.v.) or for induction of anesthesia

Table 12.5. Characteristics of inhaled anesthetics

Name	Formula	Biotransformed %	Partition coefficients Blood/gas	Fat/ blood	Vapor pressure mmHg @ 20°C	MAC (sea level)
Diethyl ether	$CH_3-CH_2-O-CH_2-CH_3$	20	12	5	440	1.9
Enflurane	$CH FCl-CF_2-O-CHF_2$	2	1.9	36	172	1.63
Methoxyflurane	$CHCl_2-CF_2-O CH_3$	50	12	49	23	0.16
Halothane	$CF_3-CHClBr$	20	2.5	51	243	0.75
Isoflurane	$CF_3-CHCl-O-CHF_2$	0.2	1.4	45	238	1.15
Desflurane	$CF_3-CHF-O-CHF_2$	0.02	0.42	27	669	6.6
Sevoflurane	$(CF_3)_2-CH-O-CFH_2$	2	0.6	48	157	1.8
Nitrous oxide	N_2O	0	0.47	2.3	38,770	105
Xenon	Xe	0	0.12			56

The partition coefficients are reported for 37°C.

(1–2 mg/kg i.v. or intramuscularly 5–10 mg/kg). To minimize the frequency of delirium, we give it together with one of the benzodiazepines and to decrease secretions, we add an anti-sialogogue.

Inhalation anesthetics (Table 12.5)

Before discussing the agents one by one, we need to deal with the question of the uptake and distribution of inhaled drugs.

Uptake and distribution of inhaled anesthetics

Behind this bland title lurks a concept that has baffled students for years, yet it is fairly straightforward.
   Here are the facts:

(i)   Solubility of the anesthetic gas in blood has nothing to do with its potency. Indeed, anesthetic effectiveness has to do with the partial pressure of the drug and not with the amount of drug in solution.

(ii)   Anesthetics taken up by the blood flowing through the lungs are distributed into different body compartments, depending on the blood flow these compartments receive, the volume of the compartment, and the solubility of the anesthetic agent in that compartment.

(iii)   The partial pressure exerted by a vapor in solution has nothing to do with the ambient pressure, but has much to do with the temperature of the solution.

Let us take these three items one by one:

(i)   Solubility of the anesthetic in blood has nothing to do with its potency.
   Table 12.5 tells the story. At equilibrium, you will find 12 times as much ether (when we say "ether" we refer to diethyl ether; some of the halogenated anesthetics are chemically also ethers, but we call them by their given name, e.g., sevoflurane and desflurane) in blood than in the overlying gas (blood/gas partition coefficient). The blood practically slurps up the ether, but

it is the portion in the overlying gas that can cross into the brain and exert its benumbing effects. Every breath that brings in more ether dumps its load of the anesthetic into the blood perfusing the lungs. It takes breath after breath to deliver enough ether for the blood to come into equilibrium with the alveolar gas.

At equilibrium, the partial pressure (but not the concentration per unit of volume) of ether in alveolar gas will be the same as in the blood.

We have picked ether (no longer used in the West but still available in the developing world) because of its extraordinary solubility in blood at body temperature. In comparison, look at sevoflurane. Ether is 20 times more soluble in blood than is sevoflurane. We can quickly bring enough sevoflurane into the alveoli to establish an equilibrium between alveolar gas and blood. For ether, it will take many, many breaths laden with ether to fill the blood compartment and to reach equilibrium between alveolar gas and blood. Yet, diethyl ether and sevoflurane have almost identical MAC values. MAC stands (neither for a computer nor for a truck) for minimal alveolar concentration, namely the concentration in alveolar gas at which 50% of patients no longer respond to a painful stimulus. Thus, when we have attained MAC values for ether and MAC values for sevoflurane, there will be much, much more ether dissolved in the patient than will be true for sevoflurane. It will be quicker to get the patient to sleep – and have him wake up again – with sevoflurane than with ether.

Observe in Table 12.5 that, at equilibrium, you will find five times as much ether in fat than in blood and 45 times as much isoflurane in fat than in blood … which brings us to the next point.

(ii) Anesthetics taken up by the lungs are distributed into different body compartments, depending on the blood flow these compartments receive, their volume, and the solubility of the anesthetic agent in that compartment.

Figure 12.3 shows the relationships. Observe the low blood flow and large volume of the fat compartment (not even assuming an obese patient!) and the small volume but enormous blood flow to the vessel rich group. These "compartments" are conceptual rather than anatomical; the vessel rich group contains heart and brain as well as kidney and liver.

You can easily imagine that during a long anesthetic, the fat compartment, despite its low perfusion, will accumulate much anesthetic agent because inhalation anesthetics are so very soluble in fat (they make excellent grease stain removers). At the end of the anesthetic, the poorly perfused fat compartment will slowly deliver anesthetic to the venous blood, causing the patient to have a protracted recovery from the anesthetic; the greater the solubility of the agent in fat, the more protracted.

(iii) The partial pressure exerted by a vapor in solution has nothing to do with the ambient pressure, but has much to do with the temperature of the solution.

Water vapor in the lungs at 37°C has a vapor pressure of 47 mmHg. At that temperature, as many molecules of water leave the blood as enter it. The vapor pressure increases with rising temperatures. At the boiling point, the vapor pressure equals ambient pressure (at the top of the mountain you need to boil your egg a little longer because the water will boil at a lower temperature). At sea level (1 atmosphere or 760 mmHg ambient pressure), it takes 1.15% of isoflurane to render 50% of the population unresponsive to noxious (if the patient were awake the word would be "painful") stimuli. At that barometric pressure, 1.15% equals about 9 mmHg. At an altitude with a barometric pressure of 500 mmHg, these same 9 mmHg would be about 1.8% of vapor in the alveolar gas. Thus, the convention of reporting anesthetic concentrations in percent – as our vaporizers do – leaves something to be desired. In Table 12.6, we compare isoflurane MAC values in two cities of very different altitude that happen to have the same name. Remember that about half of our patients will be responsive, i.e., with a movement but not necessarily conscious, at 1 MAC. In order to have almost 100% of patients unresponsive to noxious (painful) stimuli, we need to expose them to 1.3 MAC. Also, remember that most patients have been given other CNS depressants; MAC values change with age (down they go); and distribution of the anesthetic agents also depends on the patient's

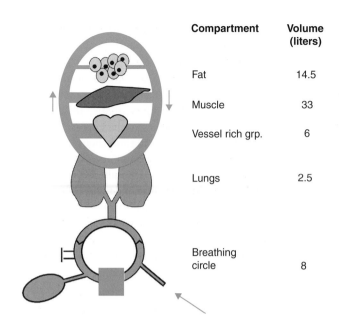

Compartment	Volume (liters)	% Cardiac output
Fat	14.5	0.06
Muscle	33	18
Vessel rich grp.	6	76
Lungs	2.5	100
Breathing circle	8	

Fig. 12.3 Conceptual compartments for agent distribution. Drugs are first distributed to the vessel rich group, which receives the majority of the cardiac output. Equilibration here is rapid (both during induction and emergence). The much larger fat compartment receives a much lower blood flow and therefore takes much longer to equilibrate with the agent concentration in blood. While agent in this compartment serves no purpose, resolution of the resulting depot maintains agent in the bloodstream for an extended period of time following discontinuation of drug administration.

Table 12.6. Comparison of MAC values for isoflurane at various altitudes

Name of city	Altitude in ft (m)	MAC in % of ambient pressure
La Paz, Bolivia	11 735 ft (3577 m)	1.8%
La Paz, Mexico	33 ft (10 m)	1.15%

cardiac output. For example, in a shock state with very low cardiac output, pulmonary blood enjoys additional time in contact with the alveolus to equilibrate with the anesthetic gas more rapidly. Furthermore, nearly all cardiac output is sent to brain and heart in this state.

We can anticipate that many CNS depressants will lower MAC. Intuitively not so obvious, however, are reports that hyponatremia, metabolic acidosis, alpha methyldopa, chronic dextroamphetamine usage, levodopa, and alpha-2 agonists can lower MAC, as does pregnancy. We find elevated MAC values in hypernatremia, hyperthermia, and in patients taking monoamine oxidase inhibitors, cocaine and ephedrine. The administration of a sympathomimetic can sometimes lighten anesthesia. Because we always titrate anesthetics to a desired effect and because patients vary greatly in their response to drugs – anesthetics as well as others – these differences in MAC rarely influence our anesthetic practice.

The gases

Only two anesthetic gases (as opposed to vapors) deserve to be mentioned: nitrous oxide and xenon. Cyclopropane and ethylene are two explosive gases used in the past.

Nitrous oxide

Nitrous oxide has been around for centuries and is still widely used. Yet you will often hear it said that, if nitrous oxide were to be introduced today, it would never pass the FDA's muster. For this jaundiced view, we can cite several reasons.

(i) The gas is a weak anesthetic with a MAC of 105%. Thus, it would require a hyperbaric chamber to administer that concentration with enough oxygen to make it safe. In concentrations up to 70% in oxygen, it is an analgesic rather than a reliable anesthetic.

(ii) Because it is such a weak drug, in the past people tended to give high concentrations of it, which is another way of saying that it was given with marginal concentrations of oxygen. Modern anesthesia machines will not let you give less than 25% oxygen, but many patients with ventilation/perfusion abnormalities require a higher FiO_2.

(iii) It does some peculiar things to some important enzymes. By oxidizing vitamin-B12-dependent enzymes (methionine and thymidylate synthetase), it inhibits formation of myelin and thymidine (important in DNA synthesis). Prolonged exposure to nitrous oxide has caused neuropathy and megaloblastic changes as well as leukopenia. A decreased white count was noticed in tetanus patients requiring prolonged mechanical ventilation during which nitrous oxide was used continuously as an analgesic sedative. Attempting to use this effect to advantage, subsequent experiments with nitrous oxide in leukemic patients confirmed the observation that the gas could reduce the white count. Unfortunately, the effect did not last and upon discontinuation of the gas, the cell counts rose back to their pathologic level. The neuropathic effect of nitrous oxide was observed by a neurologist who saw dentists complaining of different degrees of apraxia, ataxia, and impotence. Exposure to nitrous oxide was the common denominator in these patients. These effects are not observed during the relatively brief use (minutes or hours instead of repeated use or days of exposure) of nitrous oxide in patients undergoing surgical anesthesia.

(iv) Despite its low blood solubility (blood/gas partition coefficient of 0.47), the high concentration of N_2O administered (50–70% in oxygen) causes many liters to dissolve in the body during a lengthy anesthetic. Because it diffuses readily into air-containing bubbles, nitrous oxide can increase the volume of air in the cuff of an endotracheal tube, the gas in the bowel, a bleb in the lung, or gas in the middle ear. The volume of a closed air space, e.g., pneumothorax, will double in just 10 minutes if 70% nitrous is breathed! The doubling time for bowel is *much* slower (hours).

(v) We might also mention that it supports combustion, almost as well as oxygen.

(vi) For neurosurgical procedures, even low-dose and brief exposure to nitrous oxide affects evoked potentials – which we monitor to keep an eye on the integrity of the spinal cord, among other things (see Chapter 7).

(vii) Based on questionable epidemiologic data and on animal experiments, nitrous oxide has been accused of causing spontaneous abortion in personnel repeatedly exposed to trace concentrations of the gas. Consequently, maximal acceptable concentrations of nitrous oxide in the OR have been established by the government: OSHA calls for a time-weighted average concentration of less than 25 parts per million.

(viii) Finally, thrill seekers have extensively abused nitrous oxide, obtaining it legally (and stupidly) in the small whippet cylinders. There, the gas exists in its pure form, that is, without oxygen. The ill-informed who inhale it from such a source expose themselves to the double trouble of inhaling a hypoxic gas mixture while breathing a harmful gas.

In fairness, we have to say something positive about the gas. Because of its low solubility, it does not take much time to reach equilibrium between alveolar gas and blood, which translates into fairly rapid induction and emergence with minimal cardiovascular side effects. Some pediatric dentists like its mild analgesic effect and the fact that it is tasteless and odorless (which is why industry uses it as a propellant for canned whipped cream). In the pediatric dental practice, nitrous oxide is usually administered at concentrations between 30% and 50% in oxygen. Higher concentrations of nitrous oxide given without other agents often lead to excitement. In anesthetic practice, therefore, we administer the gas together with other CNS depressants, for example propofol or a halogenated anesthetic vapor.

Even though it has nothing to do with the pharmacology of nitrous oxide, and everything to do with the fact that we give it in high concentrations (up to 70% – whereas the halogenated agents are given in less than one-tenth that concentration), we need to mention three concepts linked to nitrous oxide: the second gas effect; the augmented inflow effect (also called the concentration effect); and diffusion hypoxia.

The concentration and second gas effects

The concentration and second gas effects are intertwined and can be confusing – which seems to make them irresistible topics for discussion (or colloquially for "pimping"). If you administer a high concentration of nitrous oxide to the lungs during induction of anesthesia, even though it has a low solubility, much of the gas will leave the alveoli and enter the blood. Consider an inspired gas composed of 70% N_2O, 28% O_2, and 2%

isoflurane. Imagine an alveolus containing exactly 100 molecules of this gas, adjacent to a pulmonary venule containing 17% oxygen and no nitrous or isoflurane. If half of the N_2O (35 molecules) is absorbed from the alveolus (along with about 6 oxygen and 1 isoflurane for each to equilibrate), we find that the concentration of N_2O in the alveolus falls to 60% ($[35/(35 + 22 + 1)] *$ 100). But we are not done yet. The movement of a volume of N_2O out of the alveolus and into the blood causes a vacuum of sorts, and sucks additional mixed gas of the original (70/28/2) mixture from the bronchiole into the alveolus (termed "augmented inspired ventilation"). When that volume is added to the concentrated gases left in the alveoli, we find the concentration of N_2O becomes higher still: 64% and significantly *concentrated* from 35%. This concentrating continues until the next breath brings new fresh gas.

The second gas effect is exactly the same idea as the concentration effect, except it applies to the *other* gases given along with the predominant gas (i.e., N_2O). Most often we think of the actual potent inhalational agent when we discuss this, rather than the O_2. If we take the same example but look at what happens to the isoflurane, after initial equilibration we would have just one molecule in our alveolus above, but with the "loss" of nitrous that one molecule is actually concentrated to 1.7% ($[1/(35 + 22 + 1)] * 100$). When we also factor in the effect of the augmented inspired ventilation, we settle at a final concentration of 1.8%, a substantial enhancement. If someone asks the question: raise your hand.

Diffusion hypoxia

After hours of anesthesia with nitrous oxide, many liters of the gas go into solution in the body. At the end of anesthesia, when the patient no longer inhales nitrous oxide, the liters of nitrous oxide in solution will follow their concentration gradient and be delivered to the lung where the gas will dilute other gases – including oxygen. Thus, we give oxygen for a few breaths at the end of anesthesia to prevent diffusion hypoxia.

Xenon

This noble gas is even less soluble than nitrous oxide (blood/gas partition coefficient of 0.12) and about twice as potent (MAC = 56%). In addition, it appears to have no major depressant effects on the cardiovascular system. We do not know how it produces anesthesia, being a noble gas (we don't really know how the other not so noble agents do it, either). Xenon would make a desirable anesthetic, were it not for its high cost (about $17/L). Not currently used in the USA, most studies of the gas come from abroad.

The anesthetic vapors

Ethers

Anesthetic vapors exist as fluids at ambient conditions. They have low vapor pressures, and the vapors overlying the liquid phase have anesthetic properties. It all started with diethyl ether, the great granddaddy of anesthetic vapors. Over the past 150 years, uncounted chemists have rearranged the structure of these substances and, by adding halogens, have developed a host of promising anesthetics. Each has distinctive vapor pressures, blood/gas partition coefficients, potencies (see Table 12.5), and side effects, e.g., upper airway irritation, bronchodilation, cardiac irritability.

With the arrival of the non-flammable agents, i.e., halothane (Fluothane®) and the halogenated ethers, we were able to retire from clinical use the highly flammable diethyl ether. Methoxyflurane (Penthrane) was abandoned because of its extensive biotransformation, which led to the liberation of enough fluoride ions to damage the kidneys, causing a vasopressin-resistant high output renal failure. The much less extensive biotransformation of enflurane (Ethrane®) and sevoflurane (Ultane®) also liberates fluoride ions but in such small concentrations that renal problems have not been a cause for concern. Initial worries over nephrotoxicity from sevoflurane's degradation by CO_2 absorbent in the anesthesia circuit (forming the dreaded "Compound A," also known as pentafluoro-isoprenyl fluoromethyl ether) appears to lack clinical relevance (unless anesthetizing a rat).

Halogenated aliphatic compounds

So much for the halogenated ethers. Now to a different class, the halogenated aliphatic compounds, the ancestor of which, chloroform ($HCCl_3$), dates back to 1847 when it was first shown to be an anesthetic. While neither irritating nor combustible (a big problem for diethyl ether), it eventually fell out of favor because of its propensity to cause arrhythmias and hepatic damage. A number of other halogenated aliphatic compounds came and went, until finally in the mid 1960s, halothane appeared and was soon widely used. It is still available outside the USA, and has had its lumps and bumps. It sensitizes the heart to arrhythmias triggered by catecholamines and has been accused of an injurious impact on the liver.

Halothane hepatitis

Soon after the introduction of halothane, worrisome reports of "halothane hepatitis" appeared. Fever, malaise, and evidence of liver damage as seen in the elevation of serum aminotransferases pointed to liver damage. Not the halothane molecule itself but the products of its biotransformation cause the trouble. Halothane falls prey to a reductive and an oxidative break-up, the former exaggerated in the presence of hypoxemia, the latter, in some patients, causing an immune response that can set the stage for severe halothane hepatitis at a future exposure to halothane. Hepatitis after halothane anesthesia is rare (perhaps 1 in 30 000) and much rarer after the other halogenated anesthetics. The extent of biotransformation of the drug might play a role: halothane stands out with 20–46% of the agent undergoing biotransformation as compared to isoflurane (0.2–2%) and desflurane (0.02%). The products of biotransformation of sevoflurane (2–5% metabolized) appear to cause no harm to the liver.

Comparing effects on heart, lung, and brain

All anesthetic vapors affect consciousness and have analgesic effects. They depress ventilation, as judged by decreasing minute ventilation and increasing levels of arterial carbon dioxide, with increasing depth of anesthesia. A few words about generally subtle differences between these drugs:

Inhalation induction

The older halothane and the newer sevoflurane have established for themselves a special niche because they are less irritating to the upper airway than the others. Particularly in children, who abhor needlesticks (and whose veins are more easily cannulated when the child is asleep), anesthesia can be induced quite gently by inhalation of nitrous oxide/oxygen together with either one of these two drugs.

Cardiovascular effects

All volatile agents depress myocardial contractility and cause peripheral vasodilatation. As long as baroreceptors function normally, heart rate will increase in response to hypotension. In deep anesthesia, this compensation will not suffice to prevent a drop in cardiac output. Here, halothane occupies an unusual position. It inhibits the baroreceptor; consequently, we see less tachycardia (even bradycardia in deeply anesthetized children) during halothane-induced hypotension and a greater drop in cardiac output than is true for the other agents at comparable levels of anesthesia. Another oddity regarding halothane anesthesia: otherwise well-tolerated levels of circulating catecholamines, whether injected or liberated by the body, trigger arrhythmias in the presence of halothane.

Respiratory effects

Under very deep anesthesia, ventilation stops, usually before the heart arrests. Thus, a respiratory arrest from an inhalation anesthetic overdose need not be fatal if discovered in time, and if ventilation of the (still perfused) lungs with oxygen can remove the volatile anesthetic.

In surgical anesthesia, spontaneous ventilation will still be maintained IF the patient was not given other drugs that depress ventilation – such as opiates – and IF the patient is not paralyzed by neuromuscular blocking drugs, so commonly used in order to relax striated muscles and thus ease the surgeon's job.

In general, all halogenated inhalation anesthetics decrease minute ventilation by decreasing tidal volume. The compensatory increase in respiratory rate is insufficient to prevent a respiratory acidosis (and hypoxemia when breathing room air) because of the increased ventilation of deadspace. Respiratory depression and tachypnea are less pronounced with desflurane (Suprane®) and sevoflurane than with halothane, with isoflurane (Forane®) lying somewhere in between.

Under inhalation anesthesia, patients respond only sluggishly to rising arterial carbon dioxide levels (= respiratory depression). Even low concentrations of the inhalation agents also depress the chemoreceptor response to hypoxemia.

Central nervous system effects

The inhalation anesthetics depress, in a dose-dependent manner, CNS function – as shown by clinical findings starting with a state of somnolence, during which the patient can still respond, to coma, in which external noxious stimulation elicits no visible response. This sentence was carefully chosen, because invisible CNS responses are detectable by electroencephalography and evoked potentials; these persist long after motor responses have been abolished. Eventually, they too vanish in deep anesthesia. Halogenated inhalation agents tend to increase cerebral blood flow, which is not a desirable effect in patients at risk of brain swelling. In

Table 12.7. Relative potencies of commonly used opioids

	Relative potency	Protein binding (%)	Duration (h)	$T_{1/2}$ (min)
Morphine	1	30	2–3	114
Hydromorphone	8	8	2–3	150
Meperidine	0.1	75	2–4	200
Fentanyl	100	85	1–2	200
Sufentanil	1000	92	0.5	150
Alfentanil	10	90	0.25	85
Remifentanil	200	70	0.1	5

Comparison of the opioids commonly used in anesthesia. $T_{1/2}$ is the time at which one-half of the drug has been eliminated from the body. Clinical duration, however, refers to the approximate duration of drug effect after an intravenous bolus injection. This includes a peak effect (dependent on factors such as lipid solubility [including ionization and pK], volume of distribution, and flow to the effector site) followed by a gradual waning over minutes to hours (redistribution, ion trapping, metabolism). Protein binding significantly affects the volume of distribution, and changes the drug's effectiveness in settings of altered protein binding.

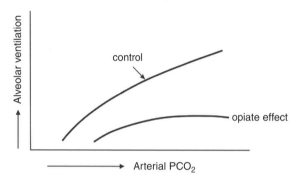

Fig. 12.4 Carbon dioxide response: effect of opioids. Rising carbon dioxide blood levels cause ventilation to increase. In very high concentrations, carbon dioxide becomes a depressant and even anesthetic. Opiates typically shift the carbon dioxide response curve to the right and flatten it. The degree of shift depends on the drug and the dose. Very high doses stop ventilation altogether, as seen all too often in "dead on arrival" victims of heroin overdose. In anesthesia, we sometimes give narcotics to the point of causing apnea (and intense analgesia) – while maintaining normal PaCO$_2$ levels by providing mechanical ventilation.

neurosurgical anesthesia, we rely greatly on intravenous techniques, using the inhalation agents only in low doses and as adjuncts.

The opioids (Table 12.7)

Today, narcotics play a major role in general anesthesia. Their advantage lies in their potent ability to abolish pain without depressing the heart. Their principal side effect remains powerful respiratory depression resulting in a decreased respiratory rate and finally respiratory arrest (Fig. 12.4). This side effect can be tolerated if we are prepared to ventilate the patient's lungs, as we do routinely when patients receive neuromuscular blocking drugs and thus require mechanical ventilation. Unchecked respiratory depression and elevation of arterial carbon dioxide can reduce resistance in the arterial bed of the cerebral circulation, leading to increased intracranial pressure. Chemoreceptor depression by opioids reduces the respiratory response to hypoxemia; however, the administration of oxygen to a hypoxemic patient may further depress ventilation, demonstrating that chemoreceptor activity still contributes to the respiratory drive.

At this time in anesthesia, we have no useful opioid that would spare the μ-2 receptors responsible for respiratory depression, while exerting a full effect on the receptors apparently involved in analgesia (μ-1, δ-1, δ-2, and κ-3 for supraspinal analgesia, and μ-2, δ-2, and κ-1 for spinal analgesia). As mentioned earlier, to be eaten alive by a lion may not be painful, presumably because the endogenous opioid polypeptides (the enkephalins, endorphins, dynorphins, and neoendorphins) kick in – evidently without causing fatal respiratory depression but presumably allowing for a gasp. We tend not to rely on this physiologic response to gourmand lions, even with the most fearsome of surgeons at work.

Opioids exhibit many side effects other than respiratory depression. Interesting to anesthesia are the depressant effects on the autonomic nervous system with a decrease in sympathetic tone and a preponderance of vagal activity, leading to bradycardia and a reduction in blood pressure. The observed hypotension after large doses of opioids gives evidence of venous pooling (exaggerated in patients with a reduced

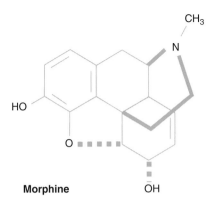

Morphine

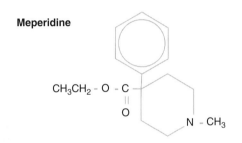

Meperidine

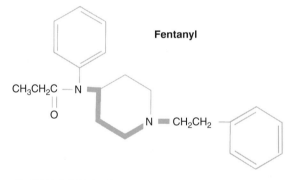

Fentanyl

Fig. 12.5 Opioid structures.

to changes in mood (either euphoria or dysphoria, depending on the setting and the patient). Some of these effects have their origin locally (constipation), others centrally (chemoreceptor stimulation triggering nausea).

By now the opioids have amassed quite a retinue of narcotic compounds, some of which appear to have unrelated chemical footprints. While heroin, codeine, and many relatives show their kinship with morphine, others are classified as piperidines and phenylpiperidines, comprising meperidine and the different fentanyl drugs.

Morphine

Morphine (Fig. 12.5) has a long tradition as an analgesic for wound pain with a typical i.m. dose of 10 mg for a 70 kg patient. Despite its propensity to stimulate histamine release, we make extensive use of i.v. morphine for management of acute pain, as an intraoperative analgesic and adjunct to general anesthesia, and post-operatively as the most common drug for patient-controlled analgesia (PCA). We also commonly administer morphine neuraxially (epidural or subarachnoid) to obtain 18–24 hours of post-surgical analgesia, though delayed respiratory depression remains a concern. One of its metabolites, morphine-6-glucuronide, retains much of morphine's activity and has been implicated in prolonged respiratory depression observed in patients with renal failure.

Hydromorphone (Dilaudid ®)

A semisynthetic derivative of morphine, hydromorphone is about 8 times more potent and reaches peak effect more quickly (20 min vs. 90 min) than morphine. This latter fact may explain hydromorphone's unwarranted reputation for less nausea and vomiting. With a 6–10 minute lockout on a PCA (patient-controlled analgesia) pump, morphine may be effectively overdosed, thereby increasing its side effects. In fact at equianalgesic doses the side-effect profiles of the drugs are the same.

Meperidine (pethidine, Demerol®, Dolantin®, Pethadol®)

Another synthetic opioid, meperidine, deserves to be mentioned, though in anesthesia we use it less today than before the arrival of its chemical grandchildren, the fentanyls. Meperidine (Fig. 12.5), with one-tenth

blood volume) rather than a direct depressant effect on the heart. Meperidine, having vagolytic effects, behaves somewhat differently.

During a cholecystectomy, we need to be aware that opioids can increase the tone of the sphincter of Oddi, thereby increasing pressure in the biliary system and interfering with a surgeon's attempt to perform a cholangiogram.

Additional side effects of opioids range from miosis (the infamous pinpoint pupils – again meperidine is the exception), itching, constipation, and nausea, the potency and shorter duration of action than morphine, occupies a unique spot among opioids in its antimuscarinic activity. Patients receiving meperidine do not develop the "pinpoint pupils" we expect with other opioids; they may also become tachycardic and complain of a dry mouth. The drug is associated with higher rates of nausea and vomiting as well. Most importantly, it should not be given to patients taking monoamine oxidase inhibitors because severe respiratory depression, excitation, and even convulsions can be the consequence (serotonin syndrome). Meperidine's main metabolite, normeperidine, lasts for days ($T_{1/2}$ elimination = 15–40 h). Particularly in the setting of impaired renal function, the accumulation of normeperidine can cause myoclonus and seizures. As of this writing, meperidine has lost its place among opioid analgesics in the USA. Its only role at present is in the treatment of post-operative shivering and rigors. Even in that role it faces formidable competition from tramadol, nalbuphine, and even magnesium.

Fentanyls

Fentanyl (Sublimaze®) (Fig. 12.5), with a potency 100 times that of morphine, has even more potent offspring. The differences among the fentanyls reside primarily in the onset and duration of action since, in general, the respiratory depressant effect runs parallel with the analgesic effectiveness. There are small differences in the onset of action after an intravenous bolus, with fentanyl and sufentanil (Sufenta®) taking about 6 minutes for the peak effect to set in while alfentanil (Alfenta®) and remifentanil (Ultiva®) reach their peaks in about a minute. Remifentanil, an ester, deserves special mention as the only narcotic that falls prey to nonspecific plasma esterases that hydrolyze the drug, thus rapidly curtailing its effect. The other opioids have to rely on liver blood flow and hepatic biotransformation. A comparison of each of the commonly used opioids may be of help (Table 12.7).

Finally, let us mention that narcotic addiction has not spared anesthesia and nursing staff. Easy access to narcotics has been blamed for the higher frequency of addiction among anesthesia personnel than other healthcare workers.

Opioid receptor antagonism: naloxone (Narcan®)

Opioids are antagonized by naloxone, chemically related to morphine and competing for receptor sites

Table 12.8. Opioid antagonist

Agent	Trade name	i.v. dose	Comments
Naloxone	Narcan®	0.1–0.4 mg	Duration 1–2 hours; may elicit withdrawal syndrome in addicts; reverses analgesia as well

occupied by the agonists (see Table 12.8). In the adult, we usually start with 40–100 mcg naloxone intravenously, expecting to see a response within a minute. The half-life of the drug is around 40 minutes. Thus, patients who had been depressed by the longer-acting drugs, such as morphine, must be observed for at least an hour in order not to miss recurring respiratory depression. In addicted patients under the influence of and tolerant to large doses of a narcotic analgesic, a larger dose of naloxone can trigger a stormy withdrawal reaction, as can administration of some of the mixed agonist-antagonist drugs, among them butorphanol (Stadol®) and nalbuphine (Nubain®). These latter agents have a ceiling effect on respiratory depression, a property considered vital in obstetrics where they are commonly used – never mind that the patient's pain is not much relieved by these agents!

Now appearing are peripheral opioid antagonists including subcutaneous methylnaltrexone (Relistor®) and oral alvimopan (Entereg®). These agents reverse peripheral opioid effects, particularly of the GI tract, but mounting evidence suggests reduced nausea and vomiting, urinary retention, and pruritus might also be achieved. Additional effects prompting research interest include reversal of opioid-induced vascular permeability and tumor recurrence. Approval at present limits use of these drugs to advanced illness and palliative care.

Non-opioid analgesics in anesthesia

Multi-modal analgesia has become the refrain for anesthesiologists. Any reduction in opioid requirement brings the welcome lessening of side effects. Furthermore, as discussed in Chapter 4, pain itself is multi-modal with numerous opportunities to interrupt the signals. In addition to consideration of regional and local anesthetic options, agents that work at other receptors deserve mention.

– Non-steroidal anti-inflammatory drugs (NSAIDs), and particularly intravenous ketorolac (Toradol®), reduce pain and inflammation, though damage to GI mucosa, interference with coagulation, and renal toxicity limit their use in some patients and some operations. The COX-2 (cyclooxygenase) selective NSAIDs have largely disappeared with concerns of prothombotic tendencies. Celecoxib (Celebrex®) alone remains, and the research into its utility for peri-operative analgesia has come into question.

– Ketamine's affinity for NMDA receptors provides excellent adjunctive analgesia at non-psychogenic doses.

– Gabapentin (Neurontin®) and its younger brother pregabalin (Lyrica®) appeared as seizure medications (and are sedating) but demonstrate excellent analgesia for neuropathic pain. Recently they have found use as preemptive analgesics, though for best effect they should be continued for several days after surgery. Despite their generic names, the analgesic effect of these drugs is not related to the GABA receptor, but involves calcium channel antagonism at the level of the spinal cord.

Clinical perspectives on the use of analgesics

In the chapter on post-operative care (Chapter 6), you will find a discussion of how to assess the severity of pain. Many different drugs find use in the treatment of pain. The following tables are not intended to guide therapy, but are presented here for the sake of orientation. We do not offer a discussion of these drugs and urge the reader to consult pharmacologic texts and the information offered by the manufacturers. For moderate to severe pain (VAS 5 to 7), you may see one of the drugs in Table 12.9 prescribed. For mild pain we often use one of the common oral, non-narcotic analgesics that are available over the counter (Table 12.10).

Neuromuscular blockers and their antagonists (Table 12.11)

Even though the title presents the official name, we will call them muscle relaxants with the understanding that we are talking about drugs used in anesthesia to facilitate tracheal intubation and to ease the

surgeon's work. The good news about muscle relaxants is that they affect only striated, voluntary muscles, but not the myocardium and the smooth muscles under autonomic control (including the uterus). Being quaternary ammonium compounds, all muscle relaxants carry a charge and thus do not readily cross the blood–brain barrier (no effect on the brain) or the placenta (no effect on the fetus). The bad news is that the relaxants do not spare the muscles of ventilation. That fact has cost many lives when partially paralyzed patients became hypoxemic because inadequate ventilation persisted during and particularly after anesthesia. Do not forget that muscle relaxants have no anesthetic effect; that a patient paralyzed by muscle relaxants has no way of signaling that he is in pain, uncomfortable or short of breath, a fact not lost on those patients suffering intra-operative awareness. There are far too many reports of recall of intra-operative and ICU events when muscle relaxants were employed. Note also that even the pharmacological reversal of the effect of muscle relaxants has undesirable side effects. Whenever muscle relaxants are used, we assume great responsibility for the safety of the patient. Many procedures do not require muscle relaxants and they should not be pressed into service to cover for inadequate anesthesia. When no muscle relaxants are used, the patient can breathe spontaneously, which they tend to do very well indeed as long as we are not heavy handed with CNS depressants. Muscle relaxants are usually divided into depolarizing and non-depolarizing drugs.

Depolarizing muscle relaxants

Succinylcholine (Anectine®) is the only depolarizing drug still in use. It has been around for 60 years and has served us well because of two characteristics: it is rapid in onset and short in duration, being hydrolyzed by plasma cholinesterases. Indeed, perhaps as much as 90% of the intravenously injected drug is hydrolyzed before reaching the effector site at the neuromuscular junction. Patients deficient in plasma cholinesterase will be paralyzed for several hours from a standard intubating dose of 1 mg/kg, which should last for only 5 minutes or so.

Cholinesterase deficiency can be genetic or acquired. One in 3200 patients (less often in Oriental and African people) may be homozygous for atypical cholinesterase. When we suspect this because of a family history or a previous anesthetic complication, we can test the patient's plasma *in vitro*, using dibucaine

Table 12.9. Analgesics for moderate to severe pain (VAS 5 to 7) in adults

Generic name	Equivalent dose	Duration	Dose	Found in trade name products
Codeine	100 mg p.o.	3–4 hours	0.5–1.0 mg/kg q4 h max 60 mg/dose	60 mg codeine with acetaminophen in Tylenol #3®
Fentanyl	50 mcg i.v.	1–2 hours	0.5 mcg/kg i.v. PCA: 0.3 mcg/kg with 6 min lockout	Sublimaze®. Also available as Duragesic® transdermal patch
Hydrocodone	15 mg p.o.	3–4 hours	5–15 mg p.o. q4–6 h	2.5–7.5 mg hydrocodone with acetaminophen in Vicodin® and Lortab®
Hydromorphone	0.75 mg i.v. 3.75 mg p.o.	2 hours	2–4 mg p.o. q4–6 h 0.5–2 mg i.v. PCA: 0.005 mg/kg with 6 min lockout	Dilaudid®
Meperidine Pethidine	150 mg p.o.	1–3 hours	50–150 mg p.o. q3–4 h 25 mg i.v. PCA: 10 mg with 15 min lockout	Demerol®, Pethadol®
Morphine sulfate immediate release	5mg i.v. 15 mg p.o.	2–4 hours	10–30 mg p.o. q4 h 0.04 mg/kg i.v. PCA: 0.02 mg/kg with 6 min lockout	Roxanol®
Oxycodone immediate release	10 mg p.o.	3–4 hours	0.05–0.15 mg/kg p.o.	Roxicodone® 5 mg oxycodone with acetaminophen in Percocet®, Roxicet®, and Tylox® 4 mg oxycodone with aspirin in Percodan®
Tramadol[a]	100 mg p.o.	4 hours	50–100 mg q4–6 h, max 400 mg/day	Ultram®
	2 tablets p.o.	4 hours	2 tabs q4–6 h, max 8 tabs/day	37.5 mg tramadol with acetaminophen in Ultracet®

[a] Tramadol is a centrally acting, non-opioid analgesic, though it has some activity at μ receptors. It also inhibits the reuptake of norepinephrine and serotonin. Unlikely to be equianalgesic with the opioids.

Table 12.10. Oral Analgesics for mild pain (VAS <5) in adults

Generic name	Trade name	Dose	Duration
Acetaminophen	Tylenol®	650–1000 mg q4–6 h max 4000 mg/day	4 hours
Ibuprofen	Motrin®; Advil®	200–800 mg q6–8 h max 3200 mg/day	6 hours
Ketorolac	Toradol®	20 mg load then 10 mg q4–6 h max 40 mg/day for 5 days	4 hours
Naproxen	Naprosyn®	250–500 mg twice daily	8 hours
Naproxen sodium	Alleve®	550 mg twice daily	

Table 12.11. Non-depolarizing muscle relaxants by duration of action

Generic name and class	Trade name	Intubating dose[a]	Biotransformation/ excretion	Comments
Benzylisoquinolines				
Intermediate acting:				
Atracurium	Tracrium®	0.4 mg/kg	Hoffman elimination and esterases	Histamine release
Cisatracurium	Nimbex®	0.2 mg/kg	Hoffman elimination and esterases	
Long acting:				
Doxacurium	Nuromax®	0.06 mg/kg	Renal (80%)	
Steroid nucleus				
Intermediate acting:				
Vecuronium	Norcuron®	0.1 mg/kg	Hepatic (80%)	
Rocuronium	Zemuron®	0.8 mg/kg	Hepatic (70%)	
Long acting:				
Pancuronium	Pavulon®	0.1 mg/kg	Renal (80%)	Tachycardia
Pipecuronium	Arduan®	0.085 mg/kg	Renal (60%)	

[a] A higher dose is often used for rapid sequence induction.

(Nupercaine®), a local anesthetic. Dibucaine strongly (80%) inhibits normal or "typical" plasma cholinesterase but not the atypical cholinesterase (20%). A report of a "dibucaine number" of 80 is good news, suggesting that the patient is homozygous for typical plasma cholinesterase. A dibucaine number of 20 or so would be found in a patient homozygous for atypical plasma cholinesterase, who would have an abnormally protracted effect from succinylcholine. Dibucaine numbers between these extremes suggest a heterozygous genetic make-up. In the patient heterozygous for normal plasma cholinesterase, the succinylcholine effect is likely to be doubled or tripled (10–15 minutes). Incidentally, patients homozygous for atypical cholinesterase are quite asymptomatic – as long as no one gives them succinylcholine or other drugs dependent on hydrolysis by plasma cholinesterases. We see the acquired deficiency – characterized by decreased blood levels of normal plasma cholinesterase – in patients exposed to organophosphates (chemical warfare and pesticides) and those on echothiophate (for glaucoma), who would also more slowly break down some other esters such as local anesthetics of the ester type.

Succinylcholine does not compete with acetylcholine at the neuromuscular junction; instead, it depolarizes the muscle and in so doing, it opens ion channels, much like acetylcholine does, but the channels stay open much longer. Potassium begins to leak out and serum potassium levels can rise by 0.5 mEq/L after an intubating dose (succinylcholine 1 mg/kg). In damaged (crush or burn injuries) or degenerating muscles (after spinal cord injury or in muscular dystrophy), this potassium leakage can be exaggerated to the point where the cardiac effects of hyperkalemia become life-threatening. The risk of yet unrecognized muscular dystrophy, together with the potential for a bradycardic response, has limited the use of succinylcholine in children. Succinylcholine has several additional undesirable properties. Before paralysis sets in, it causes fasciculation of striated muscle, a feature that has been blamed for post-operative myalgia experienced by some patients and for a transient rise in intragastric and intracranial pressures. By a mechanism not well understood, intra-ocular pressure also rises briefly after an intubating dose. Therefore, we do not use the drug in patients with an open eye lest the patient lose vitreous. In the past, succinylcholine was often used as a continuous infusion. In that application, it loses its advantage of a short-acting depolarizing blocker because the patient will develop a so-called phase II block that looks as if the patient had been given a non-depolarizing muscle relaxant (see Chapter 7).

When tracheal intubation fails and the succinylcholine effect wears off, we might be tempted to administer a second dose of succinylcholine within a few minutes of the first dose. This is dangerous, possibly causing severe bradycardia and even asystole presumably triggered by cholinergic effects of the second dose. Therefore, always administer i.v. atropine or glycopyrrolate (0.6 mg or 0.4 mg, respectively, for the average adult) before giving a second dose of succinylcholine.

Non-depolarizing muscle relaxants

The South American Indians did not know that they were delivering a non-depolarizing drug in their blowpipes when hunting monkeys. We might wonder if they were astonished that they were not weakened or paralyzed when eating the curare-poisoned monkey meat. Being a quaternary, bulky molecule, D-tubocurare is not absorbed from the gut. Today, we have a long list of non-depolarizing muscle relaxants, which act by competing with acetylcholine at the neuromuscular endplate. They are either benzylisoquinolines (like the original D-tubocurare) or steroid derivatives. We can roughly classify them as intermediate-acting (between 30 and 60 minutes), and long-acting (over 1 hour). Since the discontinuation of mivacurium (Mivacron®), no representative of the "short-acting" category currently exists. Duration is affected by the dose and by how we define duration. For example, an intubating dose (a lot of relaxation!) of a short-acting drug might provide adequate surgical relaxation (soft abdominal muscles) for only half an hour; however, even after these 30 minutes, the patient might not be capable of maintaining normal blood gases without assisted ventilation. Table 12.11 provides a short list of some of the currently used drugs with certain of their characteristics. For each drug we give an "intubating dose."

Muscle relaxant reversal

We do not reverse the effect of succinylcholine with an antagonist. Instead, we unwearyingly ventilate the patient's lungs until the block has worn off, even if that takes hours in a patient homozygous for atypical cholinesterase. This differs from the non-depolarizing drugs. An excess of acetylcholine, the physiologic transmitter substance at the neuromuscular junction, will compete with the non-depolarizing relaxant for access to the endplate. Thus we give a cholinesterase inhibitor, prolonging the life of acetylcholine so it can better compete. Because these inhibitors not only act on the neuromuscular apparatus but also generate an excess of acetylcholine at autonomic sites, we add an anticholinergic drug that acts primarily on the autonomic (muscarinic) receptors. Thus, atropine or glycopyrrolate (Robinul®) can prevent the unwanted autonomic effects of the cholinesterase inhibitors, such as excessive salivation, bradycardia, and intestinal cramping.

The most commonly used cholinesterase inhibitors are neostigmine (Prostigmin®) and edrophonium (Tensilon®). Both are quaternary ammonium compounds that do not cross the blood–brain barrier, and both are potent cholinesterase inhibitors. While they show small differences in their action, either one can serve when the weakening effect of a muscle relaxant must be reversed. Neostigmine takes up to 10 minutes after an intravenous dose to reach its peak effect; edrophonium is much faster. Reversal of neuromuscular blockade cannot be achieved unless a few receptors are unblocked to give acetylcholine a fighting chance. Using a "twitch monitor" (see Chapter 7), we do not administer reversal agents until we detect at least a small response to stimulation (indicating that no more than 90% of receptors are blocked).

Typical reversal doses are:

neostigmine up to 0.08 mg/kg or edrophonium up to 1 mg/kg

with

atropine or glycopyrrolate up to 15 mcg/kg.

These doses must be adjusted to meet the patient's requirements (see Table 12.12).

A new category of drug, the cyclodextrins, has emerged from clinical trials with impressive results. Sugammadex (Bridion®) is a selective relaxant binding agent that encapsulates rocuronium molecules, effectively removing them from circulation and delivering them to the kidney for excretion. Affinity for vecuronium is substantially less, but the drug can still be effective, eliminating the need for anticholinesterases and anticholinergics (and removing their side effects). More importantly, reversal is more rapid and can be accomplished regardless of the "twitch" level.

Chapter 7 details assessment of neuromuscular blockade and muscle strength.

Dantrolene

Dantrolene (Dantrium®) finds use as an oral medication in the treatment of muscle spasms in multiple sclerosis, cerebral palsy, stroke, or injury to the spine. It affects skeletal muscles directly, i.e., beyond the neuromuscular

Table 12.12. Antagonists to neuromuscular blocking agents

Agent	Trade name	i.v. dose	Comments
Cholinesterase inhibitors; administer with atropine or glycopyrrolate to prevent bradycardia			
Edrophonium	Tensilon®	1 mg/kg	Duration 70 min
Neostigmine	Prostigmin®	0.08 mg/kg	Duration 60 min
Pyridostigmine	Mestinon®, Regonol®	0.2 mg/kg	Duration 90 min
Physostigmine	Antilirium®	1 mg	Duration 60 min; crosses blood–brain barrier; counteracts central cholinergic syndrome
Cyclodextrins			
Sugammadex	Bridion®	4 mg/kg	Duration 100 min

Table 12.13. Local anesthetics

Agent	Trade name	Relative potency	Duration	Maximum dose for infiltration
Esters				
Chloroprocaine	Nesacaine®	4	Short	800 mg
Procaine	Novocain®	1	Short	1000 mg
Tetracaine	Pontocaine®	16	Long	100 mg
Amides				
Bupivacaine	Marcaine®	4	Long	175 mg
Etidocaine	Duranest®	4	Long	300 mg
Lidocaine/lignocaine	Xylocaine®	1	Short	Plain: 300 mg (4.5 mg/kg)
			+ epi: Moderate	+ epi: 500 mg (7 mg/kg)
Mepivacaine	Polocaine®, Carbocaine®	1	Moderate	400 mg
Ropivacaine	Naropin®	3	Long	300 mg

junction. In the treatment of malignant hyperthermia, we count on its ability to re-establish a normal level of the dangerously elevated ionized calcium in the myoplasm. We start with a bolus of 1–2 mg/kg, repeated every 5–10 minutes as necessary, to a maximum of 10 mg/kg. The drug comes in vials containing 20 mg dantrolene and 3000 mg mannitol. This has to be dissolved (with difficulty) in 60 mL sterile water. To administer 2–3 mg/kg to an adult will require many vials and an extra pair of hands to prepare and administer the drug.

The local anesthetics (Table 12.13)

Instead of flooding the whole system, from head to toe, with an inhalation or intravenous anesthetic, we can inject an anesthetic locally; directly on a nerve; place it into the epidural or subarachnoid space, catching several nerves at once; or paint or spray it on mucous membranes as a topical anesthetic. Local anesthetics come in two chemical classes: esters and amides, with tetracaine (Pontocaine®) being a well-known ester and lidocaine (Xylocaine®) an even better known amide (Fig. 12.6). A trick for remembering the class of local anesthetics: if there is an 'I' before the "caine" it is an amIde. The trick to the trick, though, is this only works for the *generic* name of the drug, e.g., bupivacaine is an amide, even when found in a bottle labeled Marcaine®.

Local anesthetics interfere with nerve conduction by blocking ion fluxes through sodium channels.

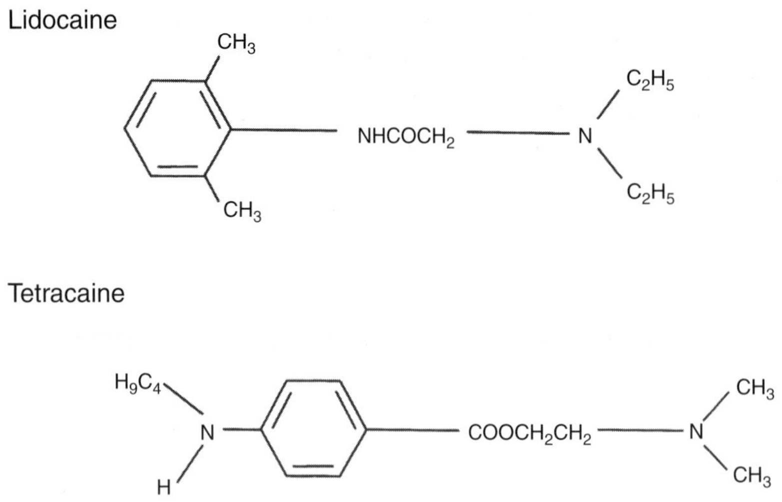

Lidocaine

Fig. 12.6 Local anesthetic structures.

Tetracaine

This blockade occurs from the inside of the cell. Local agents are weak bases with pK_b (pH at which half of the base is ionized) values between 8 and 9; at a lower pH, more of the drug will be ionized and vice versa. Only the lipid-soluble, non-ionized form can penetrate cell membranes. Once inside, the cationic form of the drug is favored because the interior of the cell tends to be more acidic than the outside. This is fortuitous, since the cationic form will go to work on the ion channel. In general, an acidic medium – for example, inflamed tissue – will favor ionization and thus delay penetration of the drug, while an alkaline medium (such as adding bicarbonate to a highly acidic commercial preparation of lidocaine) can hasten the movement of the drug through membranes.

Different nerves exhibit different sensitivities to local anesthetics. We see the clinical evidence of this during spinal anesthesia where the block for cold sensation and sympathetic activity extends to higher dermatome levels than for other sensations and motor activity. This is commonly attributed to resistance to blockade provided by the thick, heavy myelin sheath coating the motor (Aα) fibers, which is lacking on the skinny non-myelinated preganglionic sympathetic (B) fibers and postganglionic sympathetic and dorsal root (C) fibers. However, the picture is quite complex. The sensitivity will also be influenced by the position of the nerve in a nerve bundle exposed to the local anesthetic, the speed of nerve conduction, and by how much of the nerve must be exposed to the anesthetic to block it.

Once injected or applied to a membrane, the drug will be picked up and carried away by the blood. To delay this, we often add epinephrine to the local anesthetic, which constricts nearby blood vessels, thus decreasing tissue perfusion and prolonging the local anesthetic effect. It does not take much epinephrine. Solutions of as little as 1 to 800 000 have been found to do the trick. However, frequently we add epinephrine (adrenaline) in a concentration of 1 to 200 000 (5 mcg/mL) so that if we inject into the bloodstream (rather than around the nerve), the patient will get a little tachycardic, alerting us to stop the injection immediately. Greater epinephrine concentrations will not further prolong the local anesthetic effect, but will cause more tachycardia (experienced by patients as "butterflies in the stomach," headache, and apprehension). The drugs are metabolized according to their structure: the esters fall prey to plasma cholinesterase and undergo hydrolysis. Microsomal enzymes in the liver go to work on the amides. Occasionally, the products of biotransformation of local anesthetics cause mischief; for example, some patients are allergic to *para*-aminobenzoic acid, which forms during ester hydrolysis. Methemoglobinemia (and reduced oxygen-carrying capacity) has been observed after the use of prilocaine (Citanest®) and benzocaine, the latter a topical anesthetic (with a sad history of causing allergic contact dermatitis) found in some sprays and lozenges.

Lidocaine has seen widespread use as an antiarrhythmic drug. Its mechanism of action as a local anesthetic also works on the heart muscle, where it blocks cardiac sodium channels. This can explain its effect on phase IV depolarization, decreasing excitability and automaticity. The therapeutic effect of small intravenous doses of lidocaine (1 mg/kg as a bolus or 40 mcg/kg/min as an infusion – up- or down-titrated to effect) alerts us to the fact that local anesthetics do have cardiac effects, not all of which are welcome. Dangerous cardiac toxicity (hypotension, A–V block, ventricular fibrillation) has been triggered by bupivacaine mistakenly injected intravenously. All local anesthetics can have such cardiac toxicity; however, it is a particular problem with bupivacaine as its duration of binding with sodium receptors is much longer than that of other agents. Importantly, victims of bupivacaine-induced cardiac toxicity have survived after *prolonged* resuscitation. Lipid rescue of the patient with local anesthetic toxicity has saved numerous lives in just the last several years. Discovered serendipitously during animal experiments on fatty acid transport, delivery of large doses of lipid drastically increased the lethal dose of local anesthetics. The mechanism may relate to the sopping up of local anesthetic into a "lipid sink." Effects on myocardial fatty acid oxidation may also play a role. Dose recommendations continue to evolve but currently report 20% intralipid: 1.5 mL/kg bolus then 0.25 mL/kg/min for 30–60 minutes.[5]

Local anesthetics will also affect the central nervous system when injected intravenously or when a large peripheral dose is rapidly absorbed. Thus, both procaine and lidocaine have been used as intravenous anesthetics. However, their margin of safety is too narrow to recommend their routine use. With overdose, convulsions are common. As many as 4 out of 1000 patients might exhibit some CNS excitation during a regional local anesthetic. Typically, the patients complain of numbness around mouth and tongue, dizziness, tingling, and tinnitus, and they often become restless before seizing. We treat seizures with manual ventilation with oxygen and a small intravenous dose of, for example, thiopental (20–50 mg bolus for the average adult) or midazolam (1 mg bolus).

We have a large selection of local anesthetics available. The drugs differ primarily in their duration of action. Depending on dose and concentration, we have at our disposal everything from the long-acting tetracaine (Pontocaine®), bupivacaine (Marcaine®), and etidocaine (Duranest®), to the short-acting chloroprocaine (Citanest®) and procaine (Novocain®). Lidocaine and mepivacaine fit into the intermediate category.

Additives

Bicarbonate

As mentioned above, we add bicarbonate to those drugs prepared at a particularly acidic pH (lidocaine, chloroprocaine) to speed onset of anesthesia (it also reduces burning when making a skin wheal).

Epinephrine

We might add epinephrine to the local anesthetic solution to (i) prolong the duration of anesthesia, particularly for vasodilating agents such as lidocaine; (ii) reduce peak plasma concentration of the local anesthetic, also more important for vasodilating drugs; (iii) increase the density of regional anesthetic blocks (by an unknown mechanism); and (iv) as a marker for intravascular injection. Because of epinephrine's instability in an alkaline environment, commercial local anesthetic preparations containing epinephrine are highly acidic. We can add bicarbonate, and/or use plain local anesthetics to which we add epinephrine ourselves. Remember that 1:200 000 epinephrine is only 5 mcg/mL – use a tuberculin syringe and measure carefully! Important note: because we fear necrosis of the tip we do not add epinephrine to blocks placed at an "end organ," e.g., digits, penis, nose, ears.

Clonidine (Catapres®)

Through unclear mechanisms, small doses of clonidine enhance and prolong regional anesthesia. One mcg/kg added to the local anesthetic for a Bier block appears to delay the onset of tourniquet pain. In epidural and spinal anesthesia, 50–75 mcg clonidine has been found to augment the effect of both local anesthetics and opioids.

Opioids

We add opioids to neuraxial anesthetics to prolong the analgesic effect. Manageable side effects include itching, nausea, and vomiting. Respiratory depression, though less common, concerns us greatly, and we often employ pulse oximetry on the post-surgical ward. Neuraxial morphine carries a risk of delayed respiratory depression, so we continue to monitor about 24 hours after the last dose.

Bronchodilators

Bronchospasm, a common problem, whether related to asthma or chronic obstructive lung disease, can be treated with bronchodilators. These include primarily beta-adrenergic and muscarinic-anticholinergic drugs.

Among the β_2-adrenergic bronchodilators, albuterol (Ventolin® and many others) and terbutaline

(Brethaire®) find common use for inhalation. Albuterol has a longer duration of action (up to 6 hours) than terbutaline (up to 3 hours). Even though they are β_2-agonists, some patients develop β_1 effects, such as tachycardia and arrhythmias. Therefore, caution should be exercised in administering them to cardiac patients in whom tachycardia would be dangerous.

Ipratropium (Atrovent® and others), an anticholinergic, decreases contractility of bronchial smooth muscle and mucus secretion. As a quaternary amine the drug cannot diffuse into the blood, limiting systemic side effects.

Given pre-operatively to patients with a history of asthma, nebulizers might be superior to metered-dose inhalers. For management of intra-operative bronchospasm, we must ensure the drug does not attach itself to the walls of the ETT; thus nebulizers or other delivery devices find use.

Cardiovascular drugs

The anticholinergic drugs

While numerous anticholinergic drugs exist, in anesthesia we deal almost exclusively with atropine and glycopyrrolate, and occasionally with scopolamine. All three drugs act on the autonomic nervous system, blocking the effect of acetylcholine at postganglionic nerve endings. Thus, they accelerate heart rate (particularly if sympathetic tone is present), bronchodilate, cause mydriasis (thereby increasing intra-ocular pressure), inhibit salivation (and in the process dry secretions in the upper airway), inhibit sweating (by blocking the effect of postganglionic sympathetic cholinergic stimulation), and exert a variety of effects on the GI and genitourinary systems. In anesthesia we use atropine or glycopyrrolate to counteract bradycardia, salivation, and intestinal cramping, all of which are side effects of neostigmine.

Atropine and scopolamine are tertiary amines and thus capable of crossing the blood–brain barrier. In the elderly, scopolamine often causes delirium. Both drugs cross the placenta, and atropine has been observed to accelerate fetal heart rate. Both drugs have a dual effect – in addition to their well-recognized peripheral anticholinergic effect, they have a stimulating central vagal effect. With scopolamine, we sometimes see bradycardia when the central stimulating effect outlasts the peripheral blocking effect of the drug. Glycopyrrolate is a quaternary, charged compound and thus largely prevented from crossing the blood–brain barrier or the placenta.

Drugs to raise blood pressure (Table 12.14)

Hypotension is initially treated with intravenous fluids, lightening of anesthesia, and asking the surgeon not to compress major vessels such as the vena cava (if that was responsible for reducing preload). Sometimes elevating the legs and thereby increasing venous return can help to improve cardiac output and arterial blood pressure. In addition, several drugs are available to improve myocardial contractility, increase arterial resistance, and decrease venous capacitance through adrenergic effects (Table 12.14).

Ephedrine

The old standby still finds common use. We rely on its three-armed effects, alpha and beta stimulation as well as a release of norepinephrine (NE) from postganglionic sympathetic nerve terminals; 10–20 mg intravenously will increase heart rate and arterial pressure and stimulate the CNS, which we usually do not observe when we give the drug during anesthesia. It has a duration of action of about 20 minutes. Ephedrine's indirect activity prompts careful titration in patients using cocaine (NE-reuptake inhibitor), where it may have no or a dramatic effect depending on frequency and time of last use.

Epinephrine/norepinephrine

Epinephrine (adrenaline in Britain) and norepinephrine (and noradrenaline) are the two catecholamines we find circulating in blood. Norepinephrine is liberated from sympathetic nerve terminals and the adrenal medulla, while epinephrine comes only from the adrenal gland. Chemically, these two transmitter substances are identical but for a methyl group on the amine gracing epinephrine but not *nor*epinephrine (NOR = N Ohne [German for "without"] Radical). The drugs do what sympathetic stimulation does. Being physiologic transmitter substances, these catecholamines have a fleeting effect. Single bolus injections last only for a matter of a few minutes.

The body makes extensive use of these catecholamines when fight, fright, or flight call for cardiovascular, pulmonary, muscular, ocular, and intestinal adjustments. It is amazing how well these substances with overlapping adrenergic effects orchestrate their actions to an optimal end-result of sympathetic

Table 12.14. Drugs to raise blood pressure

Drug	Receptors	Effects	Infusion mixture	Infusion rate	Notes
Amrinone		↑contractility ↓SVR	500 mg in 500 mL = 1 mg/mL	5–10 mcg/kg/min	Initially bolus with 0.5–2.0 mg/kg; phosphodiesterase inhibitor; may cause thrombocytopenia
Calcium chloride		↑contractility			Slow bolus 1–10 mg/kg; direct action on myocardium; arrhythmogenic, particularly with hypokalemia
Digoxin		↑contractility ↓HR in SVT			Slow bolus 0.125–0.25 mg; delayed onset and low therapeutic safety ratio
Dobutamine	β_1	↑HR (slight) ↑contractility	500 mg/250 mL = 2 mg/mL	1–20 mcg/kg/min	Greater increase in contractility than HR, despite β_1 mechanism
Dopamine	α_1 β_1	↑HR (slight) ↑contractility bronchodilation ↑SVR (high dose)	400 mg/500 mL = 800 mcg/mL	1–20 mcg/kg/min	Direct and indirect; <10 mcg/kg/min: β_1 >10 mcg/kg/min: $\alpha_1 > \beta_1$
Ephedrine	α_1 β_1 β_2	↑HR ↑contractility bronchodilation			Mixed direct and indirect; duration 10–60 min
Epinephrine	α_1 α_2 β_1 β_2	↑HR ↑contractility bronchodilation ↓SVR (low dose) ↑SVR (high dose)	1 mg/250 mL = 4 mcg/mL or 4 mg/250 mL = 16 mcg/mL	0.05–0.15 mcg/kg/min	Arrhythmogenic; 1–2 mcg/min: β_2 4–10 mcg/min: β_1 10–20 mcg/min: $\alpha_1 > \beta$; diverts flow from kidneys to skeletal muscle; produces uterine vasoconstriction
Isoproterenol	β_1 β_2	↑HR ↑contractility bronchodilation ↓SVR	4 mg/250 mL = 16 mcg/mL	0.025–0.15 mcg/kg/min	i.v. duration 1–5 min; arrhythmogenic
Norepinephrine	α_1 α_2 β_1	↑↑ SVR ↓CO	4 mg/250 mL = 16 mcg/mL	0.05–0.15 mcg/kg/min	Massive ↑ SVR → HTN and reflex ↓HR
Phenylephrine	α_1	↑↑SVR	40 mg/250mL = 160 mcg/mL	1–3 mcg/kg/min	Reflex ↓ HR; no vasconstriction of CNS vessels
Vasopressin[a]		↑↑SVR	100 u/100 mL = 1 u/mL	0.01–1 u/min	Bolus dose 40 u in cardiac arrest; 0.4–1 u refractory hypotension

HR: heart rate; SVR: systemic vascular resistance; CO: cardiac output; HTN: hypertension; SVT: supraventricular tachycardia.
[a] Starting vasopressin dose range for refractory hypotension is from isolated case reports. Larger doses may be required. The drug does not carry an FDA indication for this use, but has found great clinical utility.

stimulation. Clinically, we are limited to giving one drug or the other, counting on just one or the other effect. For example, low doses of epinephrine may reduce blood pressure a little through a $beta_2$ effect, while larger doses raise pressure and accelerate heart rate. With norepinephrine, we see primarily increased pressure without tachycardia – as long as the baroreceptors are active. Typical doses used in the operating room might start with 10 to 20 mcg of epinephrine as a single i.v. bolus to help the average adult patient through a spell of hypotension, for example during anaphylaxis. Usually reserved for more dire situations, we titrate a norepinephrine infusion to effect, starting perhaps with 0.1 mcg/kg/min. Epinephrine can also be given by continuous infusion. During cardiac resuscitation when we assume the body to have become very much less responsive to circulating catecholamines, doses as high as 1 mg epinephrine as a bolus have been used, though current recommendations favor vasopressin in this setting.

Dopamine

A biochemical forerunner to norepinephrine, dopamine also finds clinical use. It formerly had an undeserved reputation for renal protection and countless ICU patients received "renal dose dopamine" (1–3 mcg/kg/min) in hopes it would support blood pressure while maintaining renal perfusion and promoting diuresis. While it does those things, there are no outcome benefits. In larger concentrations, it turns into a vasopressor with renal vasoconstriction, just as norepinephrine, which it can liberate from postganglionic sympathetic terminals.

Dobutamine (Dobutrex®)

A synthetic catecholamine, dobutamine is a selective β_1 agonist with greater effect on contractility than heart rate. It improves cardiac output in patients in cardiac failure. Because of its rapid metabolism, we administer dobutamine as an infusion at 2–10 mcg/kg/min, titrated to effect.

Isoproterenol (Isuprel®)

Another synthetic catecholamine, isoproterenol activates both β_1 and β_2 receptors with great vigor (2–10 times the potency of epinephrine). We use this agent to (i) increase heart rate, (ii) decrease pulmonary vascular resistance, and (iii) rarely, bronchodilate (i.v. or as an aerosol). Typical of β_1 agonism, heart rate, contractility and cardiac output increase while β_2 vasodilation

reduces SVR. The net effect is a fall in diastolic and mean blood pressures. Isoproterenol also induces arrhythmias.

Phenylephrine (Neosynephrine®)

Another old standby, phenylephrine sees vasoconstrictive service in nose drops and as an intravenous, pure α_1 agonist. We expect to see both venous and arterial vasoconstriction with the typical i.v. bolus of 40 to 100 mcg, which should raise blood pressure for about 5 minutes. Because of its relatively short duration, we can also infuse it at a rate of about 10 to 100 mcg/min (titrated to effect). Lacking β receptor stimulation, the drug will not increase heart rate or contractile force. Instead, a baroreceptor response can lead to lower heart rates.

Vasopressin (Pitressin®)

Synthesized in the posterior hypothalamus, vasopressin's effects include osmoregulation and clotting, but its propensity for vasoconstriction presents greatest utility in anesthesia, particularly when the alternative cardiovascular control systems (sympathetic and renin–angiotensin) are blunted from anesthesia and/or medications. Mediated by V1 receptors, vasoconstriction is most prominent in skin, skeletal muscle and mesenteric blood vessels, as well as the uterus. Vasopressin now competes with epinephrine as the drug of choice during cardiac arrest.

Drugs to lower blood pressure (Table 12.15)

While deepening the anesthetic or adding opioids will correct hypertension from light anesthesia, many patients require further blood pressure control. We have many agents at our disposal, with varying mechanisms of action.

Beta-blockers

The older propranolol (Inderal®) was not selective and blocked both β_1 and β_2 receptors, thus getting some patients into trouble with bronchoconstriction. Nevertheless, when it became available it represented a major advance in the treatment of hypertension, myocardial ischemia, and ventricular arrhythmias.

Frequently used today are labetalol (Normodyne®; Trandate®) and esmolol (Brevibloc®), two beta-blockers selective for the β_1 receptors with just a weak β_2 blocking component. Labetalol has the added advantage of

Table 12.15. Drugs to lower blood pressure

Drug	Mechanism of action	Onset	Duration	Adult i.v. dosage	Comments
Esmolol	β_1 blockade → ↓CO	1–2 min	10–20 min	0.25–1 mg/kg bolus	
Labetalol	$\alpha_1 \, \beta_1 \, \beta_2$ blockade → ↓SVR and ↓CO	1–5 min	2–4 h	10–25 mg divided doses	
Nitroglycerin	Direct venodilator	1 min	10 min	0.5–10 mcg/kg/min	Drug of choice in myocardial ischemia
Nitroprusside	Direct arterial and venodilator	0.5 min	2–4 min	0.2–8 mcg/kg/min	Disrupts cerebral autoregulation; causes cyanide toxicity in high doses
Hydralazine	Direct arterial dilator	10–20 min	3–4 h	5–10 mg bolus	Often used in pre-eclampsia

CO: cardiac output; SVR: systemic vascular resistance.

some α_1 blocking effect, perhaps one-seventh as strong as its β_1 effect, thus enhancing its antihypertensive action with a little peripheral vasodilatation. It has a long duration of action, lasting several hours. Typical i.v. doses start with 10 mg for the average adult. If necessary, this dose can be repeated at 2- or 3-minute intervals, three or four times. Alternatively some prefer to escalate the dose at longer intervals.

Esmolol has two characteristics that make it especially useful: it exerts a prominent effect on heart rate and has a rapid onset and relatively short duration with a half-life of under 10 minutes. The typical bolus dose is 0.25–1 mg/kg while infusions of 50 mcg/kg/min may be used for a more sustained effect.

Beta-blockers are widely used in anesthesia where the common tachycardia secondary to surgical stimulation or with tracheal intubation can lead to a mismatch of myocardial oxygen supply (reduced time for coronary perfusion) and demand (tachycardia, particularly when matched with hypertension). In addition to its intra-operative use, several studies have demonstrated that prophylactic use of beta-blockers, e.g., metoprolol, throughout the peri-operative period reduces cardiac morbidity and mortality in select patients, e.g., those with coronary artery disease. Unfortunately the risk of stroke increases in other patients, dampening the initial enthusiasm for broad application of peri-operative beta-blockade.

Direct vasodilators

When an elevated blood pressure cannot, or should not, be lowered by beta-blockade or by deepening anesthesia, and particularly when we wish to have minute-to-minute control of blood pressure, we need agents with rapid onset of action and short duration. To meet this need routinely, the body liberates nitric oxide from the vascular endothelium, which has a fleeting effect of relaxing vascular smooth muscle. Two frequently used drugs, nitroglycerin and nitroprusside, appear to work by forming nitric oxide, so intimately involved in the tone of blood vessels. Both drugs take effect within a minute and will dissipate within 5 minutes. A direct vasodilating hypotensive agent, hydralazine (Apresoline®), finds less use because of its slow onset (up to 10 minutes) and its long duration (up to 4 hours) of action. However, its long, safe track record makes it a favorite in the obstetric suite.

Nitroglycerin

Widely used in cardiology in the treatment of angina, nitroglycerin dilates vascular smooth muscle, with a preponderance of effect on venous over arterial vessels. For angina, a typical dose might be a 0.4 mg tablet under the tongue. For induced hypotension to lessen intra-operative bleeding, we infuse nitroglycerin intravenously at a rate of 0.5–1 mcg/kg/min. It is important to permit such low doses time to show their effect

Table 12.16. Antiarrhythmic drugs[a]

Agent	Trade name	i.v. dose	Comments
Adenosine	Adenocard®	6–12 mg	To convert PSVT to sinus rhythm, if only briefly; may cause bronchospasm; Duration <10 s; administer rapidly
Amiodarone	Cordarone®	300 mg	For atrial and ventricular arrhythmias; high doses linked to pulmonary toxicity
Atropine		0.6–1.0 mg	Anticholinergic; treats bradycardia
Diltiazem	Cardizem®	20 mg	Calcium channel blocker; starting dose for conversion of PSVT, or control of ventricular rate in patients with atrial fibrillation or flutter
Epinephrine		1 mg	For cardiac arrest; high-dose epinephrine no longer recommended
Glycopyrrolate	Robinul®	0.4 mg	Anticholinergic; quaternary amine that does not cross the blood–brain or placental barriers
Lidocaine	Xylocaine®	1 mg/kg bolus or 30 mcg/kg/min	For stable ventricular tachycardia and ventricular arrhythmias
Procainamide	Procan®, Pronestyl®	20 mg/min	Alternative for lidocaine-resistant arrhythmias
Verapamil	Calan®, Isoptin®	2.5–10 mg	Calcium channel blocker to treat PSVT; may increase conduction in accessory pathways

PSVT: paroxysmal supraventricular tachycardia.
[a] Beta-blockers: Agents with activity at β_1 receptors would be included in this group, see above under Drugs to lower blood pressure.

before adjusting the dose upward (potentially up to 10 mcg/kg/min in tolerant patients) in order to avoid hypotension and a stormy up and down of blood pressure by impatiently adjusting the infusion rate.

Nitroglycerin has the reputation of relieving coronary spasm and subendocardial ischemia, and thus it finds use when ST segment depression or flipped T waves signal myocardial distress. Reduced ventricular pressure and cardiac output, without a marked rise in heart rate, help to re-establish a favorable balance of myocardial oxygen demand and supply.

Sodium nitroprusside (Nipride®)

In doses similar to those for nitroglycerin, i.e., starting an infusion of 0.5–2 mcg/kg/min and up to 10 mcg/kg/min, if needed, nitroprusside appears to have a more pronounced effect on arterial vessels and the pulmonary vascular bed than nitroglycerin. In the brain, sodium nitroprusside dilates vessels and interferes with autoregulation, which can present problems to patients at risk of increased intracranial pressure. The biotransformation of nitroprusside can lead to methemoglobinemia and, in extreme cases, to the liberation

of cyanide. To minimize the chance of this toxicity, we monitor the total dose and keep it well below 500 mcg/kg in a 4-hour period.

Clonidine (Catapres®)

Though not regularly used for its antihypertensive qualities by anesthesiologists, clonidine occupies an interesting position in the classic scheme of drugs. On the one hand, it looks a little like a catecholamine, without chemically belonging to this category; on the other hand, it stimulates alpha-adrenergic receptors – but α_2 instead of α_1. Thus, it inhibits adrenergic stimulation and decreases sympathetic influence on the heart and peripheral vascular bed, resulting in bradycardia and hypotension. As such, the drug finds use in the treatment of chronic hypertension. We are acutely aware that the sudden discontinuation of clonidine medication can trigger rebound hypertension.

Clonidine also produces mild sedation and analgesia. It has been used both orally and mixed with local anesthetics to enhance and prolong analgesia (see The local anesthetics – Additives section earlier in this chapter).

Nitric oxide (INOmax®)

This interesting gas hides behind a lengthy term, namely the "endothelium-derived relaxing (vasodilatory) factor" or EDRF for short. Its precursors reside in neurons, vascular endothelium, and macrophages. Once synthesized intracellularly, the very short-lived nitric oxide (NO) triggers a cascade of steps leading to the relaxation of vascular smooth muscle. The gas now finds application in neonatal and adult critical care. Inhalation of tiny concentrations of NO (about 20 ppm) appears to benefit neonates suffering hypoxemic respiratory failure.

Antiarrhythmic drugs (Table 12.16)

Peri-operatively, we see more tachycardias (light anesthesia) than bradycardias (which might be an ominous sign of profound hypoxemia, or in children an indication of all too deep anesthesia), and we treat them according to their etiologies. That is, we would not give beta-blockers to reduce heart rate if light anesthesia must be held responsible for the rapid rate, nor would we give atropine to treat hypoxemia-induced bradycardia.

For the treatment of arrhythmias of the atria and ventricles, we have a large selection of fairly specific drugs from which we have picked a few frequently used in anesthesia and/or cardiac life support (Table 12.16). Both atropine and glycopyrrolate can be used to treat symptomatic bradycardia. However, in patients with acute myocardial ischemia, raising the heart rate (and the consequent increase in oxygen demand) can be dangerous.

Adenosine as a drug occupies a special niche because the body itself synthesizes this fleeting byproduct of ATP. We use it primarily in the treatment of re-entrant AV node tachycardias such as paroxysmal supraventricular tachycardia (PSVT). Even if the rhythm fails to convert to sinus, the transient slowing of the tachycardia can help with a specific diagnosis.

Lidocaine and procainamide work not only as local anesthetics (lidocaine better than procainamide) but also as useful antiarrhythmic drugs in the treatment of ventricular extrasystoles. Two calcium channel blockers deserve mention: diltiazem and verapamil. Both can be used to treat a variety of supraventricular arrhythmias and, by slowing atrioventricular conduction, they can reduce heart rate in patients in atrial fibrillation.

Advanced cardiac life support

Many drugs already discussed also appear in manuals on cardiac life support, for example in the treatment of arrhythmias and hypotension. One additional drug deserves a brief mention. In the past, sodium bicarbonate was given in cardiac arrest probably more often than useful. Currently, the American Heart Association recommends it for the treatment of pre-existing hyperkalemia, in diabetic ketoacidosis, in patients overdosed with tricyclic antidepressants or cocaine, and to alkalinize the urine in aspirin poisoning. We usually start with 1 mEq/kg and then, if possible, check arterial blood gases before giving more.

Notes

1   Throughout the text we use generic names for drugs. Most drugs have several trade names of which we give at least one commonly used in the USA.

2   Time for blood plasma concentration to decline by one-half after an infusion at steady-state has been discontinued. "Context" refers to the duration of the infusion.

3   A potentially fatal syndrome consisting of heart failure, rhabdomyolysis, severe metabolic acidosis and renal failure. Associated with long-term infusions, especially when accompanied by catecholamines and /or steroids.

4   N-methyl-D-aspartate.

5   Up-to-date information can be obtained through a link at www. anest.ufl.edu/ea.

Section 3

Clinical cases

In the following 11 cases, we briefly describe anesthetic approaches, issues, and some potential complications. The reader will find many of the points discussed in the first two sections of the book applied in the management of these cases. An alternative (but not, we think, the preferred) is a problem-oriented approach, namely first to read the cases and then, primed with many questions, delve into the first two sections of the book.

Clinical talk teems with acronyms. Some abbreviations used throughout the cases include:

ABG:	arterial blood gas.
ABP:	arterial blood pressure (from an invasive arterial catheter).
ACE:	angiotensin-converting enzyme.
ACT:	activated clotting time.
AICD:	automated implantable cardioverter defibrillator.
aPTT:	activated partial thromboplastin time.
ASA:	American Society of Anesthesiology physical status classification.
BIS:	bispectral index.
BP:	non-invasive blood pressure.
BUN:	blood urea nitrogen.
CPAP:	continuous positive airway pressure.
CPP:	cerebral perfusion pressure.
Cr:	creatinine.
CSF:	cerebrospinal fluid.
CV:	cardiovascular system.
CVP:	central venous pressure.
CXR:	chest X-ray.
ETT:	endotracheal tube.
fb:	fingerbreadth (the width of an average adult's finger).
FiO_2:	fraction of inspired oxygen.
Hct:	hematocrit.
HR:	heart rate.
ICP:	intracranial pressure.
INR:	international normalized ratio for PT.
LVH:	left ventricular hypertrophy.
MAP:	mean arterial pressure.
MEP:	motor evoked potential.
NIBP:	non-invasive blood pressure monitoring.
NPO:	*nil per os* = nothing by mouth.
NSR:	normal sinus rhythm.
PAC:	pulmonary artery catheter.
PACU:	post-anesthesia care unit.
P_aO_2:	partial pressure of oxygen.
PCWP:	pulmonary capillary wedge pressure.
Plt:	platelet count.
PRBC:	packed red blood cell.
PT:	prothrombin time.
PVC:	premature ventricular contraction.
S1, S2, S3, S4:	the first through fourth heart sounds, respectively.
SpO_2:	oxyhemoglobin saturation by pulse oximetry.
SSEP:	somatosensory evoked potentials.

Breast lumpectomy under conscious sedation

The following case will emphasize conscious sedation and its potential complications.

Learning objectives:

- general pre-operative evaluation
- sedative agents
- respiratory depression: detection, management
- mask–ventilation
- monitoring
- laryngeal mask airway
- reversal of sedation.

The patient, a 40-year-old and otherwise healthy woman, comes for breast biopsy.

This procedure is usually performed in two stages: first a radiologist places a needle percutaneously into the lump. Next, the patient is delivered to the operating room for removal of the lump, pathologic confirmation of the margins, and perhaps a larger procedure depending on the circumstances.

History: She has no chronic medical problems but, during a self-examination last week, detected a lump in her right breast. Needle localization under local anesthesia was performed in radiology this morning and she now presents to the operating suite for lumpectomy.

This healthy patient requires very little additional anesthetic work-up. We ask about the following:

(i) a brief review of systems, including gastroesophageal reflux disease (negative)
(ii) past surgical procedures (none)
(iii) family history of anesthetic problems (none)
(iv) current medications, including over-the-counter herbal remedies (none)
(v) allergies, including latex (none)
(vi) habits including smoking, alcohol and drugs (none).

Physical examination, including airway: Nervous woman in no acute distress; weight 60 kg; height 162 cm. BP120/80 mmHg; HR 80 beats/min; respiratory rate 12 breaths/min.

Airway: Mallampati I, 4 fingerbreadth (fb) mouth opening, 4 fb thyromental distance, full neck extension, able to prognath.

CV: S1, S2 no murmur.

Respiratory: Lungs clear to auscultation.

Dressing with needle in right breast.

This healthy patient for this elective procedure needs no laboratory or other studies and would be classified as ASA 1.

Anesthetic preparation: We discuss the risks/benefits of the various anesthetic options. She selects i.v. sedation and we administer an anxiolytic (midazolam [Versed®] 2 mg i.v.).

The surgeon will inject a local anesthetic, blunting most of the pain from the procedure, while the anesthesiologist is present to observe and reassure the patient, administer additional anxiolytics or opioids, and treat any hemodynamic instability. Most patients prefer not to be awake and aware during such a procedure. Anesthetic options include (i) conscious sedation, in which the patient remains arousable and in control of her own airway, but free from anxiety and generally unaware of the procedure, and (ii) general anesthesia in which the airway may require support by mask, laryngeal mask airway, or endotracheal tube. After we explain the risks to the patient, she selects i.v. sedation.

Establishment of sedation: Once in the operating room, we apply standard monitors (non-invasive blood pressure, ECG, pulse oximetry), taking care to avoid the right arm for blood pressure cuff application in case axillary node dissection becomes necessary. Following a 50 mg bolus of propofol, we start an infusion at 100 mcg/kg/min. The patient's saturation declines to 95% so oxygen via nasal cannula is applied at 4 L/min and the saturation rapidly returns to 100%.

In order to obtain a therapeutic blood level rapidly, we give an initial bolus of propofol and follow it with a continuous infusion to maintain the level of sedation. When the patient is sufficiently drowsy, positioning, prepping, and draping can commence. While it should not be necessary, everyone in the room must be reminded the patient is "awake." This includes a sign on the door for those entering later. Unfortunately, the decorum of the OR is not routinely suitable for the awake patient. As in any workplace, discussions may depart from the task at hand, causing concern for a patient who is aware, and might recall irrelevant or objectionable talk.

Maintenance of anesthesia: We titrate the propofol infusion to the desired effect with a goal of arousability with slurred speech, but respiratory and hemodynamic stability.

During injection of local anesthetic into the breast, she complains of pain. We administer fentanyl 50 mcg, and increase the propofol infusion rate. One minute later the patient moans and we respond with another 50 mcg fentanyl. Fifteen minutes later the SpO_2 is falling rapidly. On examination we discover she is apneic. We start ventilation by mask, but encounter difficulty maintaining an open upper airway. When things do not get much better after placing an oral airway, we advance our level of intervention and insert a laryngeal mask airway (LMA), achieving good air movement at last. Her saturation rebounds rapidly.

Less than 2 mcg/kg fentanyl generally should not cause apnea. Alone, that is usually true, however opioids combined with sedatives act synergistically to depress ventilation. Had we been monitoring respiratory pattern/rate we would have noticed that her breathing became dangerously slow a couple of minutes after we administered fentanyl. Our detection method (pulse oximetry here) failed us because we gave so much supplemental oxygen that her PaO_2 was probably close to 200 mmHg as long as she was breathing, if slowly. Thus she had to be almost apneic for her PaO_2 to fall below 80 mmHg, where a drop in the SpO_2 would be expected (try this exercise manipulating the FiO_2 [each liter of nasal cannula O_2 increases alveolar FiO_2 by about 3%] and CO_2 using the interactive simulation at *www.anest.ufl.edu/EA*).

In this case a smaller dose of fentanyl might have been more appropriate, or perhaps the use of a shorter-acting opioid such as remifentanil. More importantly, we should monitor respiratory rate – it's not hard. A luddite might choose to maintain her in conversation (although most patients prefer to be less aware than that), or place a hand on her chin and feel the breath on his palm. Only slightly more high-tech is the precordial stethoscope (impractical for this particular surgical procedure) or a pretracheal stethoscope, through which we listen to the ebb and flow of the breathing. Much can be learned using such simple techniques – changes in respiratory rate, breath volume, and airway obstruction can guide management. However, capnography attached through the nasal cannula will almost certainly be used – we prefer this as an adjunct to the simple methods rather than as a replacement. At the first sign of over-sedation, we would have supported her breathing and decreased or even interrupted the propofol infusion until the drug effect diminished enough for her natural airway composure to be reestablished. Administering naloxone to reverse the narcotic is a quicker fix if we are particularly concerned about her respiratory status and our ability to maintain her airway. However, the side effects of reversal must also be considered, particularly in the middle of an operation.

In managing the apnea, several issues need be recognized. If the problem is central, e.g., over-sedation impairing respiratory drive, the patient's lungs will have to be manually ventilated. If soft tissue obstruction of the upper airway is to blame, we need to establish an open airway with the help of an oral airway or LMA. In this difficult phase of being neither awake nor completely anesthetized, manipulation of the upper airway can lead to laryngospasm, coughing, vomiting, and significant movement (usually much to the dismay of the surgeon). In our case the problem was central depression from the combination of fentanyl and propofol and the patient tolerated the LMA. At this point we would add nitrous oxide and increase the propofol infusion rate so she will continue to tolerate the LMA.

Emergence from anesthesia: During closure of the incision, we titrate down the propofol and eventually discontinue the nitrous oxide. When the bandage has been applied, and the patient is awake and breathing with a good respiratory pattern, we remove the LMA and then suction the patient's oropharynx if needed.

Post-anesthesia care: There should be no acute pain from this procedure as the biopsy site has been infiltrated with local anesthetic. We turn the care of the patient over to the post-anesthesia care unit (PACU) nurse with standing orders of morphine for pain (as the local anesthetic wears off), and an anti-emetic, as needed.

One advantage of the LMA is that, if the patient is breathing spontaneously but not fully awake, she can be transported to the PACU with the LMA in place, where the nurse removes it at the appropriate time.

Discharge: When the patient is fully awake and tolerating oral intake, she can be discharged home with a caregiver, prescription for an analgesic, and instructions not to drive for 24 hours.

Carpal tunnel release under Bier block

The following case will describe the use of intravenous regional anesthesia.

Learning objectives:

- pre-operative management of the asthmatic patient
- intravenous regional anesthesia
- local anesthetic toxicity
- intra-operative bronchospasm.

A 50-year-old asthmatic woman comes for carpal tunnel release.

This minor procedure is usually performed as an outpatient. That is, the patient comes in the day of surgery, and returns home afterward.

History: She has frequent painful tingling of her right hand, consistent with carpal tunnel syndrome. Her past medical history is significant only for asthma since childhood. The asthma is controlled with albuterol metered dose inhaler (MDI) three times a day and more if necessary. She has never had surgery, and gives no family history of anesthetic complications. She takes only asthma medications and hormone replacement therapy. She has no allergies, but smokes two packs a day with a 50 pack-year smoking history. She drinks socially and takes no illegal drugs.

We will ask this patient additional questions regarding her lung disease, to determine its severity, as well as whether her current medical therapy is optimal.

The patient describes chronic asthma without identified precipitating factors or seasonal variation. She has never been intubated for an asthmatic attack, but has been to the emergency room on several occasions. The last event was more than 2 years ago. She has not received steroids but has required extra doses of her MDI twice in the past week, which is about normal for her. She describes feeling that she is in her usual best condition. She has not had a cold in the last 4 weeks. She has no recent pulmonary function tests (PFTs) or chest radiographs.

Pulmonary function tests are unlikely to alter our anesthetic management for this peripheral operation and would not be requested. Her medical therapy appears to be adequate.

Physical examination: Caucasian woman in no acute distress; weight 85 kg; height 5′ 4″ (160 cm).

BP 135/80 mmHg; HR 90 beats/min; respiratory rate 16 breaths/min.

Airway: Mallampati I, 4 fb mouth opening, 4 fb thyromental distance, full neck extension.

CV: S1, S2 no murmur.

Respiratory: Lungs with mild bilateral expiratory wheezes; mildly lengthened expiratory phase; no obvious use of accessory respiratory muscles.

We require no pre-operative laboratory or other studies in this ASA II patient.

Asthmatic patients are at increased risk for intra-operative bronchospasm and post-operative pulmonary complications. Avoiding instrumentation of the airway reduces this risk, therefore we prefer local or regional anesthesia.

Anesthetic preparation: We discuss risks/benefits of local anesthesia/intravenous sedation vs. intravenous regional anesthesia (IVRA) vs. regional anesthesia (e.g., axillary block) vs. general anesthesia; the patient selects IVRA. We administer nebulized albuterol followed by an anxiolytic (midazolam 2 mg i.v.).

We will perform an IVRA.

Establishment of regional anesthesia: Once in the operating room, and after the pre-operative time-out is completed, we apply standard monitors (without using the right arm), including nasal cannula with gas sampling capability (for CO_2 and respiratory rate). We place a second i.v. in the back of her right hand, and then apply a double tourniquet to the upper arm. We squeeze out all blood currently in the arm by holding it up and tightly wrapping it in an elastic Esmarch bandage. Then we inflate the distal tourniquet to about 100 mmHg above her systolic pressure, and repeat for the proximal tourniquet to continue with the exsanguination. We then deflate the distal tourniquet. After injecting 50 mL of 0.5% plain lidocaine into the i.v. below the inflated tourniquet (NOT the other i.v.!), we remove the catheter. Her arm will appear blanched and she will first have a pins and needles sensation, then no sensation at all. We titrate propofol at 50–100 mcg/kg/min to achieve the desired sedation. This sedative is a particularly good choice in the asthmatic patient.

Tourniquet pain limits operative time under IVRA. With a double tourniquet we can treat such pain by inflating the distal cuff, which compresses over tissue anesthetized by the local, after which the painful proximal cuff can be deflated. We are careful to keep one of the cuffs inflated at all times lest the local anesthetic escape into the central circulation. After about 20 minutes of total tourniquet time we can release the pressure in a staged fashion, releasing the remaining local into the system safely.

Maintenance of anesthesia: We titrate the propofol infusion to effect, maintaining arousability to speech and an acceptable respiratory rate. Suddenly the patient complains of ringing in her ears and tingling around her mouth.

These are common early signs of local anesthetic toxicity. We check the tourniquet to insure the pressure is adequate, and perfusion of the arm has not returned. We ask the surgeons about bleeding at the surgical site and monitor the patient closely for sequelae of local anesthetic toxicity including seizures and cardiovascular collapse.

We immediately inflate the distal tourniquet cuff and the symptoms subside. After 20 minutes the patient complains of pain at the site of the distal tourniquet. She is becoming restless from the discomfort and the surgeon still needs at least another few minutes to complete the procedure.

As mentioned above, tourniquet pain is often the limiting factor in IVRA. It is difficult to manage, and with the remaining operative time, we need to do something else. We could use general anesthesia. Because instrumenting the airway is a major trigger for bronchospasm, the laryngeal mask airway (LMA) would be a good choice in this setting. Another option, if the surgical situation (time, stage, and location) permits, is local supplementation.

We inform the patient we are going to correct her discomfort, release the tourniquet in several steps, and ask the surgeon to reinforce the local anesthetic at the operative site with a small field block using 1% lidocaine with 1:200 000 epinephrine. The surgeon accomplishes this and the patient is again comfortable. We continue propofol for sedation. Ten minutes before the end of the operation we give 2 mg of morphine i.v. to minimize early post-operative pain. Three minutes later her respiratory rate has increased to 30 breaths per minute, and the end-tidal CO_2 has fallen. Lung auscultation reveals bilateral wheezing.

Morphine can cause histamine release, inducing bronchospasm. We have several options for treatment. Volatile anesthetics, and especially the non-pungent halothane and sevoflurane, work well as bronchodilators. However, halothane can sensitize the heart to the arrhythmogenic effects of sympathomimetic drugs. We begin by administering albuterol via MDI (available on every anesthesia cart) and she responds nicely.

In retrospect, if the surgeon suspected this may not be a straightforward carpal tunnel release, requiring more than 30–40 minutes, then a regional anesthetic (brachial plexus block) would have afforded a longer duration of action. The mild local anesthetic toxicity could have been much worse with a complete failure of the tourniquet.

Emergence from anesthesia: During closure of the incision, we discontinue the sedative propofol infusion.

Post-anesthesia care: There should be little pain from this procedure. We leave the patient in the PACU with standing prn[1] orders of fentanyl for pain, rather than morphine, because of her bronchospastic reaction. We also write orders for an anti-emetic drug, should it be needed.

Discharge: When the patient is fully awake and tolerating oral intake, she can be discharged home with a caregiver, a prescription for an analgesic, and instructions not to drive for 24 hours.

Note

1   prn = *pro re nata*; as the need arises.

Cataract removal under MAC

The following case will describe the use of monitored anesthetic care (MAC).

> ## Learning objectives:
>
> - pre-operative management of the elderly patient
> - methohexital
> - micro-environments
> - oculo-cardiac reflex.

> An 85-year old woman comes for removal of a cataract.
>
> History: She has suffered significant visual loss from the cataract. Her past medical history reveals that she has given birth to four children and that she had an uncomplicated cholecystectomy under general anesthesia 40 years ago. She has no family history of anesthetic complications. She takes only a daily baby aspirin which she stopped a week ago, has no allergies, and does not smoke. She drinks wine socially. She gardens daily and her activity is only limited by arthritis.

Physical examination reveals:

> Elderly woman in no acute distress; weight 65 kg; height 5'2" (155 cm).
>
> BP 150/90 mmHg; HR 90 beats/min; respiratory rate 16 breaths/min, room air SpO$_2$ 97%.
>
> Airway: Edentulous, Mallampati II, 4 fb mouth opening, 4 fb thyromental distance, full neck extension.
>
> CV: S1, S2 no murmur.
>
> Respiratory: Lungs clear to auscultation bilaterally.

No additional pre-operative laboratory or other studies are required in this ASA I patient.

Such minor eye procedures are usually performed under local anesthesia (peribulbar, retrobulbar or topical) administered by the ophthalmologist. Injection of the local is not without pain, however transient, so we usually anesthetize the patient briefly (minutes) if it is anything more than topical.

Anesthetic preparation: We discuss the risks/benefits of the anesthetic plan, giving the patient an idea of what to expect: "You will be asleep for about 2 minutes while the surgeon places numbing medicine around your eye. After you wake up you will not be able to see as there will be a drape over your face. We will blow fresh air under the drape and we will be monitoring your heart and lungs. You should feel no pain but let us know should you be uncomfortable or before you may need to cough or move."

Induction of anesthesia: The eye block may be placed in the operating room, or in the pre-operative holding area, allowing more time for it to take effect. Either way, we apply standard monitors, give the patient some supplemental oxygen, and then administer a short-acting induction agent such as methohexital (Brevital®) or thiopental. When the patient loses consciousness, the ophthalmologist places the block and tests it as soon as the patient awakens. Some patients become transiently apneic following the induction agent, and we need to support their airway (chin lift) or their ventilation with a mask until they resume spontaneous breathing.

Once the eye is anesthetized, the patient must remain still for some time. Startle responses, as may occur with sedation, can be disastrous during eye surgery, therefore following her brief anesthesia-induced respite, we administer no additional sedative and the patient remains awake for the remainder of the procedure. Exhaled CO$_2$ can be trapped under the surgical drape. Rebreathing of CO$_2$, together with a sense of claustrophobia, can cause anxiety. We can blow air under the drape and/or use a suction tube to remove accumulated CO$_2$ and pull fresh air from the room into the space under the drape. Use of nasal cannula with gas sampling allows us to evaluate for significant rebreathing. We must resist using oxygen because, coupled with a fuel (the drape) and an ignition source (a pen cautery), a flash fire is possible. While rarely employed for a cataract operation, cautery is occasionally used for other eye procedures.

If the patient's oxygen saturation is lower than we desire then the nasal cannula gas can be enriched. This is accomplished by mixing air with oxygen in a ratio of at least 7 parts air to each part oxygen so that the gas exiting the nasal cannula and potentially accumulating under the drapes is <30% oxygen, which makes the risk of flash fire less likely. Obviously we cannot then hook the nasal cannula up to the pure oxygen nipple on the anesthesia machine. In fact using just 2 L of nasal cannula O_2 per minute can easily create a highly flammable environment under the drape. In the USA there are still at least 10 on-patient fires each week and overwhelmingly they take place in a scenario like this where there is cautery, an open source of oxygen, and a paper drape. The results are very often devastating.

> Maintenance of anesthesia: No additional sedatives are administered.
>
> Complication: Suddenly the patient's heart rate falls to 30 beats/min and she complains of not feeling well.

The most likely culprit of sudden-onset bradycardia in this setting is the oculo-cardiac reflex. Traction on the eye and ocular muscles can result in a slowing of the heart via a trigeminovagal pathway.[1] The bradycardia usually resolves immediately upon removal of the stimulus. The reflex response fatigues over time, but if it prevents progress of the operation, an anti-cholinergic may be required.

> The ophthalmologist releases pressure on the eye, with immediate recovery of the heart rate to 70 beats/min. When the surgeon attempts to resume the operation, the heart rate again falls. After several attempts, we give glycopyrrolate 0.2 mg i.v. The patient's heart rate rapidly increases to 90 beats/min and the surgery proceeds.

For its lack of central effects (it is a charged molecule and therefore does not cross the blood–brain barrier) we choose glycopyrrolate over atropine.

> Post-anesthesia care: When the surgery is complete we take the patient to the PACU where she is monitored for surgical complications for a brief time, then discharged home with a companion.

Note

1   The full pathway is ciliary ganglion → ophthalmic division of trigeminal nerve → gasserian ganglion → main trigeminal sensory nucleus in the fourth ventricle → vagus nerve.

The following case will emphasize regional anesthesia and obstetric issues.

Learning objectives:

- reflux: risks, prevention
- physiology: fluid dynamics
- neuraxial anesthesia: technique, epidural hematoma risk, hypotension risk
- vasopressors: ephedrine vs. phenylephrine
- neuraxial opioids: pros/cons, risks.

A 28-year-old primiparous (first baby), pre-eclamptic woman requires a cesarean section for breech presentation of a 38-week fetus.

History: She had a normal prenatal course. This morning she complained of headache, blurred vision and swelling in her face, feet, and hands. She is hypertensive, and has proteinuria and generalized edema.

Her constellation of symptoms and findings suggest severe pre-eclampsia.[1] Simply put we and the obstetrician need to control her blood pressure, start a magnesium infusion to reduce the risk of eclamptic seizure, and deliver the baby as soon as possible.

Review of systems: Frank acid reflux symptoms, low back pain with pregnancy, and recent accelerated weight gain.

The first two are normal findings in pregnancy. Progesterone-induced relaxation of the lower esophageal sphincter, increased acid secretion, and elevated intra-abdominal pressure increase the risk of aspiration of acidic gastric contents, a dangerous and potentially fatal complication during general anesthesia for delivery. The recent weight gain is edema fluid, part and parcel of pre-eclampsia.

Physical examination: Anxious woman in mild distress (headache); weight 100 kg; height 5'6" (165 cm).
BP 160/110 mmHg; HR 100 beats/min; respiratory rate 18 breaths/min.

Generalized edema including face.
Airway: Mallampati I, 4 fb mouth opening, 4 fb thyromental distance, full neck extension.
CV: S1, S2 no murmur.
Respiratory: Lungs clear to auscultation, no râles.
Neurologic: Reflexes 4+ without clonus.

To interpret these findings, we must recognize the normal physiologic changes of pregnancy:

- increased blood volume – plasma volume increases more than red blood cell mass leading to a dilutional anemia
- vasodilation to accommodate the increased volume
- increased respiratory drive – a central progesterone effect → a decrease in baseline $PaCO_2$ to 30 mmHg → increased minute ventilation. Surprisingly (given the enlargement of the abdomen) this is achieved mostly by increasing the tidal volume.

Pre-eclampsia reverses the gestational vasodilation, leading to hypertension; and increases capillary permeability, resulting in proteinuria, reduced intravascular volume, and cerebral, peripheral, and potentially pulmonary edema.

Pre-operative studies: Urine protein dipstick 4+; hemoglobin 12 g/dL; hematocrit 36%; platelets 120 000/microL.

In all pregnant patients we inquire about a history of easy bruising or bleeding. Pre-eclampsia can progress to hemolysis, elevated liver enzymes, low platelets (HELLP) syndrome. Therefore, before placing an epidural or spinal anesthetic we obtain a platelet count. A low platelet count would raise the specter of an epidural or subdural hematoma forming, a dreaded complication of neuraxial anesthesia. Proteinuria is routinely tested in pregnancy, and is one of the diagnostic criteria of pre-eclampsia.

Anesthetic preparation: We discuss the risks/benefits of regional vs. general anesthesia, emphasizing the significant advantages of regional in this setting. She agrees and consents to regional. She drinks 15 mL of a non-particulate antacid (sodium citrate) just before moving back to the OR, where we keep her nerves in check with engaging conversation.

Anesthetic options in this ASA IIIE patient include neuraxial anesthesia (spinal or epidural) or general anesthesia. We prefer regional anesthesia for several reasons: (i) all anesthetics that reach the brain also cross the placenta, therefore if the mother is asleep, we will deliver a drowsy baby, increasing the risk of neonatal depression; (ii) the mother (and often a companion) can witness the birth; and (iii) in most cases we have no need to manage her airway (but administer the antacid just in case). We explain the risks to the mother.

Despite the more rapid onset of a sympathectomy with a spinal, dramatic hypotension rarely occurs in the pre-eclamptic patient and spinal anesthesia remains the method of choice for most cesarean deliveries for speed of onset and density of the surgical block. However, should this be a multi-multi-repeat cesarean (as occurs with the declining enthusiasm for trial of labor after cesarean [TOLAC]), we consider placing an epidural as "backup" should the operative time extend beyond that of the spinal (about 90 minutes with bupivacaine).

Because we do not routinely sedate these patients, reassuring conversation throughout the procedure is essential.

Establishment of regional anesthesia: We have the patient sit on the bed, attach standard monitors, and increase the flow rate of crystalloid (normal saline or Ringer's lactate) into her i.v. After a vigorous skin prep and aseptic draping, we gently place a lumbar one-shot spinal with hyperbaric bupivacaine and a small amount of fentanyl and duramorph. We then help the patient lie down with left uterine displacement, and monitor the anesthetic level. We can carefully manipulate the angle of the bed to achieve a T4 level. Maternal blood pressure may require support as the regional anesthetic takes effect. We administer prophylactic antibiotics.

The fluid bolus should help offset the hypotension from sudden vasodilation, but must be administered with caution as this pre-eclamptic patient is prone to pulmonary edema. A greater cause of hypotension is caval compression by the uterus. We minimize this compression by either tilting the table to the left or placing a wedge under the right hip, which moves the uterus off the vena cava located to the right of her spine. For blood pressure support, we prefer phenylephrine as it is less likely to cross the placenta causing increased fetal oxygen demand. However, in the pre-eclamptic patient we use great caution administering phenylephrine or ephedrine as many have increased sensitivity to catecholamines and can have a profound response to even a small dose … titrate!

Timing of antibiotics in cesarean delivery has changed in recent years, formerly occurring after cord clamp to prevent exposure of the baby. As of this writing, recommendations include pre-operative administration similar to non-obstetric surgical cases with use of a cephalosporin and azithromycin in non-allergic patients.

Neuraxial duramorph (long-acting morphine) has many side effects – particularly nausea, itching, and (rarely) respiratory depression – but these are far outweighed by its benefit of reduced post-operative pain.

Maintenance of anesthesia: Following delivery of the child, we start a pitocin infusion. During uterine closure the patient complains of upper abdominal pain. We apply a face mask with 50% nitrous oxide in oxygen to provide conscious analgesia/sedation.

Pitocin is routinely administered to increase uterine tone and reduce blood loss. It should be given as a rapid infusion rather than a bolus as the latter can cause pulmonary hypertension and systemic hypotension. Should the uterus remain atonic, the standard second-line agent, methergine (an ergot alkaloid), is avoided in the pre-eclamptic patient because it may exacerbate vasoconstriction and hypertension, instead we choose 15-methyl-prostaglandin F2α (Hemabate®, Carboprost®) which may cause less hypertension but might exacerbate asthma (it's never easy!).

Nitrous oxide is a fair analgesic with minimal cardiovascular effects. Because MAC (minimum alveolar concentration) is reduced 40% in pregnancy, nitrous oxide gains in effectiveness.

Post-anesthesia care: The spinal level recedes over 2–3 hours. We continue intravenous fluids, pitocin, and magnesium.

Common PACU problems include anesthesia-induced shivering (Rx: meperidine, clonidine, or tramadol), morphine-induced pruritus (Rx: nalbuphine [a mixed agonist-antagonist opioid]), nausea/vomiting (possibly morphine-induced, Rx: anti-emetics), pain (Rx: ketorolac [safe even with nursing], i.v. opioids). Pre-eclampsia and the risk of eclamptic seizure do not disappear immediately upon delivery, therefore we continue magnesium sulfate infusion and blood pressure management.

> Discharge: After we document that the block is receding, we discharge the patient to the ward for 2–3 days recuperation before letting her go home.

The neuraxial duramorph provides analgesia for 12–18 hours. Additional sedative or opioid analgesics during this time risk respiratory depression, but pain should be treated! Should additional narcotics be required, continuous monitoring by pulse oximetry enables early detection of respiratory depression – provided the patient does not receive supplemental oxygen.

Note

1   Severe pre-eclampsia is defined by, among other things, presence of headache and visual disturbance.

Gastric bypass under general anesthesia

Learning objectives:

- anesthesia for the morbidly obese patient
- obstructive sleep apnea
- fiberoptic intubation
- epidural anesthesia for post-operative pain.

A 40-year-old morbidly obese woman comes for a gastric bypass operation.

This intra-abdominal procedure involves restriction of the stomach and partial small bowel bypass to give the patient a sense of fullness even with limited oral intake and to decrease nutrient absorption. It may be performed by laparotomy or laparoscopy, and rarely involves significant blood loss.

History: She is morbidly obese despite multiple diets, one of which involved the drug Fen-Phen.

Use of Fen-Phen (fenfluramine–phentermine), a popular diet pill in the 1990s, has been blamed for the development of heart valve abnormalities and pulmonary hypertension.

Review of systems: Chronic hypertension; obstructive sleep apnea (OSA) requiring a CPAP mask at night set at 15 cmH$_2$O pressure – begun last year; adult-onset diabetes mellitus; reflux; chronic low back pain and poor exercise tolerance.

We associate all of these findings and symptoms with morbid obesity. The OSA worries us in particular because of its association with pulmonary hypertension and difficult airway management.

Medications: Calcium-channel blocker, diuretic, oral hypoglycemic, H$_2$ blocker.

We will ask the patient to take her calcium-channel and H$_2$ blockers the morning of surgery, but neither the diuretic (she will already be dehydrated from her NPO period) nor the oral hypoglycemic (without food intake, her blood sugar could fall dangerously low).

Physical examination: Morbidly obese woman in no distress; weight 484 lb (220 kg); height 5' (150 cm). Body mass index (BMI) 98.

BP 150/90 mmHg; HR 90 beats/min; respiratory rate 18 breaths/min.

Airway: Mallampati IV; 3 fb mouth opening; 4 fb thyromental distance; inability to prognath, neck extension limited by redundant tissue.

CV: S1, S2 no murmur.

Respiratory: Lungs clear to auscultation.

Obesity is an independent risk factor for difficult tracheal intubation. Though the majority of obese patients are easily intubated via direct laryngoscopy, the presence of additional risk factors suggests the need for special intubation techniques. In her these additional factors include that she is clinically severely obese, requires CPAP, and has limited lower jaw mobility (is unable to push her lower jaw forward [prognath]), which is required during traditional direct laryngoscopy. Intravenous access may be difficult and various possible sites should be examined.

Pre-operative studies: Hgb 12 g/dL; Hct 36%; Plt 250000/microL; Na 140 mEq/L; K 4.2 mEq/L; BUN 23 mg/dL; Cr 1.3 mg/dL; glucose 135 mg/dL (7.5 mmol/L).
ABG: pH 7.40; PCO$_2$ 40 mmHg; PO$_2$ 85 mmHg; bicarbonate 28 mEq/L.
ECG: normal sinus rhythm at 90 beats/min, ST segments at baseline, no right ventricular hypertrophy noted.
Echocardiogram: normal valves and RV systolic pressures.

Infrequently, laparoscopic gastric bypass can result in significant blood loss, hence we like to know the starting hematocrit. Also, should that hematocrit be abnormally high, we will look even more closely at her pulmonary and cardiac functions (we are concerned that long-standing chronic hypoxemia has caused polycythemia, pulmonary artery hypertension, and right ventricular hypertrophy). We check her fasting blood glucose level because of her diabetes, and electrolytes because of her diuretic use. BUN and creatinine values can reveal renal insufficiency from diabetes and/or hypertension. Other studies further evaluate the impact of her OSA including the arterial blood gas (ABG), which shows no CO_2 retention and a mild reduction in the PaO_2 (presumably from basilar atelectasis), and the ECG, which shows no evidence of right ventricular hypertrophy.

Preparation for anesthesia: For post-operative pain management, we offer thoracic epidural analgesia, placed awake with her in the sitting position under mild sedation carefully titrated to effect. She needs general endotracheal anesthesia for the operation. Because we worry about intubation of her airway, we plan an awake fiberoptic intubation and therefore give her glycopyrrolate.

We also order metoclopramide and bicitra.

Use of an epidural catheter for post-operative pain control in this setting (morbid obesity, incision near the diaphragm) can reduce the need for opiates and their antitussive effects and thus the threat of pulmonary complications. Sedation must be titrated to effect without compromising the patient's ventilation.

The airway exam raises many concerns, not the least of which is the limited space in the mouth to maneuver intubation equipment. It appears there is little chance we can improve our prospects by distracting the jaw or extending her head. Therefore, we prepare for an awake intubation using a fiberoptic bronchoscope. To reduce the volume of secretions that may interfere with visualization we pre-treat with an anti-sialogogue (glycopyrrolate). Were she not already taking an H_2 blocker, we might add that to her pre-operative medications, intended to reduce the risk of aspiration of gastric contents and its sequelae.

Induction of anesthesia. We place a thoracic epidural catheter, encountering some (not unexpected) technical difficulty. Once placed and tested we move to the operating room.

After topical pharyngeal lidocaine, we perform superior laryngeal and transtracheal blocks. We smoothly advance a fiberoptic scope into her trachea and advance the endotracheal tube without so much as a tiny gag. Once we detect end-tidal CO_2 on the capnograph, we induce general anesthesia with a small dose of propofol and turn on the desflurane vaporizer.

Obese patients challenge even the expert at placing epidural catheters. Persistence, a cooperative patient, and experience eventually win out. Some useful tricks to identify midline (often tricky in these patients, and facilitated by the sitting position): repeatedly ask the patient whether she feels the needle to the right or left of midline; use the needle to probe for the most superficial bony surface, which will coincide with the tip of the spinous process; or employ ultrasound to identify the same.

Obese patients desaturate rapidly with apnea because of both a reduced functional residual capacity (FRC) and increased oxygen consumption. We have cause for concern, given the likely difficulty with mask–ventilation (decreased chest wall compliance), potentially difficult tracheal intubation, and even a problem identifying tracheal rings should a surgical airway become necessary (heaven forbid!).

Maintenance of anesthesia: We maintain anesthesia with desflurane in 50% inspired oxygen in air, titrating the volatile agent to maintain hemodynamic stability and a BIS (bispectral index) between 40 and 60. After the surgeon inflates her abdomen with carbon dioxide to a pressure of 15 mmHg, she requires high peak inspiratory pressures (40–50 cmH_2O) to achieve an adequate tidal volume. Tilting the bed into a head-elevated position helps the surgeon see better in the upper abdomen and also makes it easier to ventilate her. Local anesthetics administered through the epidural catheter provide relaxation of her abdominal muscles, making the operation a little easier for the surgeon. A solid epidural block to the level of T5 also minimizes the need for volatile anesthetic agents. We re-dose the epidural with 2% lidocaine with 1:200 000 epinephrine every 60–90 minutes depending on the clinical situation.

After a lengthy operation, morbidly obese patients have a slow emergence from volatile anesthetics, which are highly soluble in the poorly perfused fat, forming a depot of anesthetics. Thus desflurane is an attractive choice, because it has both very low blood and lipid solubility compared to the other volatile agents and allows us to still have a very efficient emergence. We do not use nitrous oxide, which might expand gas in the bowel and thus add difficulties for the surgeon. Obese patients may also have increased CNS sensitivity to medications, particularly opioids. The reliance on regional anesthesia reduces the need for both volatile agents and narcotics. We allow the epidural anesthetic to wane into analgesia (minimal or no motor block) before the procedure ends so she will be able to maintain her airway, breathe deeply, and cough effectively upon extubation of her trachea.

> Emergence from anesthesia: Following conclusion of the operation the patient awakens. She is strong, following commands, has a gag reflex and has a good respiratory pattern. We extubate her trachea and transport her to the PACU with continuous pulse oximetry monitoring in transit and the epidural infusion running for post-operative pain relief. We report to the PACU physician and nurse, including plans for post-operative pain management.

All patients should meet extubation criteria before the endotracheal tube is removed: fully awake, following simple commands, able to protect the airway, breathing spontaneously, and back to full strength. Here we are particularly concerned because this patient was intubated with a special technique that may be difficult to repeat quickly. Therefore, we delay extubation several minutes (or longer), or use a "tube exchanger" – a long stylet that we place down the endotracheal tube, then leave in the trachea after extubation providing a conduit for reintubation should the need arise.

> Post-anesthesia care: We manage her pain with the epidural infusion. Should she require additional analgesics, we should be extremely cautious with those that can depress ventilation.

Common PACU complications include desaturation, hypertension due to pain, and hypotension due to inadequate fluid replacement and/or epidural-induced sympathectomy. Trouble arises should a synergistic effect of weakened muscle power from the epidural block compound respiratory depression from narcotics.

> PACU event – desaturation: After about 30 minutes the nurse calls the PACU physician because the patient's SpO_2 has fallen below 90% despite 4 L/min oxygen via nasal cannula. She is arousable, after which her saturation improves temporarily, but declines again as she falls back asleep.

We consider the many etiologies of hypoxemia, and investigate the likelihood of the most probable:

- *Narcosis*? She has received no intravenous opioids, and the concentration in the epidural infusion is unlikely to cause significant respiratory depression.
- *High epidural block with muscle weakness*? Her upper and lower extremities are strong – ruling out this diagnosis.
- *Residual neuromuscular blockade*? She did not receive any non-depolarizing muscle relaxants intra-operatively, relying instead on the epidural for relaxation.
- *Atelectasis*? Probably part of the problem, but would not explain desaturation only while asleep.
- *Obstructive sleep apnea*? This rises to the top of the list when we watch the patient breathe. She snores loudly and, though difficult to see but readily felt by placing a gentle hand over her larynx, a tracheal tug is evident with each inspiration. With some breaths she fails to move any air at all.

This patient requires CPAP to sleep at home. Lingering anesthetic effects and decreased afferent sensory input from the epidural anesthetic reduce stimulation to breathe, which might conspire with her upper airway pathology and thus worsen sleep apnea. She requires CPAP to decrease both the obstruction (evident from snoring) and the atelectasis from shallow breathing (improved SpO_2 after CPAP). We keep the patient awake until a respiratory therapist brings the necessary equipment.

> Discharge: After we confirm the epidural block is behaving as expected (return of muscle function but excellent analgesia), and are confident with her ventilation, we discharge the patient to the surgery ward with continuous pulse oximetry. We alert the surgical service of her dependence on CPAP and the need for respiratory monitoring on the ward. We also inform the acute pain service (APS) of her location so they can manage her epidural medications for the next 2–3 days, until the pain level subsides and she is able to take oral medications.

In the post-operative orders we restrict additional opioids or sedatives except as prescribed by the acute pain service. These members of the anesthesia care team will be available on call as needed and will see the patient on rounds at least twice daily to adjust dosing regimens and ensure safety.

The following case will emphasize peripheral nerve block anesthesia and risks associated with care of the diabetic patient.

Learning objectives:

- anesthetic implications of chronic renal failure
- anesthetic implications of diabetes
- regional anesthesia of the upper extremity.

A 62-year-old man comes for placement of an AV (arteriovenous) fistula for dialysis.

An AV fistula access is usually placed in the arm and typically takes less than 2 hours. We expect no significant blood loss.

History: The patient with long-standing insulin-dependent diabetes has developed progressive renal failure over the past several years, requiring peritoneal dialysis for the past 6 months (last dialysis was overnight). His diabetes is believed to be the culprit causing his renal failure.

A dialysis-dependent patient will have his hematocrit, electrolytes, and ECG checked before the operation.

Review of systems: Chronic hypertension; diabetes, now with good control on insulin (HbA1c 6.4% last month); can walk 1 mile or climb a flight of stairs without shortness of breath or chest pain; denies orthopnea or paroxysmal nocturnal dyspnea. He makes urine (but obviously of poor quality), has no history of a bleeding problem, and has one prior surgery under general endotracheal anesthesia 5 years ago to repair a knee injury with no anesthetic complications.

People with diabetes are at risk of hypertension and chronic renal failure. With diabetes, his risk for delayed gastric emptying is elevated and thus we insist that he remain NPO after midnight. However, if not allowed to eat, his blood sugar may become dangerously low

as he is on insulin, some of which may still be working the morning of surgery. If he takes his morning insulin we may compound that problem. Thus, we are very concerned with peri-operative control of his blood glucose, and therefore instruct him to take only half the night-time dose of his long-acting insulin, skip his morning insulin, and we schedule his operation early in the morning. In the pre-operative holding area we check a "chem stick" (capillary blood glucose) when we start our i.v. before surgery, and treat with insulin and/or glucose to maintain a level in the range of 100–200 mg/dL (~6.0–12.0 mmol/L). Should we be unable to schedule him as a "first start" case, we might have the patient report to pre-operative holding early to check his blood glucose and manage it as needed. While his cardiac status appears good, and the Cardiac Guidelines ("Eagle criteria") would not necessitate further evaluation, we might reasonably ask for a 12-lead ECG in the last 3 months, considering the risk of silent ischemia in hypertensive, diabetic patients.

Medications: Labetalol (for hypertension), insulin (NPH and regular), erythropoietin (for anemia), Phoslo (to bind dietary phosphorus), calcitriol (to increase dietary calcium absorption and replace vitamin D).

This is basically a standard "laundry list" of medications for the ESRD (end-stage renal disease) patient.

Physical examination: Moderately obese man in no distress; weight 100 kg; height 5'10" (175 cm); BMI is 32.
BP 170/95 mmHg; HR 90 beats/min; respiratory rate 12 breaths/min.
Airway: Mallampati II; 3 fb mouth opening; 4 fb thyromental distance; full neck extension.
CV: S1, S2, no S3, S4 or murmur.
Respiratory: Lungs clear to auscultation.
Neurologic: Sensation intact in all extremities.

The risk of peripheral neuropathy in the patient with long-standing diabetes looms large. Because we often use regional anesthesia for this operation and because regional anesthesia might be blamed for post-operative neurologic symptoms, we must obtain a baseline neurologic assessment and document any pre-existing deficits. Had we heard râles during the pulmonary examination and suspected volume overload, a chest radiograph would have been in order.

> Pre-operative studies: Hgb 12 g/dL; Hct 36%; Plt 300 000/microL; Na 145 mEq/L; K 4.8 mEq/L; glucose 110 mg/dL (6.1 mmol/L); Mg 1.7 mEq/L; Cr 8.3 mg/dL; BUN 60 mg/dL.
> ECG: NSR at 90 beats/min, normal intervals, ST segments at baseline, no Q waves, LVH.

The mild anemia that commonly coexists with chronic renal failure is mitigated by the erythropoietin therapy.

> Preparation for anesthesia: We will use normal saline as the carrier fluid for drugs, while minimizing total volume. Following informed consent, and a time-out to verify the right patient, location, and plan, we place an infraclavicular block pre-operatively in the "Block Room" under midazolam and fentanyl sedation. We use a stimulating needle and ultrasound to identify the subclavian vein and artery and adjacent nerves, and inject 35 mL of 1.5% mepivacaine with 50 mcg clonidine in small aliquots without complications.

We anticipate the patient to be normovolemic as he is still making significant though poor quality urine. We choose fluids for carrying our drugs that are isotonic. Preferably, this fluid will not contain potassium, which the patient can't clear well. This makes normal saline a natural choice.

This anesthetic choice should provide surgical anesthesia of the forearm for 4–5 hours with continued analgesia for several hours after that. While we usually also sedate patients for this procedure, the use of regional anesthesia will still place less of a drug burden on the patient than general anesthesia would have. Considering all the side effects of drugs, particularly when renal clearance is limited, a "minimalist" approach seems reasonable (though it should be noted that it has never been convincingly shown that regional anesthesia improves long-term outcome over that of general anesthesia for these [or any] patients, except possibly for cesarean delivery).

> Confirmation of anesthesia: In the OR, we test the level of anesthesia by gently scratching the skin of descending dermatome levels in the area of the planned procedure.

> Maintenance of anesthesia: With the help of a nasal cannula attached to a capnograph, we monitor respiratory rate and exhaled carbon dioxide (recognizing the number is semi-quantitative when drawn from a nasal cannula). Oxygen administration is titrated to a saturation over 90%. We titrate very light sedation with a propofol infusion to effect.

Administration of supplemental oxygen is often not necessary. The SpO_2 goal of 90% is admittedly somewhat arbitrary and some might set the target saturation a little higher while others might accept it even a little lower.

> Intra-operative event – hypertension: Approximately 45 minutes into the operation, the patient's blood pressure has climbed to 195/110 mmHg with a heart rate of 95 beats/min. He is arousable and complains of a mild headache, but is not anxious or in pain from the operation.

Intra-operative hypertension has a long differential diagnosis. Leading the list in this patient, who denies surgical pain and anxiety, are iatrogenic fluid overload and exacerbation of underlying chronic hypertension, probably from missing a dose of antihypertensive medication. A mixed alpha- and beta-blocking drug like i.v. labetalol is an attractive option here, works in just a few minutes and will lower both blood pressure via the alpha-blocking effect on the arteriolar resistance vessels and heart rate via beta-blockade. Post-operatively his blood pressure control can be refined by reinstituting his oral medications and then later by dialyzing him. We choose labetalol as he is on it chronically, it has mixed beta (mostly) and alpha (less so) effects. It also counts towards the goal of providing him with some peri-operative beta-blockade as he is (1) chronically on a beta-blocker and (2) at somewhat elevated risk of peri-operative MI given his age, diabetes history, and hypertension.

> Emergence from anesthesia: We time our sedation in anticipation of the end of surgery. Five to ten minutes is a pretty typical time to be awake after propofol sedation. We transfer the patient to the PACU for monitoring. At least partial recession of the block should be documented before discharge from the PACU. We tell the patient not to touch anything hot with the affected hand because temperature perception will be impaired longer than motor or sensory functions.

Open repair of an abdominal aortic aneurysm in a patient with coronary artery disease

The following case will emphasize the care of a patient with vascular disease for a major operation.

Learning objectives:

- pre-operative evaluation of the patient with cardiovascular disease
- cardiovascular physiology
- invasive hemodynamic monitoring
- intra-operative myocardial ischemia.

A 70-year-old man is scheduled for open repair of an abdominal aortic aneurysm.

Based on the shape of the aneurysm, he was unsuitable for an endovascular stent procedure. Instead, he requires a highly invasive, open intra-abdominal procedure that involves cross-clamping the aorta for a time, with substantial implications for blood pressure management and potential for uncontrolled blood loss.

History: The aneurysm has been followed for 3 years after incidental detection during coronary angiography. Its diameter has increased recently by 10 mm, and requires repair.

The location and extent of the aneurysm determine the level of the aortic cross-clamp. We are particularly concerned with the relationship of the clamp to the renal arteries, as supra-renal clamping requires renal protective maneuvers such as administration of mannitol. High clamp location (above the diaphragm) may also endanger perfusion of the lower two-thirds of the spinal cord, which is supplied by the artery of Adamkiewicz arising from the aorta somewhere between T8 and L4. In this case we would consider prophylactic placement of a spinal drain to reduce CSF volume and improve perfusion (see section on the brain in Chapter 11).

Review of systems: Chronic hypertension; myocardial infarction (MI) 3 years ago with subsequent three-vessel coronary artery bypass graft (CABG); 10 months

ago he underwent placement of a drug-eluting (medicated) stent into one of his native coronaries after he complained of new chest pain with exertion. He is a former smoker with 45 pack-year smoking history but none in the past 3 years. He has no complaints of chest pain at present and briskly walks 1 mile three times per week (>4 METs activity). Last CHF (congestive heart failure) episode was 10 months prior to admission. None since stent placed.

Using the "Eagle criteria" from Chapter 1, his current workup is sufficient from a cardiac standpoint. However, a patient rarely has vascular disease in only one or a few vessels and we worry about cerebral as well as additional aortic and coronary arterial disease.

Medications: ACE inhibitor, beta-blocker, spironolactone, aspirin and clopidogrel, atorvastatin.

We will ask this ASA IV patient to continue to take all his medications pre-operatively per his routine except for the clopidogrel, which we will discontinue 3 days pre-operatively.

Physical examination: Elderly man in no distress; weight 90 kg; height 6′ (180 cm), BMI 28.

BP 160/90 mmHg right arm, 172/93 mmHg left arm; HR 62 beats/min; respiratory rate 12 breaths/min. Room air oxygen saturation 98%.

Airway: Mallampati II; 3fb mouth opening; 4fb thyromental distance; full neck extension.

CV: S1, S2, no S3, S4 or murmur, no bruit heard over carotids.

Respiratory: Lungs clear to auscultation.

Lower extremities: mild edema.

In patients with vascular disease, we check blood pressure in both arms because it can vary significantly between them. We accept the higher one when there is a significant difference.

Pre-operative studies: Hgb 15 g/dL; Hct 45%; Plt 300 000/microL; Na 139 mEq/L; K 4.2 mEq/L.
ECG: NSR at 90 beats/min, Q waves present in II, III, and aVF; ST segments at baseline.

Echo (6 months old): left ventricular ejection fraction 35% (normal >50%); decreased wall motion inferiorly; normal valves. C×R no acute disease.

Not only would we like to know his starting hematocrit, we insist on a "type and cross" for four units of blood. This is for two reasons: first, because this procedure can result in significant blood loss and second, because this patient has a history of coronary artery disease and, in case of hemorrhage, he is less tolerant of a decrease in his oxygen-carrying capacity. Measurement of electrolyte levels is indicated in a patient taking diuretics, as these drugs can profoundly disturb electrolyte balance (spironolactone differs from others in that it can actually raise potassium levels). We ask for a chest radiograph to rule out pulmonary pathology given his age and smoking history.

Preparation for anesthesia: We plan to use general endotracheal anesthesia.

Because of his cardiac history and anticipated hemodynamic swings associated with aortic clamping and unclamping, we plan to place pressure catheters in his left radial artery and superior vena cava via the right internal jugular vein and to monitor cardiac function and volume status during the procedure with transesophageal echocardiography (TEE).

With the arterial catheter, we can monitor the blood pressure literally beat-by-beat. It also provides a conduit for repeated arterial blood gas and acid–base determinations. We can use the central venous catheter to assess his volume status and as a central route for drug administration. The TEE informs us about function, volume, rhythm, ischemia, and if we are very experienced we can also use it to measure RV pressure and cardiac output.

Induction of anesthesia: After completing the pre-procedure time-out questions and answers we place the arterial catheter awake with sedation and local anesthesia. Following thorough pre-oxygenation, we gently induce the patient with fentanyl, midazolam, a small dose of propofol and then vecuronium for chemical paralysis, and esmolol for heart rate control. We successfully intubate the trachea with minimal hemodynamic swings. We aseptically place a central venous catheter via the right internal jugular vein under ultrasound guidance. We "zero" the transducer at the mid-axillary line and record a central venous pressure (CVP) of 15 mmHg.

We choose a combination of narcotic, benzodiazepine, and propofol for induction to minimize cardiac depression. Vecuronium has few side effects in the patient with normal hepatic and renal function.

Next we insert the echo probe to assess baseline structure, function, and volume of the heart. When we see incision time approaching, we give 2 g of cefazolin as prophylaxis against a surgical site infection.

Maintenance of anesthesia: We maintain anesthesia with isoflurane 1.1% in air enriched with 60% oxygen combined with a fentanyl infusion, titrating the isoflurane to keep hemodynamics stable, and the BIS between 40 and 60. We try to maintain a normal volume status with fluid administration to keep the patient's cardiac end diastolic volume at baseline as determined by the TEE (using transgastric short axis view) and CVP.

Intra-operative event – cross-clamping of the aorta: We are prepared to administer a vasodilator such as nitroglycerin as needed to limit the blood pressure increase with aortic cross-clamping. Infra-renal clamp placement confers less risk of kidney problems, but still warrants consideration of mannitol. Before the cross-clamp is placed, we administer heparin 5000 units i.v. and confirm with an ACT (activated clotting time).

Cross-clamping the aorta causes a sudden increase in afterload, which often but not invariably dramatically increases the blood pressure. An anticoagulating dose of heparin prevents thrombosis below the cross-clamp. We target an ACT of >200 s (much less than the >400 s required for cardiopulmonary bypass) to confirm effective anticoagulation.

Intra-operative event – removing the cross-clamp: Surgery proceeds uneventfully, the surgeon is now ready to remove the clamp. We prepare by increasing venous capacitance with nitroglycerin, filling up this new capacity with i.v. fluids or blood. Immediately before removal of the clamp, we stop the nitroglycerin infusion, acutely decreasing venous capacitance. The resulting transient volume overload quickly dissipates following release of the cross-clamp and the reactive hyperemia (low resistance) that follows.

During the period of aortic cross-clamp, veins distal to the clamp recoil, returning much of their blood to the heart. Subsequently, local hypoxia causes both vasodilation (increasing venous capacity in this area) and the accumulation of many vasodilating and cardiac depressant metabolites. Removal of the cross-clamp opens up this large vascular bed, causing a massive shift in blood volume. A major decrease in blood pressure may follow, unless we plan ahead to either fill that space with additional fluid and/or blood or shrink its volume with a vasoconstrictor drug like phenylephrine.

Following removal of the cross-clamp, we document the presence of distal pulses via Doppler, and then administer protamine to reverse the anticoagulant effect of heparin. We test the adequacy of reversal by checking another ACT.

> Intra-operative complication – ischemia: BP 90/50 mmHg; HR 110 beats/min; SpO_2 95%.
> ST segments 3 mm downward sloping in V_5 with a new systolic wall-motion abnormality noted in the anterolateral left ventricle on the short-axis view.
> Hemoglobin 7 g/dL.

The ST segment and TEE changes suggest ischemia in the distribution of the left anterior descending coronary artery, serving the left ventricle free wall.

> Management of ischemia: We increase the inspired oxygen to 100%, quickly transfuse packed red cells, titrate esmolol to HR 70–80 beats/min, and add a nitroglycerin infusion as tolerated.

Treatment must improve the myocardial oxygen supply:demand balance by reducing heart rate (both reduced demand and increased supply by prolonging coronary perfusion in diastole) and wall tension,

increasing coronary perfusion pressure (diastolic blood pressure), and increasing oxygen-carrying capacity (transfusion). Normalization of the ST segments and systolic wall-motion abnormality indicate successful treatment.

> Emergence from anesthesia: Following conclusion of the operation we verify that the patient is strong, warm, and breathing adequately and extubate his trachea.

Transport is accomplished with continuous monitoring of oxygenation, blood pressure, and electrocardiogram. We also bring along the equipment necessary to ventilate his lungs (mask, laryngoscope, extra ETT) in case he requires respiratory support.

Though not necessary for this operation, with a suprarenal clamp endangering perfusion of the distal spinal cord, we would verify and document neurologic function of the lower extremities immediately postoperatively.

In the intensive care unit where he will spend the night, the receiving nurse takes report from us. We describe intra-operative events and the course of the operation, medications, CVP, most recent lab results, and urine production. We request a post-operative 12-lead ECG to verify no change. If it appears different then we will ask the cardiologists to help advise subsequent care, check serial enzymes, treat HR> 80 with metoprolol (beta-blocker), and make sure the Hct is kept near 30.

Learning objectives:

- anesthesia for the trauma patient
- fluid management
- increased intracranial pressure.

The Emergency Department calls regarding an approximately 40-year-old man who was an unrestrained driver and ejected from his car during an accident. He only briefly lost consciousness and was clearly intoxicated (olfactory evidence at the head of the stretcher). His initial vital signs included a HR of 118 beats/min, RR of 24 breaths/min, BP 114/86 mmHg with SpO_2 99% on a 100% non-rebreather mask with a Glasgow Coma Score (GCS, Table Trauma 8.1) of 14 (one off for verbal). Abdominal ultrasound revealed a splenic injury; he has hematuria and multiple orthopedic injuries. While in the CT scanner, the patient became more somnolent and now has a GCS of 9 (Eyes: 2, Verbal: 3, Motor: 4). The head portion of the CT scan was quickly completed but further scanning aborted, and the patient transported directly to the trauma operating room with portable pulse oximetry, ECG, and NIBP. We alert all available staff to meet us there, and confirm the blood bank is readying 8 units of type-specific blood and 4 units of fresh frozen plasma.

This case presents an acute emergency, with imminent risk to life (or limb). We have little time for preoperative evaluation. In this patient, without family around, we have no history, nor any information on medications or allergies. We cannot obtain informed consent for the operation or anesthesia. In fact such a situation mandates that we proceed in an attempt to save the patient's life, even without consent. We must evaluate his status as rapidly as possible, and then very quickly but also carefully induce anesthesia such that the operation can begin.

Centers designated to receive trauma cases maintain a "trauma operating room," always set up with the necessary equipment including rapid infusion systems for warm intravenous fluids, various vascular access devices, airway management and pressure monitoring equipment, and a selection of vasopressors.

Table Trauma 8.1. Glasgow Coma Score. Scored between 3 (worst) and 15 (best); correlates with degree of brain injury: >12 mild; 9–12 moderate, <9 severe

Best eye response (4)

1. No eye opening
2. Eye opening to pain
3. Eye opening to verbal command
4. Eyes open spontaneously

Best verbal response (5)

1. No verbal response
2. Incomprehensible sounds
3. Inappropriate words
4. Confused
5. Oriented

Best motor response (6)

1. No motor response
2. Extension to pain
3. Flexion to pain
4. Withdrawal from pain
5. Localizing pain
6. Obeys commands

To plan for this case we rely on astute observation and physical examination. The GCS tells us he has suffered at least a moderate brain injury. A full body survey might reveal tell-tale scars of past operations, for instance a sternotomy scar from heart surgery or a small lower abdominal scar from an appendectomy. Bruises suggest locations of impact and elicit concerns over specific injuries; for example, bruising over the ribs might indicate fracture and potential for pneumothorax, an impact mark over the middle of the breastbone might suggest a contusion of the heart.

Physical examination in the OR: Assessment of the ABCs (airway, breathing, and circulation) takes precedence. We find him breathing spontaneously with good air movement, reeking of alcohol, with a rapid but thready pulse. On more thorough examination we find:

A man of average build with obvious superficial trauma to face, chest, arms and legs with numerous scrapes; a hard cervical collar in place; weight ~70 kg; height ~6' (180 cm); bilateral chest tubes to water seal but without an air leak.

BP 89/50 mmHg; HR 135 beats/min; respiratory rate 28 breaths/min.

Airway: patient uncooperative, difficult to fully assess; 4 fb thyromental distance; in hard cervical collar.

CV: S1, S2 no murmur, tachycardic.

Respiratory: Lungs clear to auscultation bilaterally.

Neurologic: somnolent, moving all extremities, withdraws to pain, pupils equal and responsive to light.

Access: 18-g intravenous catheter in right antecubital fossa, right subclavian 7.5 French double-lumen central venous catheter.

This patient has suffered multiple traumatic injuries. To get a handle on where we stand we need to ask more questions of the surgeons, while simultaneously applying our OR monitors.

Further history: He has an open left femur fracture; hematuria suggesting kidney, ureter, or bladder injury; free fluid in the abdomen suggesting hemorrhage from spleen, liver, or intestines; multiple rib fractures but no evidence of pneumothorax; no obvious cervical spine fracture on X-ray or CT, but the hard cervical collar remains in place out of an abundance of caution; and a small right temporal epidural hematoma on head CT. Bilateral chest tubes were placed on arrival in the Emergency Department because of apparent rib fractures, subsequently a subclavian catheter was inserted. He received a total of 4 L Ringer's lactate, 2 units type O+, uncrossmatched blood, and 3 mg i.v. morphine in the Emergency Department.

Laboratories and studies (from 30 min prior, before blood administered):

Hgb 9 g/dL; Hct 24%; Plt 150 000/microL; Na 140 mEq/L; K 3.9 mEq/L; BUN 12 mg/dL; Cr 0.8 mg/dL; glucose 165 mg/dL (9.2 mmol/L).

PT and aPTT: pending.

Blood type: A+.

This additional history adds to our concerns. The issues with which we wrestle include the following:

- **Airway management**. We cannot rule out the presence of cervical spine instability or injury. Static radiographs cannot evaluate the quality of the ligaments that protect the cervical spinal cord from damage during head movement as occurs with traditional laryngoscopy. We consider all trauma patients to have a full stomach, with risk of regurgitation and aspiration of gastric contents. Standard application of cricoid pressure, a mainstay of aspiration prophylaxis, can displace a fractured cervical spine potentially compressing the spinal cord. In the patient with cervical spine injury we simultaneously support the posterior neck while compressing the cricoid ring, either with bimanual pressure or taking advantage of the posterior portion of the hard cervical collar. Unfortunately that collar, with its bulk, proximity, and interference with mouth opening, makes management of the airway difficult.

- **Intravascular volume status**. We find accurate assessment of volume status difficult. Significant blood can be lost into concealed spaces such as the thigh and abdomen (and into the street). If the abdomen is tense, the high pressure might curtail intra-abdominal bleeding. Upon opening of the tight abdomen, a deluge of blood might signal the release of the tamponade. Establishing appropriate vascular access is a high priority. In the presence of abdominal trauma, vascular access must be sought in the upper body, as products administered through the femoral route, for example, might be lost into the abdomen en route to the central circulation. While not the case here, frequently we find existing access of inadequate caliber requiring that we supplement it with additional catheters, or exchange one of the existing catheters over a wire using the Seldinger technique (sterilely insert a long wire through the catheter, remove the catheter, then advance a new, larger catheter over the wire). Fluid management includes consideration of hemoglobin concentration, electrolytes, and osmolality (Ringer's lactate is hypotonic). Decreasing plasma osmolality contributes to brain swelling and thus in the presence of a head injury we immediately switch to 0.9% saline as it is isotonic.

- **Pulmonary status**. Presence of rib fractures introduces the likelihood of pneumothorax and/or pulmonary contusion. While not apparent on an initial chest radiograph, decreasing pulmonary compliance evolving during positive pressure ventilation (increasing peak inspiratory pressure) could herald the development of a pneumothorax, which should be noted and treated right away, before becoming a tension pneumothorax. Evidence of chest-wall trauma discourages the use of nitrous oxide; its ready diffusion into the air-filled pneumothorax will expand its volume substantially over just a few minutes. The prophylactic placement of chest tubes helps protect against evolution of a tension pneumothorax during positive pressure ventilation. In the operating room we will also place the chest tubes on suction to ensure the interpleural pressure is negative.

- **Cardiovascular status**. With no knowledge of any pre-existing cardiovascular disease, we focus on his current state. The hypotension and tachycardia are most likely a function of hypovolemia from bleeding into the abdomen and thigh, but other causes must be considered. High on the list would be cardiac tamponade or contusion, tension pneumothorax (if a chest tube is malfunctioning), fat embolism from the femur fracture, transfusion reaction, anaphylaxis, spinal shock (unlikely given that he is able to move all extremities), and electrolyte abnormalities (especially low calcium from rapid blood transfusion, though unlikely after only two units transfused; see Chapter 3). To better sort this out we connect one lumen of his central venous catheter to a pressure transducer. A low CVP confirms low filling pressures, indicating hypovolemia in this case.

- **Neurologic status**. The fact that the patient was conscious at the scene gives reason to hope for a reasonable neurologic outcome, but his state is becoming grave. With hypotension and likely increasing intracranial pressure (ICP), we must concern ourselves with cerebral perfusion. The neurosurgeon will place an ICP monitor after evacuation of the hematoma, allowing calculation of the cerebral perfusion pressure (CPP; see section on the brain in Chapter 11). In the meantime, increasing blood pressure takes precedence; we also consider measures to reduce the ICP including hyperventilation, mannitol, avoiding a head-down position, e.g., Trendelenburg's position, administering no hypotonic fluids and avoiding those with glucose. Once an ICP monitor or ventriculostomy has been placed, we can monitor the actual CPP. The latter also introduces a new method to reduce ICP: direct removal of CSF.

> Preparation for anesthesia: We talk to the patient reassuringly as we connect our standard monitors and begin pre-oxygenation. We remove the anterior portion of his cervical collar sufficiently to view the anterior neck, while an assistant prepares the patient's left wrist for a radial arterial catheter.

In trauma cases such as this we exercise our resource management skills and encourage "parallel processing." We orchestrate several helpers performing simultaneous procedures, to facilitate a rapid beginning of the operation(s).

Despite his altered mental status we continue to speak to the patient as we would want our loved ones spoken to in a similar situation.

> Induction of anesthesia: Following adequate denitrogenation, we induce anesthesia with etomidate 21 mg (~0.3 mg/kg), fentanyl 100 mcg and succinylcholine 70 mg (~1 mg/kg). One assistant provides in-line stabilization of the spine without traction, and another applies bimanual cricoid pressure, while we perform a **gentle** direct laryngoscopy and advance an 8.0 mm endotracheal tube through the vocal cords. After confirming the presence of end-tidal CO_2 for several breaths, we secure the tube and begin mechanical ventilation with a rate of 15 breaths/min and a tidal volume of 500 mL, titrated to an end-tidal CO_2 of 30 mmHg.

We prefer a rapid-sequence induction because of aspiration risks, but find pros and cons to all available agents. We wish to limit the systemic response to intubation, reduce ICP, and decrease the cerebral metabolic rate for oxygen ($CMRO_2$), while avoiding hypotension. A larger decline in MAP than in ICP reduces cerebral perfusion pressure, further endangering the patient's brain. In the presence of hypovolemia, we prefer to limit cardiovascular depression and the loss of sympathetic tone from induction agents such as propofol and thiopental. Though often considered the preferred agent in hypovolemia due to its stimulation of the sympathetic nervous system, ketamine increases ICP and is therefore relatively contraindicated in this case. Etomidate usually causes little change in the blood pressure, and reduces $CMRO_2$. Thus in this case we choose etomidate and treat any blood pressure decrease with phenylephrine. Though unlikely in this case, we have an i.v. steroid available to treat etomidate-induced acute adrenal suppression (much more common in a patient with a coexisting infectious process). For muscle relaxation we prefer succinylcholine for a rapid-sequence induction, particularly when the airway examination is less than optimal. Should intubation of the patient's airway prove difficult, the paralysis will last only a few minutes, then spontaneous respiration should resume. Though succinylcholine can cause a small, transient increase in ICP, we can blunt the effect with an adequate induction agent and/or hyperventilation. The non-depolarizing muscle relaxant alternatives do not possess the rapid onset and offset of succinylcholine, but become useful in patients at risk for hyperkalemia (burns, crush injuries) or malignant hyperthermia.

We choose an endotracheal tube with a suction port above the cuff. Continuous suctioning of the secretions that accumulate just above the cuff has proven a valuable component of efforts to decrease the likelihood of ventilator-associated pneumonia (VAP).

We begin hyperventilation after conferring with the neurosurgeon, who also requests the administration of mannitol to provoke an osmotic diuresis to decrease brain volume and thereby ICP.

> Induction of anesthesia, continued: During the induction, an assistant placed a left radial arterial catheter for continuous blood pressure measurement. While the general surgeon prepares and drapes the abdomen, we draw blood for arterial blood gas, electrolytes, hemoglobin and platelet concentrations. We transduce the arterial and central venous catheters: ABP 85/45 mmHg; HR 140 beats/min; CVP 2 mmHg.

By employing an assistant to place catheters, we free our hands for induction and maintenance of this critically ill patient and allow activities to occur in parallel. We are happy to have the subclavian over internal jugular route for vascular access to avoid any impairment to cerebral venous drainage in this head-injured patient. We send blood for analysis of hematocrit to gauge the resuscitation and determine needs for future blood products, as these take time to acquire from the blood bank.

> Maintenance of anesthesia: We maintain anesthesia with judicious administration of opioids and isoflurane as tolerated, in 50% inspired oxygen in air. We titrate the oxygen concentration to a saturation >95%, and the volatile agent to maintain hemodynamic stability. Before the surgeon opens the abdomen, we administer a non-depolarizing muscle relaxant and prepare for rapid infusion of fluids and blood should the blood pressure suddenly fall.

For abdominal operations we also tend to avoid nitrous oxide for its propensity to increase the volume of air-containing spaces, although this takes much longer to manifest in the abdomen than in the chest. We administer a broad-spectrum prophylactic cephalosporin antibiotic and then, with vasopressors in line and ample vascular access, we are prepared for the abdomen to be opened.

> Intra-operative event – surgical incision: Upon opening the abdomen, the blood pressure falls precipitously as several liters of blood are evacuated (fortunately into a cell saver so the blood is eligible for washing, concentrating, and then reinfusion). We rapidly infuse normal saline and begin transfusing blood (already checked by nurses as to blood type, expiration date, and patient) while we await the cell saver operator to complete processing of the salvaged blood. In addition we ask the nurse to order more blood and fresh frozen plasma from the blood bank. The blood gas analysis includes a hemoglobin reported as 7.2 g/dL. The surgeon identifies a splenic rupture and successfully clamps the supplying artery. We administer two more units of blood based on the laboratory results and anticipated continued bleeding from the femur fracture.
>
> Meanwhile the neurosurgeon performs a small frontal craniotomy, draining about 75 mL blood, then places an ICP monitor so that the CPP can be measured (target: 60–80 mmHg).
>
> Once the abdominal bleeding is stopped and the hemodynamics stabilized at 110/60 mmHg with a heart rate of 90 beats/min and a CVP of 8 mmHg, the surgeon closes the abdomen to make room for the orthopedic surgeon to work on the femur fracture. Suddenly the blood pressure plummets again.

Careful evaluation of the findings can narrow the numerous potential causes for hypotension in this setting. An increased central venous pressure might accompany cardiac contusion, ischemia, tamponade, pulmonary embolism, or tension pneumothorax; the latter is also associated with increased peak inspiratory pressures during mechanical ventilation. Abdominal bleeding can be ruled out by direct inspection. Continued hemorrhage concealed in the pelvis, retroperitoneal space, or thigh cannot be similarly ruled out, but should not cause such sudden instability.

> We place a transesophageal echo (TEE) probe and find the left side of the heart virtually empty, and a

fluid-density mass compressing the right ventricle. We diagnose cardiac tamponade and the surgeon proceeds to insert a needle into the pericardial sac via the diaphragm, draining the pericardial blood with rapid improvement in venous return as observed by TEE.

The patient now appears clinically stable; we confer with the surgeons and agree to proceed with correction of the open femur fracture. This proceeds with much less fanfare.

When the cause of hypotension remains unclear, a direct view of cardiac structure and function as provided by TEE can prove quite helpful.

Emergence from anesthesia: Following conclusion of the operations we leave the patient paralyzed and sedated with his trachea intubated for transport to the ICU. He will suffer major fluid shifts over the next few hours, with possible pulmonary edema and airway swelling. Furthermore his neurologic status is unclear. The sedative and paralytic drugs will be discontinued to allow assessment of his neurologic status in the ICU.

Transport of this patient requires mechanical ventilation, ideally with a small transport ventilator, but absent that a hand-powered Mapleson or self-inflating Ambu bag system will suffice. Transport also requires an oxygen source and continuous monitoring. We bring along equipment to both mask–ventilate and reintubate his trachea, should that become necessary; we also have at hand the vasoactive agents we have required recently. In the ICU we give a report to the nurse and physician, including updates on the procedures, the surgical findings, interventions made, and recent laboratory values. We remind them that the subclavian catheter has not been radiographically evaluated, nor has the cervical spine been medically cleared.

We return to follow up on the patient several times over the ensuing weeks. Expected to make a full recovery eventually, he is discharged to a rehabilitation center after three weeks.

Liver resection under general anesthesia

Learning objectives:

- management considerations for intra-operative bleeding and venous air embolism
- monitoring and vascular access considerations for anticipated major hemorrhage
- post-operative pain management in the coagulopathic patient.

A 35-year-old woman is scheduled for a partial right (posterior) hepatectomy to remove an arteriovenous malformation (AVM) that has provoked several contained intrahepatic bleeds resulting in significant abdominal pain and the potential for rupture into her abdomen.

This operation will take 4–6 hours and carries the risk of substantial blood loss (from one-half to several liters) and the concomitant potential for coagulopathy. The liver can be resected via a laparoscopic approach or more commonly via an open procedure that is in essence a large upper abdominal laparotomy. The right lobe of the liver drapes partially over the inferior vena cava (IVC) and has a large vein that drains it into the IVC. The lobe receives its blood supply largely from a branch of the portal vein and, to a much lesser degree, from the right hepatic artery. Though the hepatic arteries provide little blood flow, they provide the majority of the liver's oxygen supply. The anatomy and its relationship to surrounding structures can best be appreciated by using a 3-D interactive model from the University of Toronto (link available on our site: *www.anest.ufl.edu/ea*).

History: Her AVM has been followed for several years. Removal is now indicated as it has become increasingly symptomatic and has grown in size.

Fortunately the liver is an organ that regenerates itself – much like a salamander will grow a new tail – thus this operation should be curative with no long-term health consequences.

Review of systems: Excellent health, one hospitalization 3 years ago for uneventful labor and delivery. Good exercise tolerance. No drug allergies. She will accept blood transfusions.

In virtually all surgical patients, but especially in those where a transfusion is likely, we must establish whether they have religious or other objections to receiving human blood products. For those who refuse blood, we question further about blood salvage devices.

Medications: Occasional multivitamin.

Physical examination: Calm woman in no distress; weight 74 kg; height 162 cm.

BP 112/60 mmHg, but reports it is often as low as 88/60 when checked at home; HR 74 beats/min; respiratory rate 16 breaths/min.

Airway: Mallampati I; 3 fb mouth opening; 4 fb thyromental distance; full neck extension.

CV: S1, S2, no S3, S4, or murmur.

Respiratory: Lungs clear to auscultation bilaterally.

Easily visible peripheral veins.

With a BMI of 28, she is overweight but not obese (BMI >30). She appears to be an otherwise healthy young woman. With knowledge of her low normal blood pressures we might adjust our target range under anesthesia. We are reassured by her benign airway exam and do not expect any difficulties placing the endotracheal tube.

Pre-operative studies: Hgb 11 g/dL; Hct 33%; Plt 195 000/microL; K 3.8 mEq/L, others are normal; activated PTT 32 s and PT 13.5 s (INR 1.1); type and crossmatch for 4 units of blood; urine pregnancy test negative.

We frequently check hematocrit and hemoglobin levels in pre-menopausal women, who are often mildly anemic; the levels are further indicated to establish a baseline for an operation with the potential for significant blood loss. We will tolerate her hematocrit dropping into the low to mid 20s and use her pre-operative hematocrit to calculate the allowable blood loss (see Chapter 3). Her estimated blood volume (EBV) is 60 mL/kg × 74 kg = 4440 mL. For every 10% of her EBV that is lost and replaced with i.v. fluid, we expect a 10% drop in Hct.

We checked her platelet count and coagulation status to ensure she can mount an effective hemostatic response. This large operation will leave raw surfaces on the remaining edge of the liver which must clot. Establishing a baseline value also allows future comparison if clinical suspicion about clotting arises.

Unless the patient has menstruated in the last week or so, we frequently confirm lack of pregnancy in women of child-bearing years.

> Preparation for anesthesia: We plan to use a general anesthetic and then i.v. patient-controlled analgesia (PCA) for post-operative pain relief. In pre-operative holding we discuss with the patient the possibility of a post-operative epidural block, then titrate midazolam for anxiolysis.

We cannot offer pre-operative placement of an epidural catheter for post-operative analgesia as we have some concern she might develop a coagulation disorder in the course of the operation, which raises the specter of an epidural hematoma should we nick a vessel during catheter placement. We explain this to her and offer the epidural as a post-operative option should the PCA prove inadequate and her coagulation normalize. Only after this discussion do we begin sedation.

Because the operative field involves neither cancer nor infection we plan to harvest blood during the surgery, process it, and reinfuse it. This requires advance planning with the perfusionist for equipment set-up. We will also confirm immediate availability of the 4 units of typed and crossmatched PRBCs.

> Induction of anesthesia: Following application of routine monitors, checking baseline vital signs, and performing a pre-anesthesia time-out to verify we are undertaking the correct operation on the intended patient, we induce anesthesia (after pre-oxygenation of course) with propofol and vecuronium. We intubate with a special endotracheal tube – one that includes a separate lumen for aspirating secretions from just above the ETT cuff and below the vocal cords. After we have confirmed proper positioning of the breathing tube, we add a left 20-g radial arterial catheter using aseptic technique, and a 14-g left antecubital

> i.v. catheter. Then we place a double-lumen 7.5F 15 cm right internal jugular (IJ) catheter under ultrasound guidance, again adhering to strict sterile technique and secure it at 14 cm inserted depth.

We choose propofol because it is well tolerated and helps reduce nausea (compared to sodium thiopental) in a young woman having an intra-abdominal procedure. For neuromuscular blockade, neither speed of onset nor duration of effect is critical, thus vecuronium is selected for its relatively lower cost.

Because of an increased risk of continued intubation following the operation, we use the special ETT. Frequent suctioning of the trachea between vocal cords and ETT cuff reduces the incidence of ventilator-associated pneumonia (VAP).

The arterial catheter facilitates obtaining blood specimens for lab analyses and provides beat-to-beat blood pressure data – in valuable for operations near major blood vessels such as the IVC, which can bleed massively and abruptly, or can be compressed during the procedure, interrupting cardiac filling. The central venous catheter helps guide intra-operative fluid management and helps the surgeon. You wonder how this helps the surgeon? The highly vascular liver contains mostly venous blood with direct connection to the IVC. The latter is in valve-less continuity with its "superior" brother, where we are monitoring the central venous pressure (CVP). If the CVP is high it stands to reason that incisions in the liver will bleed more. Conversely if the CVP is too low we worry that air can get into the circulation via the operative site, wreaking havoc with cardiac function, etc. Thus we have a goal for the CVP to be on the low side, typically around 5 mmHg. We alter the CVP by manipulating preload with fluids, or pharmacologically with nitroglycerin-induced venodilation to reduce the CVP. We strive to position the tip of the central venous catheter above her heart and not within it. A useful formula to achieve that from a right IJ approach is: (patient height in cm/10) – 2 cm = desired insertion depth.

> Intra-operative management of anesthesia: We maintain her anesthetic using isoflurane in an air/oxygen mixture and will titrate narcotic near the end of the case to facilitate her transition to the PCA and post-operative analgesia. For efficiency, we coordinate with the surgeon and use the same narcotic ordered for her post-operative PCA, in effect loading her for the PCA even before leaving the operating room. We keep her

chemically paralyzed during the operation, monitoring her neuromuscular function via a twitch monitor applied over the ulnar nerve of her left wrist. The i.v. fluids administered though her largest i.v., i.e., the 14-g, are run through a warmer to help preserve her body temperature. We use forced air warming over her exposed upper body and legs. To prepare for a massive bleeding event we have a "rapid infusion system" on-hand at the head of the bed but not connected to our patient (the tubing is costly) as we know our surgeon and generally the blood loss replacement is very manageable. An orogastric tube is inserted to decompress the stomach. We confirm that a prophylactic antibiotic against a surgical site infection was administered within the 60 minutes before incision to ensure efficacy.

Intra-operative event: As the surgeon is resecting the liver parenchyma the capnograph suddenly alarms and we observe a fairly abrupt decrease in $ETCO_2$ from 38 to 30 mmHg. The mean arterial pressure also decreases by 16 mmHg from 92 to 76. Curiously the CVP actually increases from 4 to 7 mmHg.

What happened? At this point there had been about 1200 mL blood loss, much of which was soon to be available from the cell saver blood salvage system (it must first be washed and prepared for reinfusion). In waiting for this we fell slightly behind in fluid replacement while the surgeon was cutting across the liver. The resulting hypotension allowed entrainment of air into the IVC via the surgical site. The air traveled to the heart and then the pulmonary circulation. In the lungs the air bubbles create some vasoconstriction (which explains the rise in CVP) and also deadspace by interfering with blood flow. Hence the decline in exhaled CO_2.

We alert the surgeon, who floods the field while we administer additional i.v. fluid to raise the hepatic venous pressure. We support cardiac function with ephedrine, and switch the inspired gas to 100% oxygen. The entire event lasted just a minute or two.

Both flooding the field and raising hepatic venous pressure will prevent further air entrainment. Raising the inspired oxygen facilitates air (nitrogen) resorption from the pulmonary vasculature. Events such as this remind us of the importance of setting (and enabling) tight alarm limits on all monitors. Without the early warning, this event could have been much more serious.

Emergence: After closure of the abdominal fascia, we reverse the paralytic and allow the patient to resume spontaneous ventilation with some pressure support programmed into the ventilator. Because the total bleeding was less than 1500 mL and 2 units of cell saver (roughly equivalent to 1000 mL blood loss) were returned to the patient, no transfusion of banked blood was needed. A respiratory rate of 22 prompts us to administer a little more hydromorphone. By the time skin closure is complete her respiratory rate has fallen to 14 with a blood pressure of 100/65 mmHg, suggesting adequate analgesia. With the isoflurane eliminated from the breathing circuit 5 minutes later our patient opens her eyes and meets all our usual extubation criteria. We apply suction to the orogastric tube while gently removing it, thus suctioning posterior pharynx and mouth. We remove the endotracheal tube and ask about pain. She describes it as 3/10 and tolerable. We transport her to the ICU with oxygen and airway support devices available. There she will be closely monitored for any bleeding. We order a chest radiograph to verify proper position of the central venous catheter (that the catheter tip is level with the takeoff of the right mainstem bronchus) and to rule out iatrogenic pneumothorax (very much less likely after a jugular placement than a subclavian). After giving a complete report to the ICU care team, we leave her in their capable hands.

The importance of a thorough handoff cannot be overstated, especially for critically ill patients. With modern computerized electronic records, we can easily follow up the chest X-ray and post-operative laboratory results even after officially handing over care. Taking ownership of his patient is the responsibility of every physician.

Post-anesthesia care: As we are leaving the ICU, the nurse calls to say our patient's biggest complaint is the sensation she needs to void. We return to the bedside and notice some urine in a dangling loop of tubing with an air column that is bigger on the patient side of the system than on the collection bag side. We straighten the Foley catheter tubing to remove the fluid level in a dependent tubing loop. A large volume of urine drains and the patient experiences immediate relief.

The principle is simple – if there is a meniscus visible in the tubing (actually two menisci, one at each end of a column of urine in the tube) pressure will accumulate in the drainage system on the patient side. Since the bladder is readily distensible it takes little obstructing pressure for the bladder to fill up, giving the patient a sense of urgency to void.

Learning objectives:

- treatment of patient with chronic pain syndrome undergoing anesthesia
- management considerations for patients with AICD
- optimization of conditions for intra-operative neurological monitoring.

A 62-year-old truck driver has a history of chronic back pain for which he underwent L1–L4 instrumentation and fusion 3 years ago. After a year of improvement, his pain returned with a vengeance. He has been on disability for 18 months and is now diagnosed with "failed back syndrome." He is scheduled for removal of spinal hardware and a T10-sacrum posterior spinal instrumentation and fusion.

Regarding the procedure itself, extensive repeat operations on the spine tend to be bloody – in the 2+ liter range. We will plan for replacing blood loss. The patient may have donated blood several weeks before and even perhaps started on erythropoietin to stimulate reticulocytosis, or have had family and friends donate blood (donor-directed units). If his starting hematocrit is above about 38%, we will consider performing acute normovolemic hemodilution, where, at the start of the operation, we collect high-hematocrit blood from the patient while replacing that blood volume with colloid and crystalloid solutions. With this strategy, slightly anemic blood will be lost intra-operatively, resulting in less total red cell loss. Then, after the majority of the blood loss has occurred, we transfuse back the patient's own fresh whole blood with platelets and clotting factors included! One caveat is the operation can't last so long that the blood (which is delicious nourishment to any bacteria) has been at room temperature for longer than six hours. In addition, the surgeon will use a cell-scavenging system to recycle non-infected blood.

The bottom line: Before the surgeon cuts skin, we confirm availability of blood for transfusion, be it homologous packed red blood cells, or autologous blood from prior donation. We order platelets and fresh frozen plasma only for specific concerns about coagulation

and not in advance of the operation. Understanding the high probability for transfusion, we place sufficient vascular access cannulae. He will be positioned prone with arms in "surrender" position (arms abducted at the shoulders, elbows bent with hands raised above his head) on arm boards. We must take special care that the ulnar nerves, especially at the elbows, are under neither stretch nor direct pressure. If he has many visible veins in his arms, we do not feel compelled to place a central venous catheter (with the attendant risks), because the arms are easily accessible to us during surgery and we will simply add any additional peripheral access needed to manage unexpectedly heavy bleeding.

A fluoroscope for intra-operative imaging (or, other newer and even bigger intra-operative surgical navigation systems) will most often be "stored" towards the patient's head between uses. After each use we must ensure the device does not contact the arms. We cannot neglect the risk to ourselves either, and wear lead gowning for protection from radiation exposure.

History: Prior to his work-related injury, the patient was in good health and an active sportsman. When his pain worsened following the original surgery, his physician chose a multi-modal medical management approach involving significant doses of narcotic.

We must include in our intra-operative planning, appropriate replacement of his daily oral intake of narcotics with the equivalent dose of intravenous narcotics (see Table Back 10.1). Furthermore, we must address the added acute pain of the surgery. His history of chronic narcotic use raises concern for tolerance and/or an opioid-induced hyperalgesia. We consider pre-operative administration of acetaminophen, a non-steroidal anti-inflammatory (which we would only administer after consulting the surgeon as many worry about their interference with bone morphogenetic protein, which might hinder bony fusion formation), ketamine, and/or gabapentin to reduce narcotic requirements, and might discuss with our surgical colleagues the placement of epidural catheters while they have direct access to the epidural space during the operation. Effective epidural analgesia can dramatically reduce the need for narcotic beyond the

Table Back 10.1. Rough equivalency table for common narcotic drugs prescribed for chronic pain and anesthetic narcotics used intra- and post-operatively. Half-lives depend upon rate of metabolism, volume of distribution and elimination so we must be especially cautious of not over-dosing patients with hepatic and renal impairment

Drug	Route	Equianalgesic doses (mg)	$T_{1/2}$ (h)
Codeine	p.o.	200	3
Hydrocodone	p.o.	30	4
Oxycodone	p.o.	20	3
Methadone (chronic)	p.o.	3	24
	i.v.	2	
Morphine	i.v.	10	2
Hydromorphone	i.v.	1.5	2.5
Alfentanil	i.v.	1	1.5
Fentanyl	i.v.	0.1	3.5
Sufentanil	i.v.	0.01	2.5
Remifentanil	i.v.	n/a	0.1
Carfentanil[a]	i.v.	0.001	8

[a] Carfentanil is of ultra-high potency and used primarily to dart and sedate large animals (think, sedating a ½ ton bear or a 2 ton rhinoceros!) but is believed to have been used in aerosolized form in 2002 to subdue terrorists (and hostages) who had seized a theatre in Moscow. There were 127 fatalities of approximately 800 captives.

chronic doses and may additionally reduce the number and severity of associated side effects: respiratory and cognitive depression, pruritus, urinary retention, and constipation.

> Review of systems: History of viral cardiomyopathy requiring automatic implantable cardioverter defibrillator (AICD) placement. His AICD has never discharged. His ejection fraction by echocardiogram two years ago was 0.25–0.3.

Presence of an AICD represents a serious anesthetic concern. The AICD monitors ventricular electrical activity in order to defibrillate appropriately. Electrocautery used during surgery may camouflage the native ECG masquerading as a shockable rhythm in the view of the AICD. If a shock is induced on a T wave, real fibrillation may ensue. This risk worries us enough that we choose to disable the AICD function. Placement of a magnet over the generator is the most commonly used method for deactivating an AICD because with removal of the magnet, the AICD recovers full functionality. However, in this patient, who will be placed prone, we would be worried that the magnet might unintentionally slip off and that tissue trapped between the magnet and the generator would necrose. Therefore, we ask a cardiologist colleague to turn off the AICD function. Of equal importance, we must ensure the patient remains continuously monitored until the AICD is reactivated following surgery. Of note, many AICDs provide the additional function of cardiac pacing, which we usually continue if the patient is pacer-dependent.

With regard to his history of cardiomyopathy, we refer to the ACC/AHA Peri-operative Guidelines (see Chapter 1). With the "intermediate risk" of the surgical procedure, non-invasive testing (e.g., repeat echocardiography) is indicated as it could change our management with regard to fluids and monitoring.

> Medications: Methadone 12 mg orally, twice daily; amitriptyline, lisinopril, and carvedilol.

The daily dose of methadone 24 mg is equivalent to 12 mg from time of NPO till expected surgery end. We account for the difference in intravenous and oral potency of narcotics and will cover his chronic pain needs with 2/3 * 12 = 8 mg methadone i.v. every 12 hours. Amitriptyline is a tricyclic antidepressant and an inhibitor of serotonin-norepinephrine reuptake. We would advise the medicine be taken as usual before surgery, but recognize that direct-acting sympathomimetic agents may produce hemodynamic responses exceeding expectations, while indirect-acting drugs, specifically ephedrine, may produce an astonishingly meek response.

The cardiac medications are for hypertension, rate control, and afterload reduction; since he has a cardiomyopathy all should be continued the day of surgery.

> Physical examination: Overweight man in no acute distress; weight 87 kg, height 5'8" (170 cm).
>
> BP 146/84 mmHg; HR 63 beats/min; respiratory rate 12 breaths/min.
>
> Airway: Mallampati II; 4fb mouth opening; 4fb thyromental distance; full neck extension.
>
> CV: S1, S2, no S3, S4, or murmur.
>
> Respiratory: Lungs clear to auscultation.

We appreciate that this patient is overweight, deconditioned, mildly hypertensive with a normal heart rate. We remember that patients with chronic pain syndromes on high doses of narcotics may not respond to all painful interventions with typical stress responses of tachycardia and hypertension.

> Pre-operative studies: Hgb 12 mg/dL; Hct 38%; Plt 210 000/microL.
>
> Electrolytes: Na 137 mEq/L; K 4.8 mEq/L; BUN 17 mg/dL; Cr 1.5 mg/dL.
>
> ECG normal sinus rhythm at 72 beats/min; nonspecific ST changes, LVH, occasional PVC.
>
> Echo (completed 1 week ago): Normal size chambers, global moderate hypokinesis, thick left ventricular wall, normal valvular function without regurgitation, ejection fraction 0.3.
>
> CXR AP view: AICD, left pectoral region with intact leads in the right atrial appendage and right ventricular apex, cardiac silhouette with mild cardiomegaly, lungs normal.

The repeat echo demonstrating stable cardiac function reassures us greatly. As noted above, we will ensure we have units of blood crossmatched and available prior to transport to the OR.

> Preparation for anesthesia: We plan to use a general endotracheal anesthetic. After standard induction with propofol and vecuronium, we place a 14-gauge i.v. catheter and a left radial arterial catheter. We connect either of these catheters aseptically to a citrate (anticoagulant)-containing blood collection bag positioned well below the level of the heart, and drain 450 mL of the patient's blood into the collection system with an automatic cutoff so we don't overfill the collection bag, exceeding our citrate's capacity and producing a giant blood clot. We take care to replace the volume being collected with hetastarch solution so as to keep the patient isovolemic. Prior to flipping prone we attach external cardioverter pads to his chest.
>
> Intra-operative management of anesthesia: To facilitate evoked potential monitoring we maintain anesthesia with total intravenous anesthesia (TIVA) combining remifentanil and propofol. BIS monitoring helps guide anesthetic depth.

The operation will be extensive and may stress the heart and threaten the spinal cord. With the AICD deactivated, we place external cardioverter pads. The surgeon has requested intra-operative somatosensory-and motor-evoked potential monitoring (SSEP/MEP) (see Chapter 7). These modalities assess spinal cord function and integrity, but MEP monitoring precludes use of muscle relaxants after induction, which will abolish motor responses. MEPs can also be compromised and become uninterpretable with the use of potent inhalational anesthetics. Therefore, we design a plan based on TIVA, including an opioid for analgesia, and a sedative/hypnotic such as propofol. These shorter-acting agents facilitate intra-operative wake-up tests, which might be necessary after an evoked potential change, and allow for a reliably early post-operative neurological exam. Because these drugs also tend to decrease blood pressure through afterload reduction, we are prepared to infuse phenylephrine to defend cerebral and spinal cord perfusion pressure. We will use BIS monitoring to help assure that our chronic-pain patient is asleep. In the face of hypotension, however, a falling BIS value concerns us greatly as it may reflect ischemia rather than deep anesthesia. Expectation of extensive blood loss, possible hypotension requiring vasoactive support, and the prone position further raise concerns for post-operative visual loss (POVL). To reduce this risk we raise the head of the bed slightly to decrease venous congestion in the eyes. An arterial catheter facilitates serial hematocrit and blood gas assessments. Our goal is to maintain the Hct $\geq$30. Finally, we start a fourth infusion of ε-aminocaproic acid, an anti-fibrinolytic agent.

Emergence from anesthesia: As the surgeons close the back wound, the epidural catheters are placed and the ends given to us for dosing. With 30 minutes left until we can flip our patient supine and extubate, we turn off the propofol and reduce the narcotic infusion rate. We bolus our epidural catheters and begin the basal infusions our acute pain management service colleagues suggest. As we prepare to turn the patient supine, we turn off our anesthetic infusions. Once supine, we extubate if the usual criteria are met.

Preparation for surgery end includes discontinuation of all infusions. We purposely designed an anesthetic technique to produce a rapid emergence and make nearly immediate neurological assessment possible. However, because the analgesic effect from remifentanil will be metabolized away just minutes after discontinuation, we administer longer-acting narcotics prior to emergence, titrating them to effect (respiratory rate and ETCO$_2$) as the patient begins responding and breathing. The necessary doses are greatly diminished if an epidural technique (which in ideal circumstances is capable of producing a pain-free wake-up) complements the intravenous narcotics.

Pediatric inguinal hernia repair under general anesthesia

Learning objectives:

- peri-operative management of the pediatric patient
- inhalation induction of general anesthesia
- caudal block.

An otherwise healthy 14-month-old boy comes for outpatient bilateral inguinal hernia repair. We see the child and parents for the first time in the pre-operative area where they are watching a children's cartoon.

Within a relatively short period of time we must build rapport with our patient and his parents, obtain a history, perform a pertinent physical exam, formulate an anesthetic plan, explain it to the parents, request consent and fill out some paperwork (pre-operative anesthesia evaluation form and anesthesia consent). Not a small task!

History: The hernias were identified by the baby's pediatrician. He has no other medical history. There is no family history of anesthetic problems. No recent runny nose, cough, or fever.

Physical examination: Agitated child; weight 13 kg; normal appearing pediatric airway; normal breath and heart sounds but difficult to hear; no apparent upper respiratory infection.

No additional pre-operative laboratory or other studies are required in this ASA I child. His agitation stems from hunger according to his mother. Too sleepy to drink when they left home, he awoke less than two hours prior to surgery and could not have his morning juice. He also has some stranger anxiety.

Preparation for anesthesia: We gain the child's trust using our best impressions of cartoon characters, though we also take advantage of the sedating properties of oral midazolam (0.5 mg/kg) in sweet syrup. To everyone's relief he drinks it down without complaint and returns to his cartoon. We gently apply a pulse oximeter probe to his toe and leave the family alone for 15 minutes to let the midazolam work its magic.

From this point on we ask that a parent hold the boy as he will soon lose coordination and become slightly sedated. While we return to the OR to complete preparations, the pre-operative nurse keeps an eye on the child. We return to find him sedated, sleepy, and agreeable to proceed to the operating room without a fuss.

There is an art to achieving the trust of children and their parents; we (and they) benefit greatly if we develop a varied repertoire. The response to midazolam is somewhat more predictable, though many children balk at the drink. However thirsty, they just don't trust much at a hospital. Intranasal administration (0.3 mg/kg) can also be effective, though it does not engender the trust we seek. While amusing to watch, a staggering child is clearly unsafe and admonishing the parents to keep the child on the stretcher or their lap is mandatory.

OR preparation for a pediatric case obviously differs from adult cases in the sizes of equipment and doses of drugs, but also in the precautions we take. We choose an i.v. fluid bag of only 250 mL (typically around 20 mL/kg) to prevent inadvertent over-hydration, and carefully remove all air bubbles from the tubing to remove the risk of paradoxical emboli, as children may still have a patent foramen ovale and it requires much less air in the child's venous system to wreak havoc. For all medications we draw up "unit doses" based on the child's weight, again as a safety measure.

Anesthesia induction: We ask if a parent wishes to come to the OR with their child for induction but both refuse, concerned they will become too emotional. So, we distract him with a game and swiftly take our patient away, allowing him to take his stuffed animal to the OR. The walls and ceiling of our outpatient pediatric surgical center are decorated with cartoon characters and animals, entertaining our ward during transport. His dazed state and rapture with the animals also ease the parents' anxiety. In the OR we reconnect the pulse oximetry probe and quickly proceed with induction.

We apply a face mask through which he breathes sevoflurane vapor in oxygen, quickly rendering him unconscious. Meanwhile we apply blood pressure cuff at a 1-minute cycle, and ECG leads. Once our patient has achieved a stable level of general anesthesia with a spontaneous, regular respiratory rate, we begin i.v. placement. The i.v. may be placed by the anesthesiologist, nurse, or surgeon as long as they are comfortable with pediatric venipuncture.

We administer a small dose of propofol (e.g., 1 mg/kg i.v.) to briefly deepen the anesthetic, then place an appropriately sized LMA (laryngeal mask airway). After observing the capnogram and listening for breath sounds to ensure proper placement and ventilation, we check for a leak around the LMA. We protect the child's airway and prepare for placement of a caudal block.

Babies (and parents) prefer i.v. placement after anesthetic induction. We comply when there are no additional safety concerns, such as an unusual airway, high risk of aspiration (e.g., pyloric stenosis or severe reflux disease), or concerns for hemodynamic instability during induction. For healthy children we can safely perform a mask induction with only a pulse oximeter for heart rate and oxygenation, followed quickly by the other standard monitors. A frequent choice for inhalation induction is sevoflurane, which lacks the pungency of its competitors and is therefore well tolerated. As the child continues inhaling the anesthetic vapors, the brain concentration of sevoflurane increases and we observe the progression of the anesthetic from light to deep. We use clinical signs such as eye movement and respiration pattern to determine the stage of anesthesia. We do not do anything painful such as i.v. placement until the baby is sufficiently asleep to tolerate it without responding to the needlestick. Excessive stimulation during the brief excitation stage that occurs during the transition from light to deep anesthesia may trigger vomiting or laryngospasm. While we carefully plan to avoid such complications, we have immediately available an appropriately dosed succinylcholine/atropine mixture for intramuscular administration in case we need to intubate emergently. Fortunately modern inhalational anesthetics allow us to go through this stage rapidly. Unfortunately, deeper planes of anesthesia bring other problems. Not uncommonly relaxation of oropharyngeal muscles leads to airway obstruction requiring manual maneuvers or insertion of an oral airway. Excessive anesthetic vapors ultimately depress respiration and the cardiovascular system so we carefully watch the amount delivered (end-tidal agent and carbon dioxide concentrations on the gas analyzer), provide assisted ventilation if needed, or lighten the anesthetic if the blood pressure falls. Securing the eyes

closed should be accomplished before risk of corneal abrasion. Many will do this prior to i.v. placement or LMA insertion.

Though the entire anesthetic could be done with anesthetic vapors alone and blood loss during many pediatric cases is minimal, i.v. access is an extremely important safety measure in pediatric anesthesia. With the exception of brief and superficial operations, such as ear tube placement, rarely would we consider skipping the i.v. Unfortunately though, cannulating a pediatric vein can be quite challenging; we are grateful for the venodilation offered by our inhaled anesthetics. We secure pediatric i.v.'s carefully as they are often unwelcome (not to us or the nurse, but the child) when he awakens.

Similarly, the entire case could be accomplished with vapors administered via face mask; however, this generally ties the hands of the anesthesiologist. Instead we choose to place an LMA. An endotracheal tube would also suffice, but the added stimulation would require still deeper anesthesia, and often the addition of a muscle relaxant (e.g., rocuronium 0.6 mg/kg) for intubation.

Caudal block placement: We position the patient on his side and palpate the sacral hiatus and cornua (see Fig. Pediatric 11.1). We clean the skin in the injection area with a chlorhexidine isopropyl alcohol scrub and allow it to dry while we don sterile gloves. Ropivacaine 0.2%, 12 mL (1 mL/kg) should achieve a T10 block level; we add 12 mcg clonidine to our solution to prolong analgesia. When we place the 22-gauge needle in the caudal space, we gently aspirate on the syringe looking for blood or CSF to make sure we are not intravascular or intrathecal. Then we gently inject our mixture in several increments 30–60 seconds apart, observing for ECG changes after each aliquot. Upon completion of the block we place an approximately 40 mg/kg acetaminophen suppository rectally to reinforce post-operative analgesia.

Caudal blocks provide excellent analgesia for hernia and other lower abdominal and perineal procedures. As always, aseptic technique is vital. Intrathecal injection would result in a much denser and higher dermatome block with hypotension and possibly respiratory arrest depending on the dose administered. Intravascular injection would first be recognized on the ECG by a T wave rise and QRS widening. Despite a negative aspiration, we monitor closely and abort the injection immediately if we see such signs to prevent catastrophic local anesthetic systemic toxicity which would occur if the full dose were delivered intravascularly.

> Incision: We return the baby to the supine position and allow the surgeon to start preparing and draping the surgical field. We place a temperature probe and maintain a warm environment, as children have a larger body surface area in relation to their size than adults and lose body heat more quickly through the skin in a cold operating room. We switch from sevoflurane to isoflurane, increase to about 1.3 MAC and administer 1 mcg/kg fentanyl prior to incision. As the surgery progresses we titrate the agent and fentanyl, assisting ventilation where necessary to maintain a near-normal end-tidal CO_2.

Children exhibit "emergence delirium" (agitation) seemingly more commonly with sevoflurane than isoflurane, yet the latter is too pungent for mask induction, so the intra-operative use of each in turn is commonplace in pediatric anesthesia. Because our caudal block may take 20–30 minutes to reach full strength, we augment our anesthetic prior to surgical incision with small doses of fentanyl and increased sevoflurane. Signs of "light anesthesia" such as increases in heart rate, blood pressure, and respiratory rate, or movement in response to surgical stimulation prompt additional interventions.

> Emergence: The operation proceeds uneventfully. About an hour after incision the surgeon is nearly done so we turn off the vaporizer and increase fresh gas flow just above three times the patient's minute ventilation to limit rebreathing of the isoflurane and expedite its washout. In case there is airway management difficulty on emergence we use 100% oxygen (same as we did for induction) to increase the pulmonary oxygen reservoir and to prolong the time from airway obstruction to severe desaturation. When the surgeon is done with wound closure and dressing/sealant we position our patient on his side in the "recovery position," pull the LMA and gently suction his oropharynx, immediately checking for airway patency and adequate respiration. Once we confirm he is stable and comfortable with a normal room air oxygen saturation we transport him to the PACU, intermittently feeling for the reassuring warmth of his exhaled breath.

Some anesthesiologists remove the LMA during deep anesthesia (especially with younger children) and others only when the patient is fully awake. Even though an LMA is less irritating for airways, and we

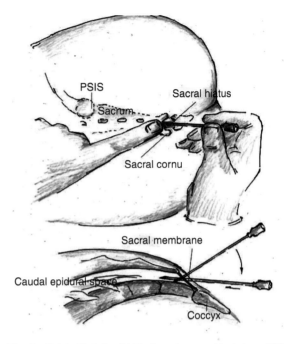

Fig. Pediatric 11.1 Caudal block anatomy and technique. PSIS, posterior sacroiliac spine. Drawing by B. Ihnatsenka, MD.

see much less coughing, straining, and breath holding on emergence than with an ETT, we remain vigilant and prepared to diagnose and treat laryngospasm, for example.

> PACU: We help the recovery nurse attach monitors, give our report, confirm the patient is stable, and swiftly move to our next case. As soon as he is settled, the recovery nurse calls for the child's parents to pacify him. An hour later the child is drinking liquids and meets discharge requirements (see Chapter 6). We come by between cases for our final assessment and sign him off for the trip home. The nurse removes the i.v. and provides some final instruction to the parents.

His agitation on arrival in the PACU is not a response to pain, but some delirium from the wake-up, as well as unfamiliar surroundings and continued hunger. Nothing parents cannot overcome. The caudal block with clonidine will provide up to 6–9 hours of good pain control, and by this time the rectal acetaminophen has also started working.

Anesthetic drugs, especially vapors, nitrous oxide, and narcotics, can cause nausea and vomiting so we are cautious with oral intake at first.

Index

Note: page numbers in *italics* refer to figures and tables